# Cystic Fibrosis—Current Topics

Volume 2

# Cystic Fibrosis—Current Topics

Volume 2

**Edited by**

**J. A. Dodge**
The Queen's University of Belfast, UK

**D. J. H. Brock**
The University of Edinburgh, UK

**J. H. Widdicombe**
University of California Medical School, San Francisco, USA

JOHN WILEY & SONS
Chichester · New York · Brisbane · Toronto · Singapore

Baffins Lane, Chichester,
West Sussex PO19 1UD, England

Telephone: National Chichester (0243) 779777
International +44 243 779777



*Other Wiley Editorial Offices*

John Wiley & Sons, Inc., 605 Third Avenue,
New York, NY 10158-0012, USA

Jacaranda Wiley Ltd, 33 Park Road, Milton,
Queensland 4064, Australia

John Wiley & Sons (Canada) Ltd, 22 Worcester Road,
Rexdale, Ontario M9W 1L1, Canada

John Wiley & Sons (SEA) Pte Ltd, 37 Jalan Pemimpin #05–04,
Block B, Union Industrial Building, Singapore 2057

*Library of Congress Cataloging-in-Publication Data*

Cystic fibrosis—current topics.

Includes bibliographical references and index.
1. Cystic fibrosis. I. Dodge, J. A. (John A.)
II. Brock, D. J. H. III. Widdicombe, J. H.
[DNLM: 1 Cystic Fibrosis. WI 820 C9765]
RC858.C95C87 1993 616.3′7 92-15773
ISBN 0-471-93101-2 (v. 1)
ISBN 0-471-95166-8 (v. 2)

*British Library Cataloguing in Publication Data*

A catalogue record for this book is available from the British Library

ISBN 0 471 95166 8

Typeset in 10/12pt Times by
Mathematical Composition Setters Ltd, Salisbury, Wiltshire
Printed and bound in Great Britain by Biddles Ltd, Guildford, Surrey

# Contents

# List of Contributors

ERIC W. F. W. ALTON *Ion Transport Laboratory, National Heart and Lung Institute, Manresa Road, London SW3 6LR, UK*

HERBERT A. BERGER *Howard Hughes Medical Institute, Department of Internal Medicine, University of Iowa College of Medicine, 500 EMRB, Iowa City, IA 52242, USA*

JOACHIM BIWERSI *Departments of Medicine and Physiology and the Cardiovascular Research Institute, University of California—San Francisco, San Francisco, CA 94143, USA*

NEIL A. BRADBURY *Department of Physiology and Biophysics and Gregory Fleming James Cystic Fibrosis Research Center, University of Alabama at Birmingham, Birmingham, AL 35294, USA*

ROBERT J. BRIDGES *Department of Physiology and Biophysics and Gregory Fleming James Cystic Fibrosis Research Center, University of Alabama at Birmingham, Birmingham, AL 35294, USA*

DAVID J. H. BROCK *Human Genetics Unit (WGH), The University of Edinburgh, Western General Hospital, Edinburgh EH4 2XU, UK*

NATASHA J. CAPLEN *Department of Biochemistry and Molecular Genetics, St Mary's Hospital Medical School, Norfolk Place, London W2 1PG, UK*

JACQUELINE CARRÈRE *Groupe de Recherche sur les Glandes Exocrines, Faculté de Médecine, 27 Boulevard Jean Moulin 13385, Marseille, Cedex 05, France*

SENG CHENG *Genzyme Corporation, 1 Mountain Road, Framingham, Massachusetts 01701, USA*

JONATHAN A. COHN *Departments of Medicine and Cell Biology, Box 3378, Duke University, Durham, NC 27710, USA*

CARLA COLOMBO *Department of Pediatrics, University of Milan, Via Commenda 9, Milan 20122, Italy*

CHARLES COUTELLE *Department of Biochemistry and Molecular Genetics, St Mary's Hospital Medical School, Norfolk Place, London W2 1PG, UK*

GARRY R. CUTTING *Center for Medical Genetics, Johns Hopkins University Hospital, CMSC 1004, 600 North Wolfe St, Baltimore, MD 21287, USA*

JOHN A. DODGE *The Queen's University of Belfast, The Nuffield Department of Child Health, Grosvenor Road, Belfast BT12 6BJ, UK*

JULIA R. DORIN *Molecular Genetics Section, MRC Human Genetics Unit, Western General Hospital, Crewe Road, Edinburgh EH4 2XU, UK*

THOMAS M. EGAN *Division of Cardiothoracic Surgery, University of North Carolina School of Medicine, 108 Burnett-Womack Building, CB #7065, Chapel Hill, NC 27599-8065, USA*

CATHERINE FIGARELLA *Groupe de Recherche sur les Glandes Exocrines, Faculté de Médecine, 27 Boulevard Jean Moulin 13385, Marseille, Cedex 05, France*

W. E. FINKBEINER *Cardiovascular Research Institute and the Department of Pathology, University of California—San Francisco, San Francisco, CA 94143, USA*

LUIS JUAN VICENTE GALIETTA *Servizio di Genetica Molecolare e Laboratorio di Citogenetica, Istituto Giannina Gaslini, 16148 Genova, Italy*

STEPHEN L. HART *Department of Biochemistry and Molecular Genetics, St Mary's Hospital Medical School, Norfolk Place, London W2 1PG, UK*

PETER W. HIATT *Baylor College of Medicine, Department of Pediatrics, Pulmonology Section, 1 Baylor Plaza, Houston, TX 77030, USA*

PETER G. MIDDLETON *Ion Transport Laboratory, Royal Brompton National Heart and Lung Institute, London, UK*

S. S. MILLER *School of Optometry and Department of Cell and Molecular Biology, University of California—Berkeley, Berkeley, CA 94720, USA*

ANGELA M. O'RAWE *The Queen's University of Belfast, The Nuffield Department of Child Health, Grosvenor Road, Belfast BT12 6BJ, UK*

MARIA LETIZIA PETRONI *Istituto di Scienze Biomediche (Ospedale San Paolo), University of Milan, Milan, Italy*

DAVID J. PORTEOUS *Molecular Genetics Section, MRC Human Genetics Unit, Western General Hospital, Crewe Road, Edinburgh EH4 2XU, UK*

GIOVANNI ROMEO *Servizio di Genetica Molecolare e Laboratorio di Citogenetica, Istituto Giannina Gaslini, 16148 Genova, Italy*

DENNIS J. SHALE *Section of Respiratory Medicine, University of Wales College of Medicine, Llandough Hospital, Penarth, South Glamorgan CF64 2XX, UK*

ALAN E. SMITH *Genzyme Corporation, 1 Mountain Road, Framingham, Massachusetts 01701, USA*

SUE M. TRAVIS *Howard Hughes Medical Institute, Department of Internal Medicine, University of Iowa College of Medicine, 500 EMRB, Iowa City, IA 52242, USA*

CHARLES J. VENGLARIK *Department of Physiology and Biophysics and Gregory Fleming James Cystic Fibrosis Research Center, University of Alabama at Birmingham, Birmingham, AL 35294, USA*

A. S. VERKMAN *Departments of Medicine and Physiology and the Cardiovascular Research Institute, University of California—San Francisco, San Francisco, CA 94143-0532, USA*

MICHAEL J. WELSH *Howard Hughes Medical Institute, Department of Internal Medicine, University of Iowa College of Medicine, 500 EMRB, Iowa City, IA 52242, USA*

J. H. WIDDICOMBE *Cardiovascular Research Institute and the Department of Physiology, University of California—San Francisco, San Francisco, CA 94143, USA*

ROBERT WILLIAMSON *Department of Biochemistry and Molecular Genetics, St Mary's Hospital Medical School, Norfolk Place, London W2 1PG, UK*

OLGA ZEGARRA-MORAN *Servizio di Genetica Molecolare e Laboratorio di Citogenetica, Istituto Giannina Gaslini, 16148 Genova, Italy*

# Preface to Volume 1

Cystic fibrosis has fascinated scientists and clinicians for half a century. Historically, its clinical complexity has been followed by increasing genetic complexity and in the three years since the faulty gene was pinpointed and sequenced, and its product described in structural terms, more than 150 separate mutations have been identified. The precise nature of the physiological defect(s) in the cell still awaits a complete and generally agreed understanding at the time of writing, and we have just begun to talk realistically of gene—or targeted pharmacological—therapy. Increasing longevity and new conventional treatments have uncovered new problems.

Several excellent clinical textbooks of cystic fibrosis are in existence and widely used, but extensive recent developments suggested that a new book with international authorship was needed, which would bring together the clinical features of the disease and their molecular and physiological basis in a format that would be of value to clinicians, geneticists and cell physiologists alike. The main problem we faced is that such a book would be out of date before publication. Hence, this volume is the first of a series. Some chapters should remain authoritative and suitable for consultation for many years. Others will quickly become obsolete as new developments occur. It is the editors' intention to produce a series of volumes at approximately one to two year intervals, which will build up into a comprehensive source of reference. We have our own plans and ideas for future chapters, but would welcome readers' suggestions for topics which they would like to see treated in depth by acknowledged experts. We hope that this first volume will whet your appetite for more.

J. A. Dodge
D. J. H. Brock
J. H. Widdicombe

# Preface to Volume 2

In the two years that have passed since the publication of the first volume of *Cystic Fibrosis—Current Topics*, progress in cystic fibrosis research has if anything accelerated. Undoubtedly, one of the high points was the creation of a series of mouse models of cystic fibrosis (CF), using techniques of homologous recombination. The other was the tentative beginning of trials of gene therapy on affected patients, with both viral and liposome vectors. The two developments, one needing state-of-art molecular biology and the other expert respiratory physiology, illustrate the profound interdependence of science and medicine in tackling the problems of CF. Developments have proceeded apace on both sides of the Atlantic, and we make no apology for leading the second volume with these subjects. As in Volume 1, we have been fortunate in getting those at the cutting edge of this exciting research to write authoritative accounts.

No one is under any illusion that gene therapy will cure CF. Understanding of the science of chloride channels remains incomplete and Part II of this volume reviews the different approaches that are being made to the cell biology of the disorder. The driving force is the belief that further progress in our ability to manipulate the cystic fibrosis transmembrane conductance regulator may make it possible to use genetic engineering to offset most of the destructive features of CF. That is for the future. For now, those who care for patients must continue to use more conventional methods (even heart–lung transplantation is conventional in the face of gene therapy), and some of these are covered in Part III.

One of the problems confronting the editors of this second volume is that the borders between genetics, cell biology and clinical medicine are becoming blurred. For Volume 3 we will probably discard these increasingly arbitrary distinctions. As before we have plans and ideas for future chapters, but would welcome your suggestions for topics that are relevant and current.

J. A. Dodge
D. J. H. Brock
J. H. Widdicombe

# Part I

## Genetics

Chapter One

# Mouse Models For Cystic Fibrosis

Julia R. Dorin[a], Eric W. F. W. Alton[b] and David J. Porteous[a]

*[a]Molecular Genetics Section, MRC Human Genetics Unit, Western General Hospital, Edinburgh, and [b]Ion Transport Laboratory, National Heart and Lung Institute, London, UK*

## INTRODUCTION

An animal model which mimics the cardinal features of cystic fibrosis (CF) has been a long-standing aim of CF research. The unlimited availability of affected tissues at all stages of disease development and the possibility of dissecting the pathophysiology *in vivo* is a compelling prospect. Now that the gene for CF has been cloned, novel drug and in particular somatic gene therapies can be considered. However, before these exciting new advances can progress to clinical trials, the issues of safety and efficacy must be addressed. A relevant animal model would provide the most stringent test-bed. Four different genetic mouse models for CF now exist[1–4] and their applicability and respective value to CF research is discussed below.

## WHY MODEL CYSTIC FIBROSIS IN THE MOUSE?

Prudent choice of a particular species might increase the chance of the major clinical features of the disease developing. The similarity to man in lung architecture or the abundance of submucosal glands have favoured the pig and

*Cystic Fibrosis—Current Topics, Volume 2.* Edited by J. A. Dodge, D. J. H. Brock and J. H. Widdicombe

ferret, respectively. However, CF is a genetic disease with a recessive mode of inheritance, and therefore a genetic disease model will require inactivation or specific modification of the homologous gene. A random mutation screen could be considered but this is a particularly arduous strategy for recessive traits. This limits the choice to the mouse, as only in this mammal is it possible to engineer mutations in a specified gene *in vitro* and to subsequently transmit this through the germline *in vivo*. As a direct result of this technology and the

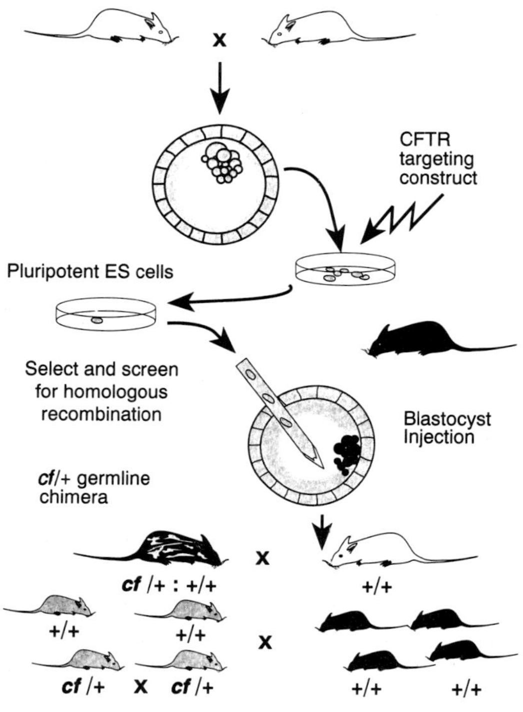


**Figure 1** This general strategy for deriving a mouse model for CF by gene targeting in ES cells begins with cells derived from an inbred mouse strain that carries a coat colour mutation(s) (shown here as a light colour). The ES cells are cultured and modified by gene targeting and cells that have the desired *Cftr* alteration are identified and reintroduced into the blastocoele cavity of a blastocyst of a different (dark) coat colour genotype. If the cells are totipotent they will contribute to all tissues of the developing mouse, including the germline. Cells that colonize somatic tissue can be visualized in the coat colour. The ES cells (light) and the host blastocyst (dark), both contributing to the coat, produce a mottled patchy coat colour. These animals are chimeric and have cells which are either +/+ or *cf*/+. Chimeras are tested for germline transmission by mating to mice that will allow detection of the ES cell coat colour mutations. Half of the ES cell-derived offspring will carry the gene-targeted chromosome and these are determined by DNA analysis. Mating of heterozygous *cf*/+ mice results in the production of *cf*/*cf* homozygotes

isolation of the *CFTR* gene, mice now exist which have mutations in the murine equivalent of the human CF gene (Figure 1).

In addition to the combination of transgenic techniques available, the mouse also has the important practical advantages of small size and considerable breeding capacity, which make it relatively cheap and easy to maintain. Despite the obvious external and anatomical differences between species, the bulk of intermediary metabolism is shared between mammals. It could be argued that differences are largely ones of detail rather than design. In support of this, relevant mouse models of several important human conditions have been identified and these include albinism, Duchenne muscular dystrophy, Gaucher's disease, aniridia, autoimmune diseases and cancers[5]. Of course species differences can also be informative in identifying prerequisites for disease development.

A further asset of the mouse is that a wide variety of inbred strains exist. Despite a huge investment of effort, the variability of the CF phenotype has proved resistant to the establishment of a clear genotype : phenotype correlation, except in terms of pancreatic disease[6]. To date, the prognosis of lung disease development cannot be ascertained on the basis of *CFTR* genotype. This implies that genetic background and/or environmental factors play a major role. The consequences of varying both genetic and environmental factors on a CF phenotype can be experimentally controlled. If positive evidence is obtained that interactive genes can affect disease progression, then these can be readily mapped in the mouse and, through synteny, indicate the location of the corresponding human loci.

The probability that a genetic mouse model for CF would mimic the clinical phenotype was given weight by the demonstration by Smith et al.[7] that the ion transport properties of wild-type mice are similar to those of normal human subjects. Isolation of the murine *CFTR* homologue was the next crucial step[8,9]. The mouse gene (*Cftr*) is present on chromosome 6 within a chromosomal region syntenic with the location of the human gene (*CFTR*) on chromosome 7[9]. The mouse gene is highly similar to the human (78% overall identity at the amino acid level). The region of the gene with the highest similarity includes exons 10 and 11, where the majority of the human mutations lie (including the most common ΔF508)[10]. This was compelling evidence to predict cross-species functional conservation and set the scene for the various labs to begin to develop their chosen gene-targeting strategies.

## GENE TARGETING IN ES CELLS

All manner of genes ($>100$) have now been disrupted in mouse ES cells and homozygous mutant allele mice have been produced from many of these cell lines. Many of the phenotypes are unexpected, revealing functional redundancy in some tissues and previously unpredicted gene involvement in others[11]. Lesch–Nyhan syndrome was the first genetic disease to be modelled in the mouse using ES cells that had been selected in culture for *Hprt* gene mutation[12,13]. The mice were not obviously mutant and by two years of age the only phenotype analogous to the self-mutilation behaviour of patients was trauma induced by over-grooming. Interestingly, using specific inhibitors of another key enzyme in the purine salvage pathway in these mutant mice resulted in the display of the self-injurious behaviour characteristic of the disease by six months of age[14]. The first human condition to be accurately modelled in the mouse by gene targeting in ES cells was Gaucher's disease[15]. Mice which are homozygous for a null allele of the glucocerebrosidase gene mimic closely the less common and more severe type 2 form of the human disorder, where patients die shortly after birth with neurological disease. These two examples demonstrate that some of the clinical aspects of human disease can be accurately reflected in a genetic model created by targeted gene mutation, but the phenotypic outcome cannot be easily predicted.

The major technical problems in the ES cell gene-targeting process are (1) identifying clones which are correctly targeted and (2) maintaining the cells in their totipotent state. ES cells are derived from the inner cell mass of 3.5-day preimplantation embryos and if cultured correctly they can be maintained so that they remain pluripotent[16]. Totipotent cells can contribute to the germline, and thus reintroduction of targeted ES cells into a host blastocyst allows the establishment of mice possessing genomic alterations created in culture (Figure 1). The technique of introducing mutations into a predetermined site in the genome utilizes homologous recombination, often referred to as 'gene targeting' or 'knockout technology'. Essentially, a transgene containing a region of the gene of interest is introduced into the cells and gene disruption occurs as a consequence of recombination into one of the endogenous copies of the gene[17]. Unfortunately random integration generally occurs at a much higher frequency than recombination at the target site. The ratio of homologous versus random integration can range from 1 : 1000 to 1 : 0.25. The factors that influence this ratio include target gene-specific properties, length of homology[18], whether or not the targeting DNA is a perfect sequence match (isogenic) for the chromosomal target[19], type of vector[20] and whether or not correct integration provides a direct biochemical selection[21].

Although numerous groups set out to 'knock out' the CF gene in ES cells, success was hard to come by. Finally, reports of ES cell lines carrying *Cftr* gene disruptions appeared[22–24]. Following this, and within a few weeks of each other, Snouwaert et al.[1] (University of North Carolina (UNC)) and Dorin et al.[2] (Human Genetics Unit (HGU), Edinburgh) reported the successful establishment of mice which were homozygous mutant at the murine CF gene. Two further CF mouse models created by ES cell gene targeting were subsequently reported, one later that same year (Colledge et al.[3] (Cambridge

(Cam), UK)) and again the following year (O'Neal et al.[4] (Baylor (Bay), Texas)). All four models are described in Table 1 and the mutant alleles are illustrated in Figure 2. The designation of the *Cftr* mutant alleles follows the nomenclature recommendations of the Committee on Standardized Genetic Nomenclature for Mice and uses abbreviations of the laboratory in which they were derived (UNC1, HGU2, Cam3 and Bay4). All four groups used slightly different targeting strategies to create mutations which differ subtly or substantially. The first three groups (those from UNC, HGU and Cambridge) all used the same isogenic source of genomic DNA. The transgenic animals created by these three groups involved disruptions of exon 10 in the murine *Cftr* gene ($cftr^{m1UNC}$; $cftr^{m1HGU}$; $cftr^{m1Cam}$); the fourth group targeted exon 3 ($cftr^{m1Bay}$). The targeting strategies employed by two of the groups targeting exon 10 ($cftr^{m1UNC}$; $cftr^{m1Cam}$) were very similar, based on the positive negative selection (PNS) 'replacement' gene-targeting scheme[25]. Correct gene targeting occurs through a double reciprocal exchange between homologous gene and vector sequences. As a consequence, the region of the endogenous gene which lies between the cross-overs is replaced. Thus there is no molecular

**Table 1** Comparison of CF phenotypes in man and mouse: residual CFTR function

| Species | Allele | Nature of mutation | Residual CFTR function |
|---|---|---|---|
| Man | R347P<br>R117H<br><br>R334W | Missense Arg to 'other' in 1st membrane-spanning domain | ~33%<br>~15% of wild-type chloride ion<br>~4% conductance |
| Man | ΔF508 | 3 bp deletion resulting in loss of a Phe residue in exon 10 of 1st nucleotide-binding domain | Functional if correctly localized, but not detectable *in vivo*[69] |
| Mouse | $cftr^{m1UNC}$ | Replacement of chromosomal exon 10 with exon 10 containing in frame stop codon S489X[22] | None detectable[1] |
| Mouse | $cftr^{m1Cam}$ | Replacement of chromosomal exon 10 with an exon 10 disrupted by the *Hprt* gene, introducing an in-frame stop codon[24] | None detectable (W. Colledge, personal communication) |
| Mouse | $cftr^{m1Bay}$ | Insertion of an intact exon 3 causing exon 3 duplication[4] | None detectable[4] |
| Mouse | $cftr^{m1HGU}$ | Insertion of a disrupted exon 10 with in-frame stop codons in plasmid sequence[23] | <10% of normal level of *Cftr* mRNA produced by aberrant splicing[28] |

mechanism for reversion to wild type and the mutations are absolute 'nulls'. Dorin et al.[2] and O'Neal et al.[4] both describe insertional gene-targeting strategies into exon 10 (*cftr*$^{m1HGU}$) or exon 3 (*cftr*$^{m1Bay}$), respectively. Insertion into the genomic target occurs without loss of sequence and therefore

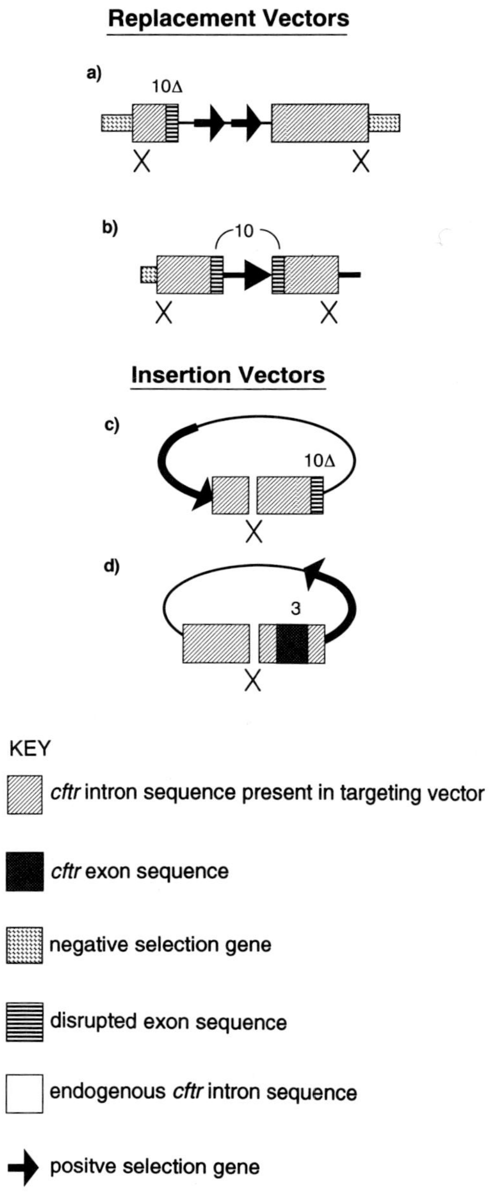

reversion to wild type by intrachromosomal recombination through the region of partial duplication is a formal possibility. Aberrant splicing around the insertional mutation can in some (but by no means all) instances result in wild-type mRNA. While *Hprt* insertional gene disruptions have been shown to be absolute 'nulls' under stringent biochemical selection[26], an insertional disruption of *N-myc* was found to be leaky[27].

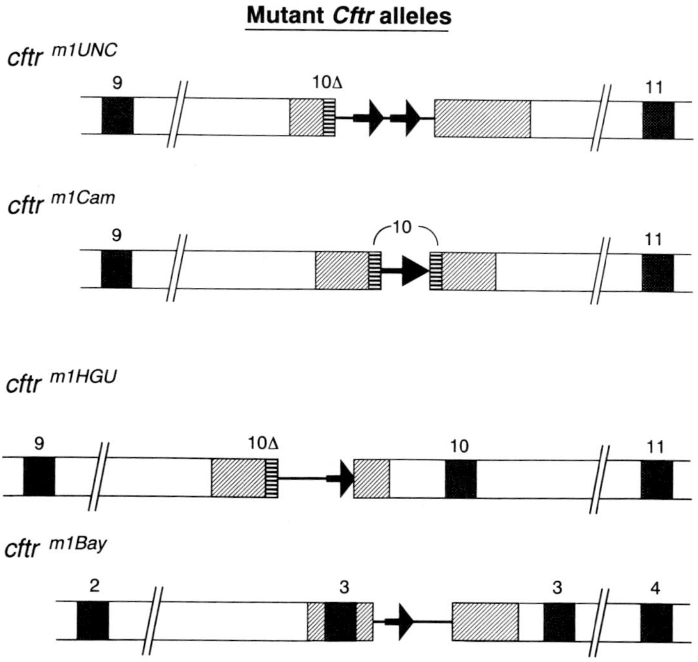


**Figure 2** (*facing page and above*) Targeting vectors and resultant genomic structure of the mutant *Cftr* alleles. The targeting strategies employed by the four groups are described in detail in the text. Koller et al.[22(a)] used a replacement vector with two *neomycin* genes (driven by two different promoters) in tandem providing the positive selection and containing 7.8 kb of *Cftr* homology. They used PNS[25] with two herpes simplex virus *thymidine kinase* (*HSV-tk*) genes to provide the negative selection and quote a targeting frequency of one in 2500 clones. Ratcliff et al.[24(b)] also used PNS with the *HPRT* gene (disrupting exon 10) providing the positive selection and one *HSV-tk* gene providing the negative selection. They report a targeting frequency of 1/1470 using 5.5 kb of homology. Dorin et al.[23(c)] and O'Neal et al.[4(d)] both employed the more efficient insertional targeting vectors[20]. The positive selection in each case was provided by a *neomycin* gene and Dorin et al.[23] used 3.5 kb of homologous DNA and quote a targeting frequency of 1/231. O'Neal et al.[4] had 6.2 kb of homology and obtained one correctly targeted clone out of every 21 G418 resistant clones. All four groups used targeting vectors containing isogenic DNA

The complete absence of *Cftr* mRNA has been demonstrated in the exon 10 *cftr*$^{m1UNC}$ replacement mice[1] and also in the *cftr*$^{m1Bay}$ exon 3 insertional mutant animals[4]. By contrast, the *cftr*$^{m1HGU}$ homozygotes display a low level of residual wild-type *Cftr* mRNA which is the result of aberrant splicing and exon skipping[28] (Table 1). The mutant mRNAs derived from the *cftr*$^{m1HGU}$ insertional mutation are not as predicted. The expected mutant mRNA cannot be detected. Instead, a novel mRNA is present. A novel 200 bp exon is derived from plasmid sequence and utilizing cryptic splice sites is incorporated between exons 9 and 11 of a mutant *Cftr*-derived mRNA. The sequence of this mRNA contains an in-frame stop at a position less than half-way into the message. This might be expected to destabilize the mRNA[29]. Mutant mRNAs which contain premature stop codons are often present at a reduced level in the cytoplasm[30]. Indeed CF patients have been described who carry nonsense mutations and display a severe deficiency of the *CFTR* mRNA derived from the allele with the premature stop codon[31]. Two models have been put forward to explain this phenomenon[32]. The 'translational translocation model' curtails entry of the mRNA into the cytoplasm by halting the normal process of the translational machinery pulling the mRNA through the nuclear pore. In the 'nuclear scanning model', pre-mRNAs are screened in the nucleus for nonsense mutations and in this case might promote skipping of the disrupted exon 10 and allow accumulation of wild-type *Cftr* mRNA in the cytoplasm. However, the exon 3 insertional mutation should also result in an mRNA with a premature stop codon because exon 3 is 109 bp and will thus create a frameshift. Perhaps the efficiency of alternative splicing in the exon 3 region of the *Cftr* gene is very low compared to the exon 10 region, and this explains why the *cftr*$^{m1HGU}$ insertion is slightly 'leaky' and the *cftr*$^{m1Bay}$ insertion is apparently not. Interestingly, alternative splicing around adjacent regions of exon 10 in the *CFTR* gene (exon 11b in the mouse[33] and exon 9 in man[34]) has previously been demonstrated. The fact that the *cftr*$^{m1HGU}$ mutation is on an outbred background whereas the *cftr*$^{m1Bay}$ mutation is on an inbred background may be another factor influencing the efficiency with which exon skipping occurs.

## ELECTROPHYSIOLOGY

Despite the different mutations all four of the CF mouse models demonstrate an electrophysiological phenotype consistent with CFTR dysfunction and can be distinguished from wild-type animals on the basis of defective chloride ion transport.

To assess how closely the four CF mouse models reproduce the bioelectric properties seen in CF subjects, their organ-specific electrophysiological properties are described below and summarized in Table 2 (respiratory tract) and Table 3 (intestinal tract).

The *in vivo* nasal epithelium of CF patients is characterized both by an increased nasal potential difference (PD) and a larger depolarization (both absolute and percentage of baseline) produced by the sodium channel blocker amiloride[35,36]. These and other studies suggest that the raised PD relates to increased sodium absorption, although how this links with the primary chloride defect is presently unknown. Nasal responses have only been reported

**Table 2** Comparison of the bioelectric phenotype of CF respiratory tract in man and mouse

| Tissue | Measurement | Man | *cftr*$^{m1UNC}$ Mouse | *cftr*$^{m1Cam}$ Mouse | *cftr*$^{m1Bay}$ Mouse | *cftr*$^{m1HGU}$ Mouse |
|---|---|---|---|---|---|---|
| Nasal epithelium | Baseline PD | ↑ | ↑ | Not reported | Not reported | ↑ |
| | Response to amiloride (sodium absorption) | ↑ | Not reported | Not reported | Not reported | ↑ |
| | cAMP-mediated chloride conductance | ↓ | ↓ | Not reported | Not reported | ↓ |
| | Calcium-related chloride conductance | Preserved | Preserved | Preserved | Not reported | Preserved |
| Lower respiratory tract | Baseline PD | Preserved or ↑ | Preserved | ↓ | Preserved (fetal) | ↓ |
| | Response to amiloride (sodium absorption) | ↑ | Not reported | ↓ | Not reported | ↓ |
| | cAMP-mediated chloride conductance | ↓ | ↓ in cultured tracheal cells<br>preserved in Ussing chamber | ↓ in Ussing chamber | ↓ in cultured fetal tracheal cells | ↓ in Ussing chamber |
| | Calcium-related chloride conductance | Preserved | Preserved | Not reported | Not reported | Preserved |

**Table 3** Comparison of the bioelectric phenotype of CF intestinal tract in man and mouse

| Measurement | Man | $cftr^{m1UNC}$ Mouse | $cftr^{m1Cam}$ Mouse | $cftr^{m1Bay}$ Mouse | $cftr^{m1HGU}$ Mouse |
|---|---|---|---|---|---|
| Baseline PD | ↓ or preserved | ↓ | ↓ | Preserved | ↓ |
| cAMP-mediated chloride conductance | ↓ | ↓ | ↓ | ↓ | ↓ |
| Calcium-related chloride conductance | ↓ | ↓ | ↓ | Not reported | ↓ |
| Sodium–glucose cotransport | ↑ | Preserved | Not reported | Not reported | Preserved |

in the $cftr^{m1HGU}$ and $cftr^{m1UNC}$ mutant animals. Both demonstrate a raised PD *in vivo* although quantitatively this is much greater in the $cftr^{m1UNC}$ mutant mice[37]. Furthermore the response to amiloride is also increased in the $cftr^{m1HGU}$ mice. *In vitro* studies in the $cftr^{m1UNC}$ animals demonstrate differences between cultured cells and native tracheae, the former showing little alteration in the amiloride response of mutant and wild-type animals, the latter demonstrating an increased response in the mutant mice[37,38]. cAMP-mediated responses are completely abolished in cultured cells from the $cftr^{m1UNC}$ mice, but the responses studied in the $cftr^{m1HGU}$ mutants *in vivo* are approximately 30% of the level in wild-type animals. Calcium-mediated responses have only been reported in the $cftr^{m1UNC}$ animals and are not altered in comparison to wild-type animals[38].

With respect to the lower airways in man, the initial *in vivo* study, in a limited number of subjects, indicated that the basal tracheobronchial PD of these patients was elevated, as in the nasal epithelium[35]. However, in a study of airway PD in CF patients following heart–lung transplantation, tracheal PD proximal to the anastomosis was not increased in comparison to that of non-CF subjects[41]. Furthermore, we have recently demonstrated that baseline bioelectric properties and radiolabelled sodium and chloride fluxes of CF bronchi are very similar to those found in non-CF subjects[42]. In the mouse models baseline bioelectric properties are unchanged in the $cftr^{m1UNC}$ and $cftr^{m1Bay}$ (fetal tissues only) mice[39,4], but reduced in the $cftr^{m1Cam}$ and $cftr^{m1HGU}$ mutant mice[39,43] in comparison to +/+ animals.

The amiloride response of human CF tracheobronchial epithelium both *in vivo*[35] and *in vitro*[42] is increased. In comparison the effect of amiloride is reduced in the trachea of both the $cftr^{m1Cam}$ mutants[44] and the $cftr^{m1HGU}$ homozygotes[39]. Thus, tracheal sodium transport appears to differ between CF subjects and the *cf*/*cf* mutant mice. The cellular composition of the lower murine trachea includes approximately 50–60% Clara cells[45]—not a predominant feature of human airways. However, the major active ion transport pathway across Clara cells is sodium[46], and therefore the reason for this anomaly is presently unclear.

As in nasal epithelium, reduced cAMP-mediated but not calcium-related chloride secretion characterizes the lower airways of both CF subjects[47,48] and the insertional mutant mice. Thus, forskolin produces a significantly smaller effect in all mutant mice. In cultured tracheae the response is completely abolished in the $cftr^{m1UNC}$ mutant mice[38] and reduced by approximately 70% in the $cftr^{m1BAY}$ mouse[4], while in Ussing chamber studies these values are approximately 75% in the $cftr^{m1Cam}$ mutants[43] and 50% in the $cftr^{m1HGU}$ homozygous animals[39] compared to wild-type animals. However, Ussing chamber studies of tracheae from the $cftr^{m1UNC}$ animals show forskolin responses indistinguishable from +/+ animals, suggested to relate to an elevation of intracellular calcium by this agent[40]. Calcium-related responses are preserved in the $cftr^{m1UNC}$, $cftr^{m1HGU}$ and $cftr^{m1Cam}$ animals[38,39,44], but have not been reported for the $cftr^{m1BAY}$ homozygous mutant mice.

The principal defect in the intestinal tissues of CF patients, as in the airways, relates to reduced cAMP-related chloride secretion[49]. In contrast to the respiratory tract, calcium-linked chloride transport also appears to be defective in CF subjects[50], suggesting that CFTR may function as a common final pathway for chloride secretion in the intestinal tract. Chloride secretion also contributes to intestinal baseline properties, and a reduced PD has been demonstrated in some studies in CF patients[51] Sodium–glucose cotransport has been suggested to be increased in the small intestine of CF subjects[52]. With respect to the CF mouse models, caecal responses have been studied in the $cftr^{m1UNC}$, $cftr^{m1HGU}$ and $cftr^{m1Cam}$ mutant animals, all showing reduced baseline properties. This is also true for each of the intestinal segments of the $cftr^{m1UNC}$ and $cftr^{m1HGU}$ animals[38,39]. However, baseline ileal $I_{SC}$ (short-circuit current) in the $cftr^{m1BAY}$ animals appears not to differ with genotype[4].

Forskolin responses are again significantly reduced in each of the mice, but are virtually abolished in the $cftr^{m1Cam}$ and $cftr^{m1UNC}$ homozygotes[43,38] and reduced by approximately 80% in the $cftr^{m1BAY}$ mutants[4] and 65% in the $cftr^{m1HGU}$ animals[39]. Calcium-linked responses are significantly reduced in the intestine of the $cftr^{m1UNC}$, $cftr^{m1HGU}$ and $cftr^{m1Cam}$ mutant animals[38,39,53]. Responses have not been reported for the $cftr^{m1BAY}$ animals. No evidence for increased sodium–glucose cotransport has been reported in the small intestines of either the $cftr^{m1HGU}$ or $cftr^{m1UNC}$ mice[38,39].

With respect to the pancreas, CF patients secrete less bicarbonate and fluid than non-CF subjects. This is likely to relate to the presence of CFTR in the apical membrane of pancreatic ductal cells, where it plays a key role in chloride/bicarbonate exchange. In the $cftr^{m1HGU}$ mice cAMP-activated chloride currents were reduced as expected, but calcium-related currents were preserved[54]. It is worthy of note that the latter were up to 11-fold larger than the former, and this coupled with the presence of some wild-type CFTR mRNA may explain the lack of pancreatic pathology in these mice[2]. To date no reports of sweat gland function or secretory response to $\beta$-adrenergic agonists in any of the CF mice have appeared, although such studies are under way.

Thus, the characteristic ion transport defect of reduced cAMP-mediated chloride secretion throughout the respiratory and intestinal tracts is present in each of the mouse models. Furthermore, many of the other abnormalities found in man are also seen, with the exception of increased sodium absorption in the trachea. This suggests that these models will be of value in furthering the understanding of CF pathophysiology and in studying the effects of novel treatments. In the virtual absence of submucosal glands and with no evidence for increased sodium absorption, development of pathology in the lungs of these CF animals would emphasize the role of chloride transport in airway surface epithelium in the causation of such abnormalities.

## HISTOPATHOLOGY OF THE CF MICE

### INTESTINAL DISEASE

Table 4 describes the survival rates of the CF mice from the four different groups. The phenotype of the mice produced by Dorin et al.[2] is significantly different from that of the animals produced by the other three groups[1,3,4]. These latter animals all have a severe phenotype in terms of the morbidity and mortality which can be largely ascribed to the severity of intestinal disease. Within one week of birth, 40–80% of these animals present with a severe gut blockage which leads to intestinal perforation, peritonitis and death. A second critical period resulting in fatality is around weaning, leaving less than 5% of these mutant animals surviving into adulthood. The intestinal site of the perinatal blockage is either immediately proximal or distal to the caecum[4,43]. The animals that die at weaning may have the constriction located in the small intestine, but it is more commonly in the large intestine.

Ten per cent or more of newborn CF infants present with ileal obstruction termed *meconium ileus* and this is practically diagnostic of the disease[55]. These babies fail to pass meconium and develop abdominal distension and this may result in perforation and peritonitis. A few CF babies have a meconium plug in the large intestine and meconium passage is delayed, but this feature is shared with several clinical entities. The intestinal disease of the 'severe' CF

**Table 4** Comparison of intestinal disease severity in mouse and man

| Species | Mouse | | | | Man |
|---|---|---|---|---|---|
| Mutant allele | $cftr^{m1UNC}$ | $cftr^{m1Cam}$ | $cftr^{m1Bay}$ | $cftr^{m1HGU}$ | >300 |
| Type of mutation | Replacement | Replacement | Insertion | Insertion | Nonsense, missense, frameshift, deletion |
| Genomic site | Exon 10 | Exon 10 | Exon 3 | Exon 10 | All exons, but predominantly MSD1–3 and NBD 1 and 2 |
| Death within 1 week of birth | ~50% | ~80% | ~40% | ~5% | 10–20% ileal blockage (meconium ileus) or obstruction in large intestine (meconium plug) in newborns* |
| Death around weaning | ~40% | ~10% | ~10% | ~2% | Distal intestinal obstruction syndrome* |
| Death after 40 days | Not reported | Not reported | Not reported | 2% | In ~20% of children and adults |
| Body weight at weaning | 10–50% reduced | 50% reduced | 70% reduced | No reduction | Failure to thrive and reduced growth rate |
| Survival to adulthood | <5% | <10% | Not reported (≪50%) | <93% | *Intestinal blockage and obstruction not fatal, owing to medical and surgical intervention |

mutant mice is thus rather similar to that observed in this minority of extreme clinical cases. Interestingly, the phenotype of the CF mice produced by Dorin et al.[2] echoes the severity of intestinal disease seen in man. Only 5% of the $cftr^{m1HGU}$ homozygous animals die perinatally from gut blockage which, when present, is of a similar nature to that observed in the other CF mice[28]. A further 2% of $cftr^{m1HGU}$ homozygotes die at weaning. Thus 93% of homozygous mutant CF animals survive to adulthood and 2% of these die from a distal intestinal obstruction similar to that observed in 20% of CF non-newborns and termed *meconium ileus equivalent* or *distal intestinal obstruction syndrome*. The low level of mRNA found in the exon 10 insertional model appears to be sufficient to result in clearance of meconium in 95% of animals perinatally and 90% of animals overall. All four of the CF mutant mice are reported as having mucin accumulation with dilatation of the crypts and engorgement and increase of goblet cells[1,2,4,43]. These gut abnormalities are displayed only in 75% of $cftr^{m1HGU}$ homozygote animals that survive weaning.

Comparison of the CF exocrine gland histology in man and mouse is detailed below and summarised in Table 5.

## BRUNNER'S GLAND

CF subjects are reported as having Brunner's gland hypertrophy and duct dilatation with mucin-filled acinar lumina. In man, these glands are found throughout the duodenum, but in mice there is only one large gland just distal to the stomach. Interestingly, the $cftr^{m1UNC}$ mutant mice are described as having pronounced and extensive gland destruction and distension[1], while the $cftr^{m1HGU}$ (J. R. Dorin unpublished data) and $cftr^{m1Bay}$ homozygotes[4] do not appear to have any Brunner's gland abnormality.

## PANCREATIC DISEASE

In man, ~85% of CF subjects are pancreatic insufficient from birth[56]. The pancreas is histologically abnormal in almost every case examined and virtually destroyed at autopsy. Obstruction of ducts by inspissated secretions is one of the first features, followed by dilatation of acini and secretory ducts and constriction of the epithelium architecture. Acinar cell loss and areas of destruction are widespread, being replaced with fibrous tissue and fat. The islets of Langerhans, however, appear to survive functionally intact for long periods of time. None of these CF-associated abnormalities are reported to the same degree in any of the four CF mouse models. The only abnormalities seen in $cftr^{m1UNC}$ mutant mice have been attributed to nutritional deficiency[1]. However, Ratcliff et al.[43] state that 50% of the $cftr^{m1Cam}$ mice which survive over 17 days have focal dilatation and blockage in several pancreatic ducts. O'Neal et al. report that the $cftr^{m1Bay}$ animals show some evidence for pancreatic atrophy, but not in all animals. The question must be asked whether the observed pathology is a direct consequence of the *Cftr* mutation or a secondary consequence of intestinal disease and peritonitis. The $cftr^{m1HGU}$ mice have no evidence of any pancreatic histological abnormality[2]. Why do the CF mice not share the hallmarks of pancreatic disease as seen in CF patients? One reason could be that the normal level of *Cftr* expression in the pancreas is markedly reduced in the mouse compared to man[57]. The $cftr^{m1HGU}$ animals are the only CF mice where the bioelectric properties of the pancreas have been examined[54]. As discussed above the high level of $Ca^{2+}$-regulated chloride conductance in the rodent pancreas may compensate for the defective CFTR regulated ion transport. The lack of pancreatic involvement evident in the 'severe' CF mice ($cftr^{m1UNC}$, $cftr^{m1Bay}$ and $cftr^{m1Cam}$) does, however, question the presumption that meconium ileus in CF babies is a consequence of pancreatic malfunction.

## LIVER AND GALLBLADDER

The histology of the liver has only been reported for the $cftr^{m1UNC}$ mutant animals and it was apparently normal. However, the gallbladder in the $cftr^{m1UNC}$ homozygotes is apparently distended or ruptured[1] whereas the $cftr^{m1Bay}$ mutants report no histological abnormality for this organ[4]. Thirty per cent of CF patients have micro-gallbladder at autopsy.

## SALIVARY GLAND

Some CF individuals are reported as having enlarged and dilated salivary gland ducts with inspissated secretions leading to atrophy[56]. The $cftr^{m1Bay}$ mice are reported to have no histological abnormality of these glands, while the $cftr^{m1UNC}$ mice have disruption of serous acini and $cftr^{m1HGU}$ mice have mild dilatation of the salivary glands in some few animals[1,2,4].

## LACRIMAL GLANDS

Ratcliff et al.[43] were prompted to examine the lacrimal glands of their CF mice ($cftr^{m1Cam}$) because they were prone to eye infections and persistent eye closure. Although no obvious mucin accumulation was present, acinar dilatation was observed in 5/7 mice analysed. The Baylor group, however, report no such abnormality in their CF mice[4]. With the small number of animals examined, it is perhaps premature to draw any firm conclusions at this stage. No lacrimal gland abnormality to our knowledge has been reported in CF patients.

**Table 5** Comparison of CF phenotypes in man and mouse: exocrine organs

| Species | Allele | Pancreas | Gallbladder and liver | Brunner's gland | Salivary gland | Lacrimal glands |
|---|---|---|---|---|---|---|
| Man | R117H | Pancreatic sufficient. Fibrosis of acini; dilatation of ductules; plugs within acini; focal acinar calcifications | Micro-gallbladder in 30% of autopsy. Fatty infiltration of liver; focal, then multilobular biliary cirrhosis | Hypertrophy and duct dilatation; mucin-filled acinar lumina | Enlarged and dilated ducts, inspissated secretions leading to atrophy in some individuals | Not reported |
| | ΔF508 | Pancreatic insufficient. Otherwise as for R117H | | | | |
| Mouse | $cftr^{m1UNC}$ | No clear abnormality, not attributable to being nutritionally compromised | Gallbladder distended or ruptured | Gland destruction and distention | Disruption of acini | Not reported |
| Mouse | $cftr^{m1Cam}$ | Focal dilatation and blockage of several ducts in 50 % of animals over 17 days | Not reported | Not reported | Not reported | Acinar dilatation but no mucus |
| Mouse | $cftr^{m1Bay}$ | Pancreatic atrophy observed, but could be attributed to being nutritionally compromised | No histological abnormality | No histological abnormality | No histological abnormality | No histological abnormality |
| Mouse | $cftr^{m1HGU}$ | no evidence of histological abnormality | Not reported | No histological abnormality | Mild dilatation in some animals | Not reported |

## FERTILITY

The vast majority of CF males are azoospermic due to aplasia of the vas deferens and epididymis[58]. Female CF subjects also display reduced fertility, with a delayed age of menarche compared to the control population[55]. Although all the *cf/cf* mice are fertile and there is no evidence of an absent vas deferens in the male mice examined, the degree of fertility is reduced (J. R. Dorin and D. J. Porteous, unpublished data).

## LUNG DISEASE

The major cause of morbidity and mortality of CF patients is lung disease. Although no histological abnormalities are present at birth, submucosal gland hypertrophy and dilated acinal and duct lumina are evident before chronic infections are established. Mucin accumulation and small airway obstruction are commonly believed to lead to bronchiolitis and chronic infection, and then extensive bronchiectasis. Infectious pathogens are commonly *Staphylococcus aureus*, followed by *Pseudomonas aeruginosa*[55,56]. The submucosal glands of the proximal airways are the only site of high-level *CFTR* expression in the respiratory tract in man[59]. *CFTR* expression in the epithelial lung cells is extremely low, with only an estimated one copy per cell of *CFTR* mRNA[60]. It has been suggested that the submucosal gland is a likely initial site of disease pathogenesis and a primary target for therapy. Mice have a relative paucity of these glands, which do not extend beyond the carina, and this has led people to question whether they could develop CF lung disease. If they do, then the submucosal gland must have a minor involvement. It should also be noted that pulmonary involvement in CF subjects begins initially in the small airways, which are devoid of submucosal glands.

In common with man, none of the CF mice present with respiratory tract disease at birth. No respiratory abnormality was reported in the $cftr^{m1Cam}$ animals up to five weeks of age[43]. (See Table 6 for a summary of the reported lung pathology evident in the *cf/cf* mice.) The $cftr^{m1Bay}$ animals are reported as having dilatation of acini and accumulation of material in the mucosal glands in the pharynx[4]. The $cftr^{m1UNC}$ animals are reported as having atrophy of serous gland tissue in the nasal dorsolateral sinuses[1]. The ducts in the nasal mucosa and proximal trachea show slight dilatation and goblet cell hyperplasia is observed in the proximal airways. As mentioned above, CF infants display no evidence of lung abnormalities at birth and it is presumed that environmental factors contribute heavily to the development of the pulmonary complications. As a result of the good long-term survival of the exon 10 insertional CF mouse model, it should be possible to address comprehensively which of many putative factors are necessary for development of CF lung disease or augment the disease process. There is a low level of wild-type *Cftr* mRNA present in the lungs of the exon 10 insertional mutant mice[28], yet cAMP-mediated chloride secretion is still markedly reduced. This finding is consistent with the recent analysis of chloride transport in CF patients with various missense mutations. Sheppard et al.[61] report that the chloride conductance of R347P and R117H mutant constructs in the vaccinia virus T7 hybrid expression system are approximately 30% and 15% of wild-type values, respectively. Individuals who are R347P/ΔF508 or R117H/ΔF508 compound heterozygotes are therefore predicted to retain approximately 15% or 7.5% of normal CFTR function, respectively. However, these individuals are still diagnosed as having CF and still develop severe lung disease although the pancreatic involvement is ameliorated. Twenty-five per cent of the *cftr*$^{m1HGU}$ mutant animals (housed in a conventional animal house) display lung abnormalities including bronchitis, bronchopneumonia, mucin accumulation, focal atelectasis and bronchiectasis. Littermate controls do not show the same level of these abnormalities (J. R. Dorin and D. J. Porteous, unpublished data). The next step is to see whether acute or chronic exposure to CF pathogens will precipitate the development of severe lung disease and whether mucin hypersecretion is

**Table 6** Comparison of CF phenotypes in man and mouse: respiratory tract pathology and lung disease

| Species | Allele | Phenotype |
|---|---|---|
| Man | R117H and ΔF508 | No histological abnormality at birth<br>Dilated acinar and duct lumina in submucosal glands before chronic infections<br>Submucosal gland and goblet cell hypertrophy into the distal airways<br>Mucin accumulation and small airway obstruction leading to bronchiolectasis and chronic infection, then extensive bronchiectasis<br>Chronic infection usually with *Staphylococcus aureus* initially and subsequently *Pseudomonas aeruginosa* |
| Mouse | *cftr*$^{m1UNC}$ | Atrophy of serous gland tissue in nasal dorsolateral sinuses<br>Dilation of ducts in nasal mucosa and proximal trachea<br>Goblet cell hyperplasia in proximal airways |
| Mouse | *cftr*$^{m1Cam}$ | No histological abnormality reported |
| Mouse | *cftr*$^{m1Bay}$ | Dilatation of acini<br>Accumulation of material in mucosal glands of pharynx |
| Mouse | *cftr*$^{m1HGU}$ | Lung abnormalities in ~25% of animals<br>Mucin accumulation<br>Focal atelectasis<br>Bronchitis<br>Lung disease after bacterial challenge |

triggered by infection. Chronic exposure of the $cftr^{m1HGU}$ mice (and littermate controls) to *S. aureus* has resulted in abnormal lung pathology in the mutant mice (D. J. Davidson et al., submitted). Is the order of exposure to CF pathogens important or not? How does the CFTR defect relate to increased susceptibility to specific infections? How does the local immune deficiency relate to CFTR function? A chronic *P. aeruginosa* infection (particularly of the CF specific mucoid form) or a *P. cepacia* infection in these animals would be of great value in searching for improved treatments of these life-threatening infections.

## PROSPECTS FOR REFINED MOUSE MODELS?

What other mouse models for CF are a priority? The phenotype of a compound heterozygote with one 'mild' $cftr^{m1HGU}$ allele and one 'severe' allele would be of great interest as a further 50% reduction in the amount of wild-type CFTR from that seen in the $cftr^{m1HGU}$ homozygotes will result in a mouse with an intestinal phenotype which is somewhere between 'mild' and very 'severe'. Of even greater interest will be mice engineered to carry clinical mutations.

## CLINICALLY RELEVANT MUTATIONS IN THE MOUSE

The value of creating clinically relevant mutations in the mouse lies in being able to compare genotype and phenotype on a controlled genetic background and also to test novel therapeutic strategies that may be specific for a particular mutant protein. The priority must be for a mouse carrying the ΔF508 mutation. This and other clinically relevant mutations can be modelled by a variety of gene-targeting strategies or by a classical transgenic approach.

## GENE-TARGETING STRATEGIES

Insertional gene-targeting vectors can be adapted simply to create precise mutations by the 'hit-and-run' or 'in–out' strategy[62,63]. For this, forward and back selectable markers are present in the vector and the targeting sequence carries the chosen mutation in the mouse gene. Correctly targeted clones ('hits') are identified and then subjected to the back selection, which will identify clones ('runs') that have lost vector sequence through intrachromosomal recombination. The genome will either revert to wild-type sequence or will be modified to include the introduced mutation depending on whether the recombination event occurs proximal or distal to the modified site.

ES cell ‘hit’ clones have been reported which carry either the ΔF508 or ΔI507 mutations targeted to the mouse *Cftr* gene[20].

Replacement gene-targeting vectors can be used to introduce specific mutations to the genome. Once again, the introduced gene sequence carries the desired mutation; the vector DNA, including a dominant selectable marker (e.g. *neomycin*), is contained within intron sequences. A correct replacement event will result in exonic sequences modified only by the mutation. The only proviso is that expression of the plasmid-derived genes must not interfere with expression of the target gene. Deng et al.[64] have reported the targeting of the ΔF508 mutation to the *Cftr* gene in ES cells by this method.

Ratcliff et al.[24] promote one final gene-targeting strategy. Their $cftr^{m1Cam}$ replacement introduced the *Hprt* gene into exon 10 of the *Cftr* gene. Biochemical selection can be used to select both for and against the presence of this gene. A region of the *Cftr* gene encompassing exon 10 and including a ΔF508 mutation could be introduced into the $cftr^{m1Cam}$-targeted ES cells and the negative selection applied. Cells surviving the back selection must have lost *Hprt* gene function. If this is as a result of homologous recombination, it will have been replaced by the ΔF508 *Cftr* sequence. The major problem with this strategy is the inefficiency of transfection and homologous recombination compared to *Hprt* inactivation by mutation.

### CLASSICAL TRANSGENESIS

An alternative approach is to use pronuclear injection of fertilized mouse oocytes to introduce a *CFTR* cDNA transgene carrying the chosen mutation into a random site. Provided this random site is not on chromosome 6, the mice carrying the transgene can be crossed to any of the existing CF mutant mice. In this way the ‘knockout’ CF mice can be engineered to express the ΔF508 protein. The transgene can be of either mouse or (perhaps more relevantly) human origin and tissue expression can be controlled by an appropriate choice of promoter. Transgenes carrying the wild-type *CFTR* gene under a gut-specific promoter might be valuable to complement the ‘severe’ intestinal phenotype in the replacement of exon 3 insertional mice and thus increase their survival.

## TESTING NEW THERAPEUTIC APPROACHES

Before the cystic fibrosis gene was cloned, treatment could be at best palliative or serendipitous. Now, there are grounds for optimism that improved therapies will be developed on two complementary fronts. A biomolecular understanding of CFTR function will certainly aid the design of rational approaches to pharmacological intervention. The availability of cloned CFTR expression constructs means that gene correction strategies can also be conceived. Both lines of investigation must benefit from the availability of appropriate animal models for testing prior to clinical trials.

## PHARMACOLOGICAL APPROACHES

Clinical trials to determine the efficacy of amiloride (a sodium channel blocker) have suggested either a modest improvement in $FEV_1$[65] or no improvement[66] and studies combining both amiloride and UTP (a chloride secretagogue that acts through a non-cAMP-mediated pathway) are currently under way. Studies of efficacy in the CF mutant mice can help in the design of improved protocols which might offer a more clear-cut clinical benefit.

The ΔF508 protein fails to become fully glycosylated and as a consequence the mutant protein is not correctly localized in the plasma membrane[67]. However, under low-temperature conditions some mutant protein is fully glycosylated (presumably because it folds correctly) and is delivered to the apical membrane[68]. Once correctly localized, chloride conductance and regulation are essentially normal[69]. This has directed attention towards possible pharmacological approaches to treatment. Can ΔF508 protein be overexpressed so that therapeutic levels of protein reach the apical membrane? Butyrate has been shown to upregulate the expression of *CFTR*, *in vitro* (A. E. Smith personal communication). Will it work *in vivo*? Even if this approach were unsuccessful in treating ΔF508 homozygotes, there is a sizeable minority of patients with mild pancreatic disease but who are still susceptible to lung disease for whom a modest upregulation of their residual CFTR function might well be therapeutic. Recent work suggests that the stability of the ΔF508 mutant protein at the plasma membrane is reduced[70]. This may suggest that even if the processing block at the endoplasmic reticulum could be overcome, correctly localized ΔF508 protein may not be able to function to restore normal chloride conductance. Is it possible to interfere specifically with inappropriate chaperone association which maintains the mutant protein in the endoplasmic reticulum? Can chloride conductance be restored by inhibiting the endocytosis of apical ΔF508 protein, without disrupting cellular functions relating to membrane trafficking? Although the focus of these strategies is on modifying the function of mutant CFTR, none are intrinsically specific to CFTR and each is likely to affect the expression of other cellular proteins. Thus, issues of safety/toxicity must be at the forefront from the outset. Gross cellular toxicity can be addressed *in vitro*, but extensive and rigorous tests will obviously be required *in vivo*. Few, if any, treatments will be without any side-effect; the clear objective will be to find a window of opportunity between toxicity and efficacy. In this regard, a genetic model is all but essential. The $cftr^{m1HGU}$ mouse, with its low level of residual CFTR activity, provides an ideal genetic model for testing many of these approaches.

In developing strategies focused specifically on the ΔF508 mutation, the mutant mice in prospect bearing this mutation will be invaluable.

## SOMATIC GENE THERAPY

Progress in our biomolecular understanding of CFTR function has increased dramatically since 1989, but there is much still to learn and understand. Cloning of the gene immediately brought into sharp focus the prospect of treatment by gene correction therapy. If a normal copy of the *CFTR* gene can be introduced into affected tissues in CF patients, then all of the downstream (and as yet incompletely understood) consequences of *CFTR* gene dysfunction would be corrected. Exciting though this prospect is, it is not without its own problems. More than ever before, issues of safety assume an overriding importance. Not even gene therapy can correct tissue damage. Ideally, therefore, treatment must start before organ damage has taken place. The lung will be the first target for somatic gene therapy as this is the organ which currently accounts for all but a small fraction of the disease morbidity and mortality. As discussed above, there is little evidence for lung disease at birth and near-maximal lung function can be maintained for as long as repeated opportunistic lung infection is prevented. Nevertheless, as CF individuals are unpredictable in their susceptibility to infection and response to treatment, in all likelihood gene therapy will need to be started in the CF child. This in itself raises important issues of informed consent and places an onerous responsibility on the scientist and physician to ensure that the proposed method of treatment will be both safe and effective for the lifetime of the CF individual. Animal testing for safety must be a prerequisite of any clinical trial and surely the preferred option must be to combine this with efficacy assessment in a relevant animal model.

So what progress has been made down the route to gene correction therapy and where have animals, in particular the CF mutant mice, played a part? Before deciding on a strategy for somatic gene therapy, several competing factors must be considered and balanced. In what form is the CFTR gene to be expressed? By what route and by which cellular uptake mechanism is the transgene to be delivered? How will these choices be influenced by the desire for efficient transfer, long-term stable expression and primary safety considerations? And what of the longer-term requirements, that the gene delivery system be produced to the standards required of a prescription drug? Many of these requirements are in mutual conflict. Application to CF apart, somatic gene therapy is itself a fledgling field. Treatment of CF by somatic gene therapy is the first proposed application where the disease is not immediately life threatening. It is therefore unreasonable to expect that any of the currently available gene transfer systems can meet all these requirements.

Focusing for the moment specifically on the lung, this objective raises both opportunities and special challenges. The lung epithelium is directly accessible through respiration. The CF physician and patient are well used to non-invasive aerosolized drug treatments and to investigation and biopsy by bronchoscopy. Set against this, the purulent secretions which characterize the diseased CF lung may constitute a serious barrier to gene delivery. Surfactant protein C promoter-driven expression of human *CFTR* in the lung and testes in transgenic mice implies that delivery of somatic gene therapy to the lung epithelia is non-toxic[71]. Once delivered, any therapeutic effect can last only for the lifetime of each terminally differentiated transfected cell. Epithelial stem cells remain elusive; xenograft rat tracheal reconstitution experiments have suggested the rare basal cell as a candidate[72]. Efficient delivery of stable transgenes to such cells is a major challenge for the future. For the moment, full advantage must be taken of the fact that the respiratory epithelium has such a slow turnover. If efficient transfer and stable transgene expression can be achieved, then the treatment might need only to be repeated at monthly intervals or less. The absence of a significant cell turnover effectively rules out retroviruses as a mode of gene delivery. Attention therefore switched to adenovirus, which is naturally tropic for the lung and which can be engineered to accommodate the *CFTR* gene. Rosenfeld et al.[73] showed that the cotton rat lung epithelium could be efficiently infected with *CFTR* recombinant adenovirus and potentially therapeutic levels of *CFTR* expression obtained. On the basis of these studies and additional studies in primates, several groups applied successfully to the Recombinant Advisory Committee and to the Food and Drug Administration in the USA for permission to undertake clinical trials. Several trials are currently under way and the first encouraging results have been reported[74]. It is premature to comment extensively on these results and before those from the other studies in progress are also available, but some key points are valid. The first is that recombinant *CFTR* adenovirus is capable of transferring the *CFTR* gene and correcting the basic bioelectrical defect but only transiently. A second consideration regarding the use of adenovirus is the propensity to elicit an inflammatory response to infection. This remains a real concern, but as bioelectrical correction was obtained at a mutliplicity of infection of 1, this caveat may be less serious than previously believed. A significant concern about the use of adenovirus is the stringent requirement that each batch be devoid of wild-type virus, to remove any possibility of accidental recombination to form an infectious particle. A gene delivery strategy which circumvents these potential problems is very attractive. Liposomes are hypoimmunogenic, chemically defined and easily mass produced to pharmacological stardard. Their disadvantages are that gene delivery is indiscriminate and less, efficient than virus infection. To date, two related experiments reporting correction of the electrophysiological defect in CF mutant mice have been published. Both used *CFTR* cDNA expression plasmids transferred to the respiratory epithelium as a complex with cationic liposome. Hyde et al.[44] reported direct tracheal instillation of *CFTR* cDNA complexed with DOTMA/DOPE, available commercially as Lipofectin. In four out of six animals reported, evidence was presented for complete correction of the electrophysiological defect in tracheal explants. The other two animals showed no detectable correction, which the authors put down to failure of delivery. Alton et al.[75] reported a larger study in which the DNA was delivered as an aerosol by nebulization. Using $\beta$-gal as a reporter gene, they observed successful transfer using DOTMA/DOPE, DOTAP (also commercially available) and DC-chol/DOPE. DC-chol/DOPE had been approved for use in gene therapy trials to treat melanoma on the basis that it showed no toxic effect on intravenous use in mice, pigs and rabbits[76]. Alton et al.[75] found no evidence for toxic effect or histological damage in mice from DOTAP, but used only DC-chol/DOPE to transfer the *CFTR* gene to the CF mutant mice. They provided evidence for partial to complete correction of the electrophysiological defect in the nose (measured *in vivo*) and in the trachea (*in vitro*). The former result is important because early clinical trials are likely to start with gene delivery to the nose, where simple measurements and drug responses can be used to measure efficacy. The latter result is important because it is the airway defect which must be corrected to be of clinical benefit. It will be important now to determine how efficient, repeatable and long lasting is the effect of liposome-mediated gene transfer. On the basis of the promising results of DNA liposome delivery by nebulization to the CF mice, permission to carry out a phase I trial involving single nasal application has been approved and is under way in the UK.

Topical application of DNA/liposomes was used to attempt to correct the electrophysiological defect in the intestinal tract, but was without a marked effect[75]. This may have been due to any number of factors, including a less favourable environment. It is, however, worthy of note that by comparison with the lung, the level of expression of *CFTR* in the intestinal crypts is much higher, as is cell turnover. Thus, it may be much more difficult to achieve gene correction by this route. Modified formulations and delivery protocols may solve the efficiency problem. Increased efficiency and a degree of specificity of cell transfection should also be possible by coupling epithelial cell surface receptor molecules, such as transferrin or influenza virus haemagglutinin, to the DNA/liposome complex[77].

Zhu et al.[78] report intravenous delivery of reporter constructs and *CFTR* complexed with cationic liposomes and present evidence consistent with systemic delivery and long-term expression, indicating that epithelial stem cells are indeed transfected. This remarkable result demands repetition and extension. If it is shown possible to consistently correct the electrophysiological defect in the CF mutant mouse by this simple procedure then this would be a major advance. It has the intrinsic appeal that not only would several affected tissues (lung, liver, intestine and pancreas) be readily accessed, but that gene delivery would be to presumptive stem cells, thus ensuring long-term, possibly even life-long correction. There is unfortunately a down side to systemic delivery as this would potentially mean that the germline would be affected.

Although the sterility of males would not be corrected unless administered *in utero* (an ethically unacceptable procedure at this point in time), the possibility of germline transmission through females would be real and again is unacceptable as legislation currently stands. Perhaps the answer lies in the intravenous delivery of DNA targeted specifically to the endothelium of affected somatic tissues. A promising step in this direction has already been made by Ferkol et al.[79], who report efficient gene transfer *in vivo* using a polymeric immunoglobulin fragment as a synthetic receptor molecule. Again, safety and efficacy tests in CF mutant mice are called for as a crucial step before considering clinical trials.

## CONCLUDING REMARKS

It is clear that the CF mutant mice collectively model many of the hallmarks of the disease in remarkable detail. There can be little doubt that basic research in cystic fibrosis will benefit greatly from the existing mutant mice and from the 'clinically relevant' mutants in prospect. Together with the instructive species-specific differences, this promises to provide many new opportunities and stimulate novel lines of investigation. Beyond the improved understanding this will bring to our basic understanding of disease pathophysiology, these mice are certain to help speed the development of safe and effective new treatments.

## ACKNOWLEDGEMENTS

J.R.D. is supported by a Caledonian Research Fellowship and E.W.F.W.A. by a British Heart Foundation Intermediate Fellowship, and the studies by the Medical Research Council, the Cystic Fibrosis Research Trust and the Association Française de Lutte Contra la Mucoviscidose.

## REFERENCES

1 Snouwaert JN, Brigman KK, Latour AM, et al. An animal model for cystic fibrosis made by gene targeting. *Science* 1992; **257**: 1083–88.
2 Dorin JR, Dickinson P, Alton EWFW, et al. Cystic fibrosis in the mouse by targeted insertional mutagenesis. *Nature* 1992; **359**: 211–15.

3 Colledge W, Ratcliffe R, Foster D, et al. Cystic fibrosis mouse with intestinal obstruction. *Lancet* 1992; **340**: 680.

4 O'Neal WK, Hasty P, McCray PB, et al. A severe phenotype in mice with a duplication of exon 3 in the cystic fibrosis locus. *Hum Mol Genet* 1993; **2**: 1561–9.

5 Porteous DJ, Dorin JR. How relevant are mouse models for human diseases to somatic gene therapy? *Tibtech* 1993; **11**: 173–81.

6 The cystic fibrosis genotype–phenotype consortium. Correlation between genotype and phenotype in patients with cystic fibrosis. *N Engl J Med* 1993; **329**: 1308–12.

7 Smith SN, Alton EWFW, Geddes DM. Ion transport characteristics of the murine trachea and caecum. *Clin Sci* 1992; **82**: 667–72.

8 Tata F, Stainer P, Wicking C, et al. Cloning the mouse homologue of the human cystic fibrosis transmembrane conductance regulator gene. *Genomics* 1991; **10**: 301–7.

9 Yorifuji T, Lemna WK, Ballard CF, et al. Molecular cloning and sequence analysis of the murine cDNA for the cystic fibrosis transmembrane conductance regulator gene. *Genomics* 1991; **10**: 547–50.

10 Tsui L-C. Mutations and sequence variations detected in the cystic fibrosis transmembrane conductance regulator (CFTR) gene: a report from the CF Genetic Analysis Consortium. *Hum Mutat* 1992; **1**: 197–203.

11 Joyner A. Gene targeting and gene trap screens using ES cells: new approaches to mammalian development. *Bioessays* 1991; **13**: 649–56.

12 Hooper M, Hardy K, Handyside A et al. HPRT-deficient (Lesch–Nyhan) mouse embryos derived from germline colonisation by cultured cells. *Nature* 1987; **326**: 292–5.

13 Kuehn M, Bradley A, Robertson E, Evans M. A potential animal model for Lesch–Nyhan syndrome through introduction of HPRT mutations into mice. *Nature* 1987; **326**: 295–8.

14 Wu C, Melton D. Production of a model for Lesch–Nyhan syndrome in HPRT deficient mice. *Nature Genet* 1993: **3**: 235–40.

15 Tybulewicz V, Tremblay M, LaMarca M, et al. Animal model of Gaucher's disease from targeted disruption of the mouse glucocerebrosidase gene. *Nature* 1992; **357**: 407–10.

16 Evans M, Kaufman M. Establishment in culture of pluripotential cells from mouse embryos. *Nature* 1981; **292**: 154–6.

17 Capecchi M. The new mouse genetics: altering the genome by gene targeting. *Trends Genet* 1989; **5**: 70–6.

18 Hasty P, Rivera-Perez J, Bradley A. The length of homology required for gene targeting in ES cells. *Mol Cell Biol* 1991; **11**: 5586–91.

19 Te Riele H, Robanus Maandag E, Berns A. Highly efficient gene targeting in ES cells via homologous recombination with isogenic DNA constructs. *Proc Natl Acad Sci USA* 1992; **89**: 5128–32.

20 Dickinson P, Kimber W, Kilanowski F, et al. High frequency gene targeting using insertional vectors. *Hum Mol Genet* 1993; **2**: 1299–302.

21 Dorin J, Inglis J, Porteous D. Selection for precise chromosomal targeting of a dominant marker by homologous recombination. *Science* 1989; **243**: 1357–60.

22 Koller BH, Kim HS, Latour AM, et al. Toward an animal model of cystic fibrosis: targeted interruption of exon 10 of the cystic fibrosis transmembrane regulator gene in embryonic stem cells. *Proc Natl Acad Sci USA* 1991; **88**: 10730–4.

23 Dorin JR, Dickinson P, Emslie E, et al. Successful targeting of the mouse cystic fibrosis transmembrane conductance regulator gene in embryonal stem cells. *Transgenic Res* 1992; **1**: 101–5.

24 Ratcliff R, Evans MJ, Dorin J, et al. Disruption of the cystic fibrosis transmembrane conductance regulator gene in embryonic stem cells by gene targeting. *Transgenic Res* 1992; **1**: 177–81.
25 Mansour S, Thomas K, Capecchi M. Disruption of the proto-oncogene *int-2* in mouse embryo-derived stem cells: a general strategy for targeting mutations to non-selectable genes. *Nature* 1988; **336**: 348–53.
26 Deng C, Capecchi M. Re-examination of gene targeting frequency as a function of the extent of homology between the targeting vector and the target locus. *Mol Cell Biol* 1992: **12**: 3365–71.
27 Moens CB, Auerbach AB, Conlan RA, Joyner AL, Rossant J. A targeted mutation reveals a role for N-Myc in branching morphogenesis in the embryonic mouse lung. *Genes Dev* 1992; **6**: 691–704.
28 Dorin JR, Stevenson BJ, Fleming S, et al. Long term survival of the exon 10 insertional cystic fibrosis mutant mouse is a consequence of low level residual wild type *Cftr* gene expression. *Mammalian Genome* in press.
29 Dear I, Maquat L. Premature translation termination mediates triose phosphate isomerase mRNA degradation. *Mol Cell Biol* 1988; **8**: 802–13.
30 McIntosh I, Hamosh A, Dietz HC. Nonsense mutations and diminished mRNA levels. *Nature Genet* 1993; **4**: 219.
31 Hamosh A, Trapnell BC, Zeitlin PL, et al. Severe deficiency of cystic fibrosis transmembrane conductance regulator mRNA carrying nonsense mutations R553X and W1316X in respiratory epithelial cells of patients with cystic fibrosis. *J Clin Invest* 1991; **88**: 1880–5.
32 Urlaub G, Mitchell PJ, Ciudada CJ, Chasin LA. Nonsense mutations in the dihydrofolate reductase gene affect RNA processing. *Mol Cell Biol* 1989; **9**: 2868–80.
33 Delaney S, Rich D, Thomson S, et al. Cystic fibrosis transmembrane conductance regulator splice variants are not conserved and fail to produce chloride channels. *Nature Genet* 1993; **4**: 426–31.
34 Chu CS, Trapnell B, Murtagh J, et al. Variable deletion of exon 9 coding sequences in cystic fibrosis transmembrane conductance regulator gene mRNA transcripts in normal bronchial epithelium. *EMBO J* 1991; **10**: 1355–63.
35 Knowles M, Gatzy, J, Boucher RC. Increased bioelectric potential difference across respiratory epithelia in cystic fibrosis. *N Engl J Med* 1981; **305**: 1489–95.
36 Alton EWFW, Currie D, Logan-Sinclair R, et al. Nasal potential difference: a clinical diagnostic test for cystic fibrosis. *Eur Respir J* 1990; **3**: 922–6.
37 Grubb BR, Vick RN, Boucher RC. Sodium hyperabsorption by airway epithelium in the CF mouse. *Pediatr Pulmonol* 1993; **9**: 211 (Abstract).
38 Clarke LL, Grubb BR, Gabriel SE, et al. Defective epithelial chloride transport in a gene-targeted mouse model of cystic fibrosis. *Science* 1992; **257**: 1125–8.
39 Smith SN, Steel DM, Middleton PG, et al. Bioelectric characteristics of the exon 10 insertional mouse model of cystic fibrosis closely mimic those found in man. Submitted.
40 Grubb BR, Clarke LL, Gabriel SE, et al. Characterization of ion transport defects in the CF mouse and the relationship to disease. *Pediatr Pulmonol* 1993; **9**: 133 (Abstract).
41 Alton EWFW, Khagani A, Taylor RFH, et al. Effect of heart–lung transplantation on airway potential difference in patients with and without cystic fibrosis. *Eur Respir J* 1991; **4**: 5–9.
42 Alton EWFW, Rogers DF, Logan-Sinclair R, et al. Bioelectric properties of cystic fibrosis airways obtained at heart–lung transplantation. *Thorax* 1992; **47**: 1010–14.

43 Ratcliff R, Evans MJ, Cuthbert AW, et al. Production of a severe cystic fibrosis mutation in mice by gene targeting. *Nature Genet* 1992; **4**: 35–41.
44 Hyde S, Gill D, Higgins C et al. Correction of the ion transport defect in cystic fibrosis transgenic mice by gene therapy. *Nature* 1993; **362**: 250–5.
45 Pack RJ, Al-Ugaily LH, Morris G, Widdicombe JG. The distribution and structure of cells in the tracheal epithelium of the mouse. *Cell Tissue Res* 1980; **208**: 65–84.
46 Van Scott MR, Hester S, Boucher RC. Ion transport by rabbit nonciliated bronchiolar epithelial cells (Clara cells) in culture. *Proc Natl Acad Sci USA* 1987; **84**: 5496–500.
47 Willumsen NJ, Davis CW, Boucher RC. Cellular Cl-transport in cultured cystic fibrosis airway epithelium. *Am J Physiol* 1989; **256**: C1045–53.
48 Widdicombe JH, Welsh MJ, Finkbeiner WE. Cystic fibrosis decreases the apical membrane chloride permeability of monolayers cultured from cells of tracheal epithelium. *Proc Natl Acad Sci USA* 1985; **82**: 6167–71.
49 Welsh MJ. Abnormal regulation of ion channels in cystic fibrosis epithelia. *FASEB J* 1990; **4**: 2718–25.
50 Hardcastle J, Hardcastle PT, Taylor CJ, Goldhill J. Failure of cholinergic stimulation to induce a secretory response from the rectal mucosa in cystic fibrosis. *Gut* 1991; **32**: 1035–9.
51 Goldstein JL, Nash NT, Al-Bazzaz F, et al. Rectum has abnormal ion transport but normal cAMP-binding proteins in cystic fibrosis. *Am J Physiol* 1988, **254**: C719–24
52 Baxter PS, Goldhill J, Hardcastle J, et al. Enhanced intestinal glucose and alanine transport in cystic fibrosis. *Gut* 1990; **31**: 817–20.
53 Cuthbert AW, MacVinish L, Hickman M, et al. Ion transport in the murine colonic epithelium of normal and transgenic cystic fibrosis animals. Submitted.
54 Gray MA, Winpenny JP, Porteous DJ, et al. CFTR and calcium-activated chloride currents in pancreatic duct cells of a transgenic CF mouse. *Am J Physiol* **266**: (*Cell Physiol.* **35**) C213–C221.
55 Mearns M. Cystic fibrosis: the first 50 years. A review of the clinical problems and their management. In: *Cystic Fibrosis: Current Topics* Vol 1 (eds JA Dodge, DJH Brock, JH Widdicombe) Wiley, Chichester, 1992, pp 217–50.
56 Boat T, Welsh MJ, Beaudet A. Cystic fibrosis. In: *The Metabolic Basis of Inherited Disease* (eds CL Scriver, AL Beaudet, WS Sly, D Valle) McGraw-Hill, New York, 1989, pp 2649–80.
57 Trezise AEO, Buchwald M. In vivo cell-specific expression of the cystic fibrosis transmembrane conductance regulator. *Nature* 1991; **353**: 434–7.
58 Kaplan E, Shwachman H, Perlmutter AD, et al. Reproduction failure in males with cystic fibrosis. *N Engl J Med* 1968; **279**: 65–9.
59 Englehardt JF, Yankaskas J, Ernst SA, et al. Submucosal glands are the predominant site of CFTR expression in human bronchus. *Nature Genet* 1992; **2**: 240–8.
60 Yoshimura K, Nakamura H, Trapnell BC, et al. Expression of the cystic fibrosis transmembrane conductance regulator gene in cells of non-epithelial origin. *Nucleic Acids Res* 1991; **191**: 5417–23.
61 Sheppard DN, Rich DP, Ostedgaard LS, et al. Mutations in CFTR associated with mild-disease-form Cl channels with altered pore properties. *Nature* 1993; **362**: 160–4.
62 Hasty P, Ramirez-Solls R, Krumlauf R, Bradley A. Introduction of a subtle mutation into the *Hox-2.6* locus in embryonic stem cells. *Nature* 1991; **350**: 243–6.
63 Valancius V, Smithies, O. Testing an 'in–out' targeting procedure for making subtle genomic modifications in mouse embryonic stem cells. *Mol Cell Biol* 1991; **11**: 1402–8.

64 Deng C, Thomas KR, Capecchi MR. Location of crossovers during gene targeting with insertion and replacement vectors. *Mol Cell Biol* 1993; **13**: 2134–40.
65 Knowles MR, Church N, Waltner W, et al. A pilot study of aerosolized amiloride for the treatment of lung disease in cystic fibrosis. *N Engl J Med* 1990; **322**: 1189–94.
66 Graham A, Hasani A, Alton EWFW. No added benefit from nebulized amiloride in patients with cystic fibrosis. *Eur Respir J* 1993; **6**: 1243–8.
67 Kartner N, Augustinas O, Jensen TJ, et al. Mislocalization of ΔF508 CFTR in cystic fibrosis sweat gland. *Nature Genet* 1992; **1**: 321–7.
68 Denning GM, Anderson M P, Amara JF, et al. Processing of mutant cystic fibrosis transmembrane conductance regulator is temperature-sensitive. *Nature* 1992; **358**: 761–4.
69 Li C, Ramjeesingh M, Reyes E, et al. The cystic fibrosis mutation (ΔF508) does not influence the chloride channel activity of CFTR. *Nature Genet* 1993; **3**: 311–16.
70 Lukaes GL, Chang XB, Bear C, et al. The ΔF508 mutation decreases the stability of cystic fibrosis transmembrane conductance regulator in the plasma membrane. *J Biol Chem* 1993; **268**: 21592–8.
71 Whitsett JA, Dey CR, Stripp BR, et al. Human cystic fibrosis transmembrane conductance regulator directed to respiratory epithelial cells of transgenic mice. *Nature Genet* 1992; **2**: 13–20.
72 Engelhardt JF, Allen, E.D. Wilson J.M. Reconstitution of tracheal grafts with a genetically modified epithelium. *Proc Natl Acad Sci USA* 1991; **88**: 11192–6.
73 Rosenfeld MA, Yoshimura K, Trapnell BC, et al. In vivo transfer of the human cystic fibrosis transmembrane conductance regulator gene to the airway epithelium. *Cell* 1992; **68**: 143–55.
74 Zabner J, Couture LA, Gregory RJ, et al. Adenovirus-mediated gene transfer transiently corrects the chloride transport defect in nasal epithelia of patients with cystic fibrosis. *Cell* 1993; **75**: 207–16.
75 Alton EWFW, Middleton PG, Caplen NJ, et al. Non-invasive liposome-mediated gene delivery can correct the ion transport defect in cystic fibrosis mutant mice. *Nature Genet* 1993; **5**: 135–42.
76 Stewart MJ, Plautz GE, Buono L del, et al. Gene transfer *in vivo* with DNA–liposome complexes: safety and acute toxicity in mice. *Hum Gene Ther* 1992; **3**: 267–75.
77 Cotten M, Wagner E. Non-viral approaches to gene therapy. *Curr Opin Biotechnol* 1993; **4**: 705–10.
78 Zhu, N, Liggitt D, Liu Y, Debs R. Systemic gene expression after intravenous DNA delivery into adult mice. *Science* 1993; **261**: 209–11.
79 Ferkol T, Kaetzel CS, Perales JC, et al. Gene transfer into respiratory epithelial cells using receptor-mediated endocytosis. *Pediatr Pulmonol* 1992; **9** 77–8 (Abstract).

Chapter Two

# Towards Gene Therapy for Cystic Fibrosis

Charles Coutelle, Natasha J. Caplen, Stephen L. Hart, Peter G. Middleton[a] and Robert Williamson

*St Mary's Hospital Medical School, Department of Biochemistry and Molecular Genetics and [a]Ion Transport Laboratory, Royal Brompton National Heart and Lung Institute, London, UK*

## INTRODUCTION

Although the idea of gene therapy was discussed before the advent of recombinant DNA techniques, there was no possibility of using normal copies of genes to treat an inherited disease until human DNA sequences could be cloned, analysed and isolated in quantity. Therefore, it has taken a comparatively long time for gene therapy to reach a stage where it can be tested in practical terms, and it is still very much in its experimental and developmental stage (for reviews see references 1–4). Somewhat unexpectedly to those contemplating gene therapy over the last 15 years, cystic fibrosis (CF) has become one of the pathfinder diseases for the application of this new form of treatment to an inherited disorder, and at present there are several phase I studies under way to explore optimal conditions for this approach.

*Cystic Fibrosis—Current Topics, Volume 2.* Edited by J. A. Dodge, D. J. H. Brock and J. H. Widdicombe

## A CASE FOR SOMATIC GENE THERAPY OF CYSTIC FIBROSIS

Somatic gene therapy for CF aims at the introduction of a normal gene sequence into cells of the affected tissues. Provided an appropriate set of control sequences is present, the expression of this DNA sequence should lead to synthesis of the normal protein, which should correct the ion transport defect and prevent the secondary organ damage caused by the cellular malfunction.

Ideally somatic gene therapy for CF should permanently replace the affected gene by its healthy counterpart in affected cells. This is, however, not a feasible strategy at present, because of the very low efficiency of such a replacement event (called homologous recombination) when the normal sequence is artificially introduced into a cell. All present strategies are therefore orientated towards complementation of the two mutant alleles by addition of the normal gene sequence.

**Table 1** Cystic fibrosis
*Clinical symptoms*

| Pulmonary | Intestinal | General |
|---|---|---|
| Chronic coughing | Meconium ileus | Failure to thrive |
| Purulent sputum | Voluminous, fatty stools | Underweight |
| Dyspnoea | rectal prolapse | Male sterility |
| | abdominal pain | |
| | (subacute obstruction) | |

*Genetics*
Inheritance: Autosomal recessive monogenic
Incidence: 1 in 2000 newborns in North/Middle-European population

*Reasons for gene therapy*
Life-threatening disease with current survival of approximately 30 years
No entirely satisfactory therapy available to date
Patients usually highly motivated by present treatment and used to active and understanding participation in trials for new forms of therapy
Progressive lung damage is major cause of morbidity and mortality
Airways are easily accessible for treatment, allowing regularly repeated application of gene therapy constructs
CFTR gene has been cloned and molecular mechanism of disease intensively analysed *in vitro* and *in vivo* including successful correction studies in cell culture and in animal models for CF
CFTR is effective at very low levels in normal lung cells. Its overproduction does not appear to be toxic
Availability of non-invasive test for efficacy in nasal epithelia

Mutations in the cystic fibrosis transmembrane regulator (CFTR) gene are the molecular basis of CF. The CFTR protein coded by this gene is an integral membrane protein. Its main physiological role is that of a cAMP-regulated chloride channel[5]. CFTR mutations which cause CF lead to a disturbance of the ion and water transport across the luminal surface of the secretory epithelia of the gut, pancreas, lung, bilary ducts and sperm ducts and to the dehydrated mucus characteristic of cystic fibrosis[6], either because the protein is not synthesized, is not translocated to the membrane, or is dysfunctional[7].

The resulting dehydrated mucus supports repeated infection which leads to chronic inflammation of the airways and gut lumen (Table 1). To date treatment of CF is symptomatic, including daily physiotherapy and antibiotics directed against respiratory infections, together with pancreatic enzyme supplementation and intensive dietary support of the otherwise chronically malnourished patient. More recently DNase and $\alpha_1$-antitrypsin have been on trial as more specific therapies, but these are still directed at symptoms rather than the underlying defect. Gene therapy has now become a promising long-term approach to treatment for CF, particularly with respect to prevention of lung disease.

## WHY CYSTIC FIBROSIS?

There are several reasons why CF is a particularly suitable candidate for somatic gene therapy. The genetics of CF is well understood; both the cDNA and the genomic DNA for CFTR have been isolated, and it is known that having the mutant gene presents no pathology provided there is a single copy of the normal gene present as well. CFTR is effective when expressed at very low levels in normal lung cells[8]. It also does not seem to need sophisticated gene regulation, since neither over-expression in cell culture[9–11] nor permanent synthesis of the human protein in transgenic mice[12] causes any cellular toxicity or organ impairment. Experiments with CF cells in culture have shown that the ion transport defect caused by the mutant CFTR gene can be corrected by introduction of a single copy of the normal CFTR coding sequence into the affected cells. It has been shown that normal CFTR expression (when corrected using a retroviral CFTR cDNA construct) in less than 10% of cells grown in co-culture with uncorrected CF cells is sufficient to generate chloride transport in the entire monolayer similar to that observed in an epithelial sheath consisting of 100% corrected cells[13]. This is probably due to ionic coupling of adjacent cells through gap junctions[14]. There are several mouse models for CF where the murine CFTR gene has been mutated, and while none of these mirror precisely the human pathology, all are appropriate models for testing somatic gene therapy. Therefore from the point of view of genetics, CF has many features making it a good choice for these approaches.

The pathophysiology and clinical course of the disease also have features which commend CF to somatic gene therapy. CF is a fairly common and serious disease, for which no satisfactory treatment is available to date. Present forms of treatment require a high degree of compliance, discipline, understanding and active participation by the patients. The handicaps are entirely physical; there is no associated mental retardation. The organ which is severely affected in most cases and for which the pathology becomes life threatening, the lung, is relatively easy to access by bronchoscopy or inhalation, which may make even regularly repeated treatment acceptable to patients. Alton and collaborators[15] have developed a non-invasive, sensitive and reliable *in vivo* method to detect the ion transport defect in CF patients by measuring the electrical potential difference in the epithelial cells lining the nose. This has become a favourite procedure to monitor the effect of gene therapy trials in patients, for use as a surrogate endpoint during clinical trials.

In the UK, there are about 6000 children and 1500 adults affected by CF (the precise number is difficult to determine, as some cases are mild and do not present until later in life, and often with atypical symptoms), and many of these are prepared to volunteer for clinical trials to develop somatic gene therapy. There is a high level of public awareness of the disease, and funding is likely to be available from government sources, the medical charities and industry. Because of this constellation of scientific, pathological and social advantages, CF is one of the first diseases for which somatic gene therapy trials have been undertaken.

## STRATEGIES TOWARDS GENE THERAPY FOR CYSTIC FIBROSIS

All approaches to gene therapy depend critically on the tissue which is to be treated. In the case of CF the lung, and in particular its bronchi and bronchioli, is the organ most efforts presently focus upon. It is impossible to remove the lung, treat it *ex vivo*, and re-transplant it; it is also unrealistic to remove cells from the epithelial layer, treat them in culture and replace them. Therefore, the strategies which have been pioneered for diseases of the bone marrow (adenosine deaminase (ADA) deficiency) and liver (low-density lipoprotein (LDL) receptor defects leading to familial hypercholesterolaemia) are not applicable to CF. On the other hand, the probability that only a relatively low level of expression in a limited number of cells is required to restore normal ion transport, and the possibility of vector delivery by inhalation to the appropriate small airways, makes a good case for *in vivo* gene application by nebulization to the lung epithelia. Approaches towards *in vivo* somatic gene therapy are presently concentrating on gene delivery by virus vectors or liposomes and different *in vitro* and *in vivo* model systems have been used to assess the various aspects of these approaches (Table 2).

Although treatment of the lung aimed at the pulmonary pathology is the first objective of all present trials towards gene therapy for CF, treatment of the epithelial cell sheet lining the intestine, pancreas and bilary ducts will be next on the agenda and will require new concepts for targeting and gene delivery to the cells of the affected tissues.

## MODEL SYSTEMS

Cell culture assays have been used to demonstrate the correction of the ion transport defect in CF cells by expression of the wild-type CFTR cDNA sequence[9,11]. Such assays have also been used to test the efficiency of different virus and plasmid vector constructions expressing CFTR cDNA under the control of a variety of different viral and eukaryotic gene promoters[9,10,16,17].

*In vivo* instillation or inhalation of constructs expressing human CFTR or marker genes into the lungs of normal rodents and primates has been used to investigate the efficiency of delivery and expression under different promoters, the duration of expression, its cellular localization and the occurrence of toxic side-effects[17–24].

**Table 2** Use of model systems in gene therapy for CF

*Cell culture*
Correction of ion transport defect in CF cells by expression of wild-type CFTR cDNA
Efficiency tests of virus and plasmid vector constructions expressing CFTR cDNA under control of a variety of virus and eukaryotic promoters
Demonstration of cooperative correction effect of chloride transport

*Normal animals*
Instillation or inhalation of constructs expressing marker genes or human CFTR into the lungs of rodents and primates to investigate:
- —The efficiency of gene delivery and expression under different promoters
- —The duration and cellular localization of expression
- —The occurrence of any toxic side-effects

*Transgenic mice*
Random integration into genome (pronuclear injection of a human CFTR cDNA):
- —No cellular toxicity or organ impairment due to the permanent expression of the human CFTR in lung and testes

Transgenic mouse models for CF (homologous recombination in embryonic stem cells:
- —Observation of variable degrees of disease pathology depending on mechanism of integration
- —Use of animals in gene correction experiments

Transgenic mice generated by oocyte pronuclear injection of a human CFTR cDNA have this gene sequence integrated at random into their genome. It has been expressed under the control of human surfactant transcriptional elements in the respiratory epithelia and testes of these animals without any indication of toxicity or organ damage[12]. Transgenic mouse models for CF have also been constructed by targeted integration of mutated gene sequences into the mouse CFTR gene using homologous recombination in embryonic stem cells[25–27]. Different degrees of disease pathology have been observed depending on whether this integration is performed by replacement[25,27,28] or insertion[26] of the targeted gene sequence. Animals generated by replacement of the normal sequence with its mutated counterpart show a severe pathology and very high perinatal mortality, mainly due to intestinal complications[25,29]. Insertion, in contrast, introduces the mutated sequence 5′ to the remaining normal gene sequence. The effects of this insertion can be overcome partially; probably by splicing out of the mutated sequence during RNA processing. These animals have a milder disease phenotype[26]. Both models have been used in gene correction experiments[17,18].

## DELIVERY SYSTEM

Three virus vector systems and liposome–DNA complexes are the delivery systems presently under test for gene therapy for CF (Table 3).

### Adenovirus vectors

Most groups using a viral strategy for gene therapy of CF are presently investigating the potential of adenovirus vectors. Adenovirus naturally infects lung epithelia. It has a genome size of about 36 kb, can infect non-dividing cells and expresses large amounts of gene product. The adenoviral vectors constructed for gene therapy are derivatives of the wild-type adenovirus types 2 and/or 5. Both belong to the subgroup C of this virus, for which no oncogenic potential has been observed in any species investigated, including man[30,31]. For use as gene therapy vectors, the E1 gene region, and in most cases the E3 gene region as well, have been deleted. Deletion of the E1 gene functions makes the virus replication deficient, and such viral vectors have to be packaged by growth in the human embryonic kidney helper cell line 293, which expresses the E1 function constitutively[32]. Adenoviral vectors of this type have the capacity to package about 38 kb DNA containing an insert of up to about 7.5 kb.

Deletion of the E3 genes does not seem to influence viral growth; however, its presence limits the insert size that can be cloned into this vector. The poorer packaging abilities of recombinant vectors containing the E3 region due to this size constraint have been cited as an additional safety feature of such constructs. The gp19 protein from the E3 region prevents presentation of the

**Table 3** Gene delivery systems discussed in context of CF

| Advantages | Disadvantages |
|---|---|
| *Adenovirus* | |
| Suitable for *in situ* application, especially lung (high efficiency of *in vivo* infection in non-replicating cells) | No integration into host genome (only transient expression) |
| Very high virus titres (up to $10^{10}$ infect.U/ml) | Complicated vector genome |
| Biology well understood | Virus proteins may cause inflammatory reactions |
| | Limited insert capacity (about 7–8 kb) |
| *Adeno-associated virus* | |
| Small genome (5 kb) | Not very well studied |
| Preferential integration into human chromosome 19 | Requires adenovirus as helper for replication |
| Humans are natural hosts | Limited capacity for foreign genes (about 4 kb) |
| Non-pathogenic, non-toxic | |
| *Retrovirus* | |
| Small and simple genome | Infects only dividing cells |
| Stable co-linear integration into host genome | Random integration (potentially mutagenic) |
| Well-known biology | Often only transient expression |
| High efficiency of transfer into replicating cells | Relatively low virus titre ($10^7$ infect.U/ml) |
| No toxic effects on host cells | May recombine with replication-competent virus |
| | Limited capacity for foreign DNA (10 kb) |
| *Liposomes* | |
| No infectious capability | No specific targeting |
| Transfer of very large pieces of DNA (up to 150 kb) | Low transfection efficiency |
| Low toxicity | Only transient expression |

MHC class 1 protein on the cell surface[33,34]. In this way, it should inhibit T cell response against cells infected with such adenovirus and reduce inflammatory reactions which might be caused by virus administration. It has, however, also been argued that removal of the E3 function will, by increasing the immune response, protect against any wild-type or replication-competent adenoviral construct.

Adenovirus vectors can be produced at high titres and show a very high level of infectivity, reaching almost 100% in cell culture and *in vivo*. Two factors contribute to this high efficiency: receptor-mediated cell attachment and entry via the integrin binding domain of the penton base, and the ability to escape the lysosome degradation pathway into which most endosomally introduced substances are directed. All major cell types of the airway epithelia of rodents[21] and primates (Pavirani, personal communication) are infected by adenovirus recombinant vectors carrying the β-galactosidase marker gene. Human CFTR and $\alpha_1$-antitrypsin cDNA have also been cloned into the deleted E1 gene region of the adenovirus genome and successfully expressed in the lung epithelium of cotton rats[19,20]. Expression of human CFTR protein was detected for about two weeks and CFTR mRNA transcripts for up to six weeks[20].

However, since the adenovirus usually does not integrate into the genome of lung epithelial stem cells, it will eventually be lost due to degradation or the regular replacement of epithelial cells. Repeated re-infection will therefore be necessary, which may cause immune reactions against this treatment. There may also be a risk of generating a replication-competent infectious virus as a result of complementation *in trans*. The viral proteins are known to induce inflammatory reactions independent of viral replication. This could pose particular clinical difficulties in the context of CF, as reduced resistance to infection and chronic inflammation are general problems in the care of CF patients.

Several different adenovirus/CFTR cDNA constructs have been prepared, with different viral sequences and promoters governing CFTR expression. The CFTR cDNA recombinant, Ad CFTR, is based on the adenovirus type 5 genome, with extensive deletions in the E1 and E3 gene regions. The entire 4.5 kb protein coding region of human CFTR is expressed under regulatory control of the adenovirus type 2 C major late promoter and its three tripartite leader sequences at the 5′ end, and the SV40 polyadenylation site at the 3′ end[20]. A similar CFTR expression vector based on adenovirus type 5, Ad.CB-CFTR, uses the chicken β-actin gene promotor[35]. The CFTR cDNA construct Ad2/CFTR-1 in which the E3 gene has been retained is expressed under control of adenovirus 2 transcription elements[36]. All three adenovirus/CFTR constructs are presently being tested in the USA in phase I clinical trials.

## Adeno-associated virus vectors

Another virus with pulmonary tropism which has been considered for *in vivo* gene therapy of cystic fibrosis is the adeno-associated virus (AAV) (for review see reference 37). It has a small genome of 5 kb and is only able to accommodate an insert of foreign DNA of about 4.5 kb. It can infect non-dividing cells and the wild-type virus has been shown to integrate specifically into chromosome 19, thereby reducing the risk of virus-induced mutagenesis and oncogenesis by random integration. However, this specificity of integration (which could also ensure long-term gene expression, especially if stem cells were targeted) does not seem to be retained in recombinant virus. Flotte et al.[16] have been able to package an N-terminal truncated CFTR cDNA–AAV recombinant. Truncation of the first 486 nucleotides of the CFTR cDNA which just cuts into the first transmembrane spanning domain of CFTR does not inhibit its cAMP-stimulated chloride transport function. Functional CFTR was therefore expressed under control of the AAV inverted terminal repeat in a human bronchial CF cell line, demonstrating that AAV has indeed a potential as vector for gene therapy of CF. *In vivo* instillation of the AAV–CFTR construct into the lungs of rabbits directed CFTR protein expression for up to six months, indicating the potential of this vector system[38].

**Retroviral vectors**

Because of their promising use in several gene therapy trials for other diseases such as ADA deficiency and several forms of cancer[2], and the potential of providing a permanent treatment by integration into the genome of stem cells, retroviral vectors continue to be explored in the context of gene therapy for CF. However, retroviral infection occurs rarely in non-dividing cells and the virus is unable to integrate into the genome in this case[39]. This places severe limitations on the use of retroviral vectors for *in vivo* gene therapy of lung epithelial cells, which divide very slowly. The main objectives are therefore directed towards increasing the efficiency of infection and the specificity of targeting with the ultimate aim of reaching all cycling stem cells during transfection. One strategy to obtain both goals is to modify the virus envelope by incorporation of targeting domains specific for distinct receptor molecules on the cells of interest. Bayle et al.[40] have obtained a 10-fold increase of *in vitro* transduction of a retroviral vector into airway epithelia by incorporating an envelope glycoprotein from a primate virus into the envelope of their vector. Up to 80% of primary airway epithelia are infected *in vitro* by use of this vector. No *in vivo* experiments have been reported so far.

**Cationic liposome–DNA complexes**

Cationic liposome–DNA complexes[41] have been used successfully in non-viral approaches for the introduction of DNA into cells *in vitro* and *in vivo*. Various expressing plasmids and even DNA of 650 kb yeast artificial chromosomes (YACs)[42] have been transferred into cells by this method. Since these DNA-lipid complexes have no replicative capability most of the health and safety concerns associated with virus vectors do not apply. Furthermore, liposome formulations containing hydrolysable bonds have been synthesized which reduce general cytotoxicity. Such liposomes are naturally degraded after fusion with the cell membrane and delivery of the complexed DNA. One of these preparations composed of 3$\beta$[*N*-(*N'*,*N'*-dimethylaminoethane-carbamoyl] cholesterol dioleoyl phosphatidylethanolamine (DC-chol/DOPE)[43] shows a high transfection efficiency and low cytotoxicity[44] (Caplen et al., in preparation). This preparation caused no acute or toxic systemic reactions when given intravenously to mice at a dose of 0.42 nmol[44]. No autoimmune reaction or transfer of DNA into gonadal cells was observed after repeated intravenous, intraperitoneal or subcutaneous injection of plasmid DNA-DC-chol/DOPE injection in mice[45]. DC-chol/DOPE has been approved for human application in cancer treatment[44,46,47].

Zhu et al.[48] also found no indications of cellular or systemic toxicity after intravascular administration of up to 800 nmol of the liposome DOTMA/DOPE (trade name Lipofectin) composed of *N*-[1-(2,3-dioleyloxy)propyl]-*N*,*N*,*N*-trimethylammonium chloride[49]/dioleoyl phosphatidylethanolamine. After intravenous administration into the mouse of up to 100 μg plasmid DNA in a 1 : 8 ratio (μg : nmol) with this liposome, CAT reporter gene expression was found in parenchymal cells of most organs, including ovaries. These authors[48] also report successful CFTR expression of large numbers of lung cells over a period of more than 150 days in mice after intravascular CFTR cDNA–liposome administration. It remains to be seen whether such massive doses of liposome–DNA complexes administered via the bloodstream are a feasible approach to gene therapy for CF, particularly in view of possible problems using airway administration which may arise due to mucus obstruction. It will be important to confirm the finding and determine the sites and numbers of parenchymal cells which take up and express the exogenous genes, and to study whether there is expression in germ cells. However, if these questions can be answered satisfactorily, intravenous administration could become a promising approach for parenchymal cell delivery, with topical targeting by catheter to defined sections of the circulation.

Instillation[17,23] and nebulization[18,22] have been successfully used to introduce different liposome plasmid DNA complexes *in vivo* into the airways of mice. Marker genes coding for luciferase, β-galactosidase[23] or CAT[22], as well as human CFTR cDNA[23], have been expressed *in vivo* in the lung of wild-type mice after delivery by DOTMA/DOPE. Lipofectin[17] and DOPE/DC-chol[18] were used to deliver and express human CFTR cDNA plasmids *in vivo* in the lung of two different transgenic CF mouse strains by intratracheal instillation and nebulization, respectively. Successful correction of the cAMP-dependent chloride transport defect in the airways of these animals was detected *in vitro* and *in vivo* by electrophysiological measurements[17,18]

Using DC-chol/DOPE for marker gene delivery, β-galactosidase expression was detected in about 40% of the airway epithelial cells of normal mice[18]. Thus would, in all probability, be sufficient to correct the ion transport defect in CF in the human lung, but is still significantly lower than transfection efficiencies obtainable with adenoviral vectors. Specific targeting to those cells in which CFTR has to be expressed, and in particular to stem cells, could enhance the efficiency and persistence of any gene therapy effect. Longer-term efforts will certainly aim at combining the best features of these approaches and of other gene delivery systems to optimize gene therapy of CF.

## PHASE I GENE THERAPY CLINICAL TRIALS OF CYSTIC FIBROSIS

Based on these extensive investigations in cell culture, tissue samples and normal and CF experimental animals, phase I clinical trials for somatic gene therapy of the pulmonary manifestations of CF have now started. Several trials using adenovirus vectors carrying CFTR cDNA sequences have been approved by the Recombinant Advisory Committee (RAC) and the Food and Drug Administration (FDA) in the USA. The use of FDA-approved liposome preparations (DC-chol/DOPE) for CFTR cDNA delivery has been approved by the UK Committee on the Ethics of Gene Therapy and the UK Medicines Control Agency (MCA). Neither the adenovirus nor the liposome trials intend to provide definitive treatment at this point, even to the very small number of adult volunteer patients involved. They aim primarily at investigating safety but also look for efficacy and dose response of the different vector and delivery systems by measuring the correction of the ion transport defect *in vivo*, as a surrogate endpoint, on a very small area of the airway epithelia of the patients. In the Iowa/Genzyme adenovirus trial, and the Royal Brompton/St Mary's/ Edinburgh liposome trial, the effect of gene administration is being monitored by measuring the changes in the electrical potential difference on the surface of nasal epithelial cells. This non-invasive procedure allows the time course of gene expression and its persistence after application to be followed. The electrophysiological data will be supported by tests for expression of normal CFTR cDNA in epithelial brushings and biopsies. Studies of the epithelial lining of the nose have the additional advantage of permitting an initial measuring period in which the baseline electrical potential differences for each CF patient can be established.

The UK liposome gene therapy trial is a collaborative study between the CF gene therapy groups at the Royal Brompton Hospital/National Heart and Lung Institute, the Department of Biochemistry and Molecular Genetics of St Mary's Hospital Medical School/Imperial College and the MRC Human Genetics Unit in Edinburgh. The first stage of this trial has involved fifteen patient volunteers; increasing doses of CFTR cDNA plasmid (10,100,300 $\mu$g) were applied to both nostrils at a DNA to liposome ratio of 1 : 5. The electrical potential differences were monitored before application and 6 h after application, followed by measurements over 28 days. All procedures were controlled using preparations which contained no CFTR cDNA, and were conducted double-blind. A limited and transient biological response was observed in the CFTR cDNA treated group (Caplen et al., submitted).

The first published adenovirus CFTR trial, performed by the teams of Welsh and Smith (Iowa/Genzyme)[50], used increasing doses of virus from $2 \times 10^6$ to $6 \times 10^7$ infectious units per cell, which were delivered to the nasal epithelia of three CF patients. All three showed a decrease of the baseline electrical potential difference and increase in the response to cAMP agonists. The correction of the potential differences lasted for about three weeks, while cAMP stimulation was only detectable for about 10 days. No adenovirus-related pathology was reported for this initial trial. In a similar unpublished investigation by Crystal's group (NIH), nasal delivery was followed one day later by bronchoscopic application into a large bronchus. This trial had to be suspended temporarily following an inflammatory reaction of one of the patients. It is not clear whether this reaction was idiosyncratic, or represented a dose which would cause difficulties in other patients. A further adenovirus trial by Wilson (Philadelphia) has started recently; no informaton on safety or outcome is yet available. Boucher (North Carolina) and Wilmolt and Whitsett (Cincinnati) have also obtained permission for similar adenovirus CFTR trials.

All protocols monitor for any signs of inflammation, migration of the constructs to other sites in the body, shedding into the environment or other adverse effects. However, over-expression of CFTR in transgenic mice and in cell culture has no adverse effects, and we are all repeatedly exposed to wild-type adenovirus during our lifetime. Provided these phase I trials give positive results, protocols for repeated application, and eventually application to the lower airways will follow, leading to real attempts to treat CF pulmonary disease within the next five to ten years.

## ETHICAL AND LEGAL CONSIDERATIONS

All present strategies for gene therapy of CF are orientated solely towards somatic gene supplementation. This aims at the correction of the functional defect in a range of somatic cells expressing the affected phenotype in a particular patient. Germline gene therapy would, in contrast, lead to correction of all cells of an individual, including the germline, and also be propagated to following generations. Clinicians, scientists and the public agree that there is presently no medical or ethical justification for manipulating human germline cells and no attempt is made towards germline gene therapy for CF. For this monogenic autosomal recessive disease, with a risk of one affected fetus in four offspring of a heterozygote couple, preimplantation diagnosis[51] (which would in any case be necessary to decide which fertilized eggs to correct) has made gene therapy at this level redundant. Gene therapy for CF, even if applied *in utero* late in pregnancy for clinical reasons, will involve somatic gene correction. Since the inadvertent introduction of a gene therapy vector into gonadal cells in the course of an *in vivo* gene therapy trial cannot be ruled out completely, analysis for prevention and risk assessment of this extremely unlikely event will be carried out along with these trials. We anticipate that this risk is much less than the accepted risk of germline alteration associated with cancer chemotherapy.

It is generally agreed that somatic gene therapy does not create new ethical problems[52]. However, since it is an experimental treatment, or research towards treatment, ethical approval for individual protocols has to be obtained. For the proposed phase I trials for CF gene therapy, approval was given for the adenovirus vector approach by the NIH Recombinant Advisory Committee (RAC) on the basis of extensive written documentation[52a,b] and a public hearing. The documents submitted to the NIH RAC by the different US groups describe the disease, its molecular and cellular basis, its current therapy and prognosis, underlining the relevance of gene therapy for CF. They describe the structure and biology of adenovirus and the rationale behind construction of the proposed CFTR cDNA recombinant. Experimental data of *in vitro* tests and *in vivo* experiments in rodents and primates supporting the efficacy and safety of these constructs and a detailed description of the production and quality control of the recombinant vectors are provided. Various safety aspects raised by the proposed use of adenovirus recombinant are commented on, in particular in relation to possible replicative, recombinatory and oncogenic potentials of adenovirus, its ability to integrate into the host genome, the possibility that it may infect germ cells or be shed into the environment and its potential to provoke adverse reactions by the host. The protocols for the proposed phase I trials are described in detail, giving an exact account of the procedures to be followed and defining the criteria for patient selection and for assessment of the results with respect to safety and efficacy. Special consideration is given to confidentiality and informed consent, follow-up of the patients and the reporting of adverse effects.

Our protocol for a liposome-based phase I clinical trial for CF was approved by the Committee on the Ethics of Gene Therapy following clarification of queries relating to patient information and consent, patient selection, information to participating staff, the assessment of safety and efficacy and the preparation of DNA. DNA for the trial was prepared at the MRC Human Genome Mapping Project Resource Centre, at Northwick Park Hospital, according to a detailed protocol agreed by the Medicines Control Agency. The liposomes DC-chol/DOPE were prepared using FDA-approved procedures by Drs Huang and Gao (University of Pittsburgh). Our experiences concerning the regulatory procedures and production of resources are described elsewhere[53].

## FUTURE IMPROVEMENTS AND DEVELOPMENTS

### TOPICAL APPLICATION

The next steps in gene therapy for CF following lung delivery will include approaches towards treatment of the hepatobiliary, intestinal and pancreatic problems associated with the disease. Topical application via endoscopy and by direct intravascular delivery could target these organs. A first attempt to correct the defect in hepatobiliary cells has been made by Yang et al.[35] using retrograde infusion of adenoviral β-galactosidase and human CFTR cDNA recombinants into the bile ducts of rats. These experiments show transfection with the β-galactosidase recombinant in all biliary cells and almost 80% of hepatocytes, while for CFTR cDNA most of the biliary cells are transfected and only few hepatocytes. For reasons unknown the transgenic expression of β-galactosidase is more stable in the epithelia of the small biliary ducts (up to 21 days) than in hepatocytes (much reduced after seven days). Such a procedure could in principle be used to target the biliary duct as well as the pancreatic duct in humans once a procedure for long-term gene correction has been developed. Delivery and uptake of the CFTR sequence into the amniotic fluid using viral or other vector systems, to achieve delivery to the enteral system and the lung, could be used for intrauterine treatment late in pregnancy.

### SPECIFIC CELL TARGETING AND EXPRESSION

A general strategy to improve the efficiency of gene therapy would involve increasing the specificity of cellular targeting and expression. In the case of CF, as with many other genetic diseases, stem cell targeting *in vivo* would be of major importance for approaches directed towards long-term cure using self-replicating vector systems. Work to identify which of the different epithelial cells in lung, pancreas and gut require proper CFTR expression and, even more, to identify the stem cells from which they originate, is still very much at its beginning. Cell-specific expression, which could be obtained by use of cell-specific promoters, does not seem to be of importance for gene therapy of CF, since endogenous expression in the relevant cells is very low and since neither over-expression nor ectopic expression seems to cause any harm[12].

Most strategies for specific cell targeting make use of the ability of cell-specific receptors to bind various macromolecules, including antibodies, hormones, growth factors and pathogens. Many of these ligands are then internalized by the process of receptor-mediated endocytosis. This involves the formation of clathrin-coated pits accumulating a high density of the specific receptors on the cell membrane, and their invagination from the membrane to form intracellular vesicles. These are then rapidly uncoated and directed to endosomes from which most of the ligands are transferred to lysosomes (reviewed in reference 54).

Receptor-mediated targeting for gene delivery has been achieved by linking polylysine complexed with plasmid cDNA constructs to ligands which recognize specific cell surface receptors. Besides acting as a binding ligand for the DNA, polylysine also causes condensation into a doughnut structure, which protects DNA against shearing and facilitates cell entry[55]. This approach has no *a priori* size constraints and was used to introduce cosmid DNA constructs with a size of about 48 kb into cells[56]. A range of different cells types has been targeted *in vitro* using transferrin ('transferrinfection')[57–59], and different gene sequences introduced in this way have been transiently expressed at a high level. Hepatocyte-specific targeting was achieved *in vitro*[60] and *in vivo*[61] using asialoglycoprotein. Receptor-mediated *in vitro* targeting of marker plasmid DNA into colon carcinoma cells and primary culture tracheal epithelia has been achieved using a polylysine–Fab fragment complex derived from antibodies directed against the polymeric immunoglobulin receptor expressed on the basolateral surface of these cells[62].

One of the drawbacks of these systems is that a significant proportion of the DNA delivered in this way is rapidly degraded in lysosomes[63]. The exact fate of DNA molecules introduced by liposomes is still poorly understood and it may well be that some of the entering DNA–liposome complexes are lost by lysosomal degradation in this case. Birnstiel and collaborators have recently pioneered an approach to avoid lysosomal degradation by using the ability of adenovirus to disrupt endosomes and prevent degradation by releasing the DNA complexes into the cytoplasm[64]. These investigators have shown that coincubation[56,64] or linking of inactivated adenovirus to transferrin–polylysine plasmid cDNA complexes[65,66] significantly increases the expression of the newly introduced genes *in vitro* and *in vivo*. This approach was successfully used by others to enhance receptor-mediated gene delivery in hepatocytes[63]. Similar lysosome disruption properties have also been demonstrated for haemagglutinin HA-2, the N-terminal fusogenic peptide of influenza virus[68] and chloroquin[59]. Some cytopathic effects have been observed with adenovirus[56], while the haemagglutinin peptide does not seem to be toxic and may be more suitable for use *in vivo*[68].

We have investigated the potential of several proteins used by bacteria or protozoa to attach and enter mammalian cells, such as invasin[69], internalin[70] and penetrin[71], for the development of novel receptor-mediated targeting and delivery systems. Invasin is the bacterial cell surface protein responsible for internalization of *Yersinia pseudotuberculosis*, which attaches with high affinity to a subset of $\beta_1$-chain integrins of non-phagocytic cells[69] and mediates cell entry of the parasite[72]. Integrins are a family of cell surface receptors which can bind extracellular ligands as well as cytoskeletal molecules. The binding activity of invasin to $\beta_1$-integrins can be competed by peptides containing the arginine–glycine–aspartic acid (RGD) sequence[72]. RGD is required by fibronectin and collagen for attachment to $\beta_1$-integrins and is also necessary for internalization of adenovirus[73].

To test the ability of such ligands to mediate cell binding and entry, we are presently working on their expression in fusion with surface proteins of the single-stranded filamentous fd phage and are monitoring binding and internalization of the modified phage into mammalian cells. Oligonucleotides encoding an RGD-containing cyclic peptide expressed in fusion with the fd phage gene VIII protein have led to the display of this peptide in many copies on the surface of this phage. The structural rigidity of the cyclic peptide increases the integrin binding affinity of the RGD domain. Our initial results with confocal immunofluorescence microscopy and co-localization analysis show that these recombinant phages are internalized by Caco-2 epithelial cells[73a].

Polylysine bridges attached to the RGD peptide and other identified targeting molecules will be used to complex DNA and internalize it together with the modified phage to deliver and express foreign genes into cells via this system. To release the DNA from the lysosome by membrane lysis after endocytosis, we plan to link inactivated adenovirus to this complex. By choosing appropriate ligands this system should enable cell-specific targeting and physiological uptake of DNA without apparent size constraints.

## MAMMALIAN ARTIFICIAL CHROMOSOMES

A long-term approach towards gene therapy is through the construction of a mammalian artificial chromosome (MAC). Such a MAC would carry and express a normal CFTR gene as part of a sequence of genomic human chromosomal DNA. In addition to the CFTR gene and its surrounding regulatory sequences, it would also carry the DNA elements required for stable replication and segregation, including a centromere, telomeres and origins of replication (Figure 1). Ultimately the MAC should be autonomously replicating and segregate non-randomly in mammalian cells. The telomere sequences would prevent integration into the host genome, avoiding the potential danger of random viral vector integration. It would also allow permanent expression and physiological regulation.

One of the main scientific problems of this strategy is the present lack of understanding of the structural and functional requirements of a mammalian centromere—the chromosomal element responsible for the correct segregation of chromosomes to daughter cells at cell division. Although several DNA sequences and proteins have been identified as centromeric components (for review see references 74 and 75) and a long-range map of the centromeric region of the Y chromosome recently constructed[76], it is still unknown which DNA sequences are essential for centromere function. One approach towards

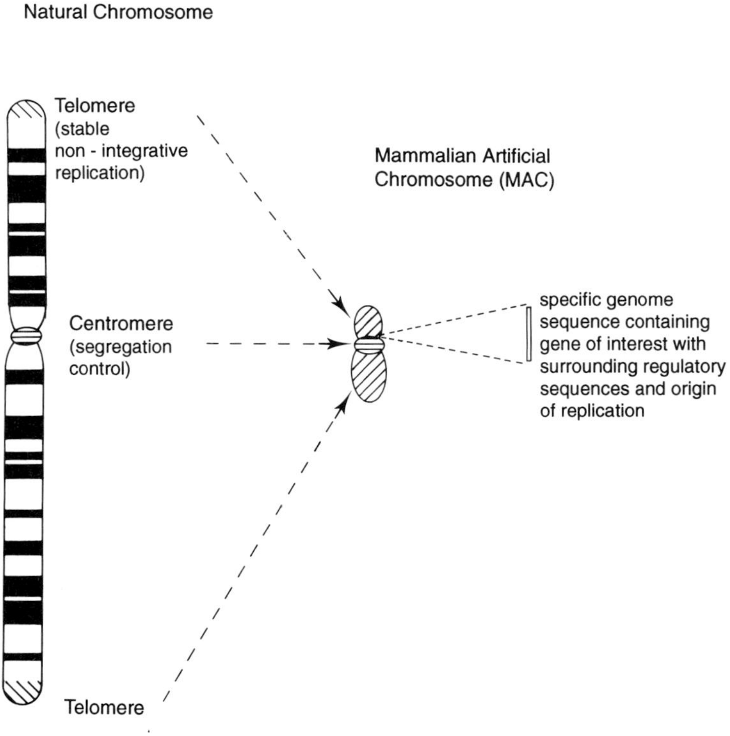


**Figure 1** Construction of a mammalian artificial chromosome

construction of a MAC is therefore to rely on the natural centromere and to truncate the unwanted part of the chromosome by seeding of a telomeric DNA sequence[77,78]. This strategy is complicated by the preferential seeding of telomere sequences close to the natural telomeres[78]. We are presently attempting to isolate relevant mammalian centromeric sequences, and are developing a test for centromere function by segregation analysis based on the observation that yeast and YAC DNAs can replicate extrachromosomally, but do not segregate after transfer to mammalian cells[79]. Isolated centromere elements will be inserted into such a test YAC, and then transferred to mammalian cells. Insertion of functional centromere DNA into the YAC should lead to correct segregation of the extrachromosomal DNA. Novel approaches to targeting and entry will be of particular interest for DNA of the size of a mammalian artificial chromosome, which will exceed the packaging capacity of any virus system. However, it should also be remembered that many cells (such as neurones) are very long lived and therefore correct segregation is not essential, and even lung epithelia have a half-life of approximately 100 days.

## FUTURE OUTLOOK

Since the outcome of these very first steps towards gene therapy for CF is unclear it is not possible to predict which of the many possible approaches will lead to a real therapeutic gain for those with the disease. Even when effective therapy is achieved, it is very likely that it will be using a combination of the best features of the different approaches, and of novel developments in the future. It should also be considered that alternative pharmacological means of treatment such as the direct administration of modified CFTR, based on knowledge of the molecular defect causing CF, could make gene therapy for this disease irrelevant. In any case the current approaches under test using somatic gene therapy for CF on an experimental basis illustrates the enormous progress which has been made since the identification of the CFTR gene only a few years ago, and indicates that we have entered into a new era in the fight against this disease and the many others for which it will be a model.

## ACKNOWLEDGEMENTS

The work of the Cystic Fibrosis Gene Therapy group at St Mary's/Imperial College is supported by the Muller Bequest, the Cystic Fibrosis Trust and the Medical Research Council. We are grateful to Dr Clare Huxley for helpful suggestions, and our colleagues from the Royal Brompton Hospital/National Heart and Lung Institute for many useful discussions in our joint programme of research.

## REFERENCES

1 Friedmann T. Progress toward human gene therapy. *Science* 1989; **244**: 1275–81.
2 Anderson WF. Human gene therapy. *Science* 1992; **256**: 808–13.
3 Roomer K, Friedmann T. Concepts and strategies for human gene therapy. *Eur. J. Biochem* 1992; **208**: 211–25.
4 Mulligan RC. The basic science of gene therapy. *Science* 1993; **260**: 926–32.
5 Bear CE, Li C, Kartner N, et al. Purification and functional reconstitution of the cystic fibrosis transmembrane regulator (CFTR). *Cell* 1992; **68**: 809–18.
6 Boucher RC, Knowles MR, Cantley L, et al. Na transport in cystic fibrosis respiratory epithelia. *J Clin Invest* 1986; **78**: 1245–52.
7 Welsh MJ, Smith AS. Molecular mechanisms of CTFR chloride channel dysfunction in cystic fibrosis. *Cell* 1993; **73**: 1251–4.
8 Trapnell BC, Chu C-S, Paakko PK, et al. Expression of the cystic fibrosis transmembrane regulator gene in the respiratory tract of normal individuals and individuals with cystic fibrosis. *Proc Natl Acad Sci USA* 1991; **88**: 6565–9.
9 Drumm ML, Pope HA, Cliff WH, et al. Correction of the cystic fibrosis defect in vitro by retrovirus-mediated gene transfer. *Cell* 1990; **62**: 1227–33.
10 Gregory RJ, Cheng SH, Rich DP, et al. Expression and characterization of the cystic fibrosis transmembrane conductance regulator. *Nature* 1990, **347**: 382–6.

11 Rich DP, Anderson MP, Gregory RJ, et al. Expression of cystic fibrosis transmembane conductance regulator corrects defective chloride channel regulation in cystic fibrosis airway epithelial cells. *Nature* 1990; **347**: 358–63.
12 Whitsett JA, Dey CR, Stripp BR, et al. Human cystic fibrosis transmembrane conductance regulator directed to respiratory epithelial cells of transgenic mice. *Nature Genet* 1992; **2**: 13–20.
13 Johnson LG, Olsen JC, Sarkadi B, et al. Efficiency of gene transfer for restoration of normal airway epithelial function in cystic fibrosis. *Nature Genet* 1992; **2**: 21–5.
14 Gilula NB, Reeves OR, Steinbach A. Metabolic coupling, ionic coupling and cell contacts. *Nature* 1972; **35**: 262–5.
15 Alton EWFW, Hay JG, Munro C, et al. Measurement of nasal potential difference in adult cystic fibrosis, Young's syndrome, and bronchiectasis. Thorax 1987; **42**: 815–17.
16 Flotte TR, Afione SA, Solow R, et al. Expression of the cystic fibrosis transmembrane conductance regulator from a novel adeno-associated virus promoter. *J Biol Chem* 1993; **268**: 3781–90.
17 Hyde SC, Gill DR, Higgins CF, et al. Correction of the ion transport defect in cystic fibrosis transgenic mice by gene therapy. *Nature* 1993; **362**: 250–5.
18 Alton EWFW, Middleton PG, Caplen NJ, et al. Non-invasive liposome-mediated gene delivery can correct the ion transport defect in cystic fibrosis mutant mice. *Nature Genet* 1993; **5**: 135–42.
19 Rosenfeld MA, Siegfried W, Yoshimura K, et al. Adenovirus-mediated transfer of a recombinant $\alpha_1$-antitrypsin gene to the lung epithelium *in vivo*. *Science* 1991; **252**: 431–4.
20 Rosenfeld MA, Yoshimura K, Trapnell BC, et al. In vivo transfer of the human cystic fibosis transmembrane conductance regulator gene to the airway epithelium. *Cell* 1992; **68**: 143–55.
21 Mastrangeli A, Danel C, Rosenfeld MA, et al. Diversity of airway epithelial cell targets for in vivo recombinant adenovirus-mediated transfer. *J Clin Invest* 1993; **91**: 225–34.
22 Stribling R, Brunette E, Liggitt D, et al. Aerosol gene delivery in vivo. *Proc Natl Acad Sci USA* 1992; **89**: 11277–81.
23 Yoshimura K, Rosenfeld MA, Nakamura H, et al. Expression of the human cystic fibrosis transmembrane conductance regulator gene in the mouse lung after *in vivo* intratracheal plasmid-mediated gene transfer. *Nucleic Acids Res* 1992; **20**: 3233–40.
24 Pavirani A. Lung specific gene therapy. *18th European Cystic Fibrosis Conference*, Madrid, 1993. Abstract S.1.2, p 85.
25 Snouwaert JN, Brigman KK, Latour AM, et al. An animal model for cystic fibrosis made by gene targeting. *Science* 1992; **257**: 1083–8.
26 Dorin JR, Dickinson P, Alton EWFW, et al. Cystic fibrosis in the mouse by targeted insertional mutagenesis. *Nature* 1992; **359**: 211–15.
27 Ratcliff R, Evans MJ, Cuthbert AW, et al. Production of a severe cystic fibrosis mutation in mice by gene targeting. *Nature Genet* 1993; **4**: 35–40.
28 Clark LL, Grubb BR, Gabriel SE, et al. Defective epithelial chloride transport in a gene-targeted mouse model of cystic fibrosis. *Science* 1992; **257**: 1125–8.
29 Colledge WH, Ratcliff R, Forster D, et al. Cystic fibrosis mouse with intestinal obstruction. *Lancet* 1992; **340**: 680.
30 Strauss S. Adenovirus infections in humans. In: *Adenoviruses* (ed HS Ginsberg) Plenum Press, New York, 1984, pp 451–96.
31 Horowitz MS. Adenoviruses. In: *Virology* (eds, BN Fields, DM Knipe) Raven Press, New York, 1990, pp 1723–40.

32 Graham FL, Smiley J, Russel WC, et al. Characteristics of a human cell line transformed by DNA from human adenovirus type 5. *J Gen Virol* 1977; **36**: 59–72.
33 Wold WS, Gooding LR. Region E3 of adenovirus: a cassette of genes involved in host immunosurveillance and virus–cell interactions. *Virology* 1991; **184**: 1–8.
34 Kvist S, Ostberg L, Persson H, et al. Molecular association between transplantation antigen s and cell surface antigen in adenovirus-transformed cell line. *Proc Natl Acad Sci USA* 1978; **75**: 5674–8.
35 Yang Y, Raper SE, Cohn JA, et al. An approach for treating the hepatobiliary disease of cystic fibrosis by somatic gene transfer. *Proc Nat Acad Sci USA* 1993; **90**: 4601–5.
36 Zabner J, Petersen DM, Puga AP, et al. Safety and efficacy of repetitive adenovirus-mediated transfer of CFTR cDNA to airway epithelia of primates and cotton rats. *Nature Genet* 1994; **6**: 75–83.
37 Carter BJ. Adeno-associated vectors. *Curr Opin Biotechnol* 1992; 3: 533–9.
38 Flotte TR, Conrad C, Afione SA, et al. Stable in vivo CFTR gene expression from an AAV vector. *Pediatr Pulmonol* 1993 (Suppl 9); 7th Annual North American Cystic Fibrosis Conference, Dallas, Texas, Abstract S2.1, pp 74–5.
39 Miller DG, Adam MA, Miller AD. Gene transfer by retrovirus vectors occurs only in cells that are actively replicating at the time of infection. *Mol Cell Biol* 1990; **10**: 4239–42.
40 Bayle JY, Johnson LG, St George JA, et al. High-efficiency gene transfer to primary monkey airway epithelia cells with retrovirus vectors using the gibbon ape leukaemia virus receptor. *Hum Gene Ther* 1993; **4**: 161–70.
41 Gershon H, Ghirlando R, Guttman SB, et al. Mode of formation and structural features of DNA–cationic liposome complexes used for transfection. *Biochemistry* 1993; **32**: 7143–51.
42 Lamb BT, Sisioda SS, Lawler AM, et al. Introduction and expression of the 400 kilobase precursor amyloid protein gene in transgenic mice. *Nature Genet* 1993; **5**: 22–9.
43 Gao X, Huang L. A novel cationic liposome for efficient transfection of mammalian cells. *Biochem Biophys Res Commun* 1991; **179**: 280–5.
44 Stewart MJ, Plautz GE, Del Bouno L, et al. Gene transfer in vivo with DNA–liposome complexes: safety and acute toxicity in mice. *Hum Gene Ther* 1992; **3**: 267–76.
45 Nabel EG, Gordon D, Yang Z-Y, et al. Gene transfer in vivo with DNA–liposome complexes: lack of autoimmunity and gonadal localization. *Hum Gene Ther* 1992; **3**: 649–56.
46 Miller AD. Human gene therapy comes of age. *Nature* 1992; **357**: 455–60.
47 Nabel GJ, Chang A, Nabel EG, et al. Clinical protocol: immunotherapy of malignancy by *in vivo* gene transfer into tumors. *Hum Gene Ther* 1992; **3**: 399–410.
48 Zhu N, Liggitt D, Liu Y, et al. Systemic gene expression after intravenous DNA delivery into adult mice. *Science* 1993; **261**: 209–11.
49 Felgner PL, Gadek TR, Holm M, et al. Lipofection: a highly efficient, lipid-mediated DNA-transfection procedure. *Proc Natl Acad Sci, USA* 1987; **84**: 7413–17.
50 Zabner J, Couture LA, Gregory RJ, et al. Adenovirus-mediated gene transfer transiently corrects the transport defect in nasal epithelia of patients with cystic fibrosis. *Cell* 1993; **75**: 1–20.
51 Handyside AH, Pattinson JK, Renketh RJA, et al. Biopsy of human preimplantation embryos and sexing by DNA amplification. *Lancet* 1989; **i**: 347.

52 Clothier CM. *Report of the Committee on the Ethics of Gene Therapy*. HMSO, London, 1992.
52a Welsh MJ, Smith AS, Zabner J, et al. Clinical protocol; cystic fibrosis gene therapy using an adenovirus vector: *in vivo* safety and efficacy in nasal epithelium. *Hum Gene Ther* 1994; 5209–19.
52b Wilson JM, Grossman M, Cabrera JA, et al. A novel mechanism for achieving transgene persistance in vivo after somatic gene transfer into heptocytes. *J Biol Chem* 1992; **267**: 11483–9.
53 Caplen NJ, Gao X, Hayes P, et al. Gene therapy for cystic fibrosis in human subjects by liposome mediated DNA transfer: regulatory process and production of resources. *Gene Ther* 1994; **1**: 139–147.
54 Smythe E, Warren G. The mechanism of receptor mediated endocytosis. *Eur J Biochem* 1991; **202**: 689–99.
55 Wagner E, Cotten M, Foisner R, et al. Transferrin–polycation–DNA complexes: the effect of polycations on the structure of the complex and DNA delivery to cells. *Proc Natl Acad Sci USA* 1991; **88**: 4255–9.
56 Cotten M, Wagner E, Zatloukal K, et al. High-efficiency receptor-mediated delivery of small and large (48 kilobase) gene constructs using the endosome-disruption activity of defective or chemically inactivated adenovirus particles. *Proc Nat Acad Sci USA* 1992; **89**: 6094–8.
57 Cotten M, Längle-Rouault F, Kirlappos H, et al. Transferrin–polycation-mediated introduction of DNA into human leukemic cells: stimulation by agents that affect the survival of transfected DNA or modulate transferrin receptor levels. *Proc Natl Acad Sci USA*, 1990; **87**: 4033–7.
58 Wagner E, Zenke M, Cotten M, et al. Transferrin–polycation conjugates as carriers for DNA uptake into cells. *Proc Natl Acad Sci USA* 1991; **87**: 3410–14.
59 Zenke M, Steinlein P, Wagner E, et al. Receptor-mediated endocytosis transferrin–polycation conjugates: an efficient way to introduce DNA into hemopoietic cells. *Proc Natl Acad Sci USA* 1990; **87**: 3655–9.
60 Wu GY, Wu CH. Receptor-mediated in vitro gene transformation by a soluble DNA carrier system. *J Biol Chem* 1987; **262**: 4429–32.
61 Wu GY, Wu CH. Receptor-mediated gene delivery and expression *in vivo J Biol Chem* 1988; **263**: 14621–4.
62 Ferkol T, Kaetzel CS, Davis BP. Gene transfer into epithelial cells by targeting the polymeric immunoglobulin receptor. *J Clin Invest* 1993; **92**: 2394–400.
63 Cristiano RJ, Smith LC, Woo SLC. Hepatic gene therapy: adenovirus enhancement of receptor-mediated gene delivery and expression in primary hepatocytes. *Proc Natl Acad Sci USA* 1993; **90**: 2122–6.
64 Curiel DT, Agarwall S, Wagner E, et al. Adenovirus enhancement of transferrin–polylysine-mediated gene delivery. *Proc Natl Acad Sci USA* 1991; **88**: 8850–4.
65 Curiel DT, Wagner E, Cotten M, et al. High-efficiency gene transfer mediated by adenovirus coupled to DNA–polylysine complexes. *Hum Gene Ther* 1992; **3**: 147–54.
66 Wagner E, Zatloukal K, Cotten M, et al. Coupling of adenovirus to transferrin–polylysine/DNA complexes greatly enhances receptor-mediated gene delivery and expression of transfected genes. *Proc Nat Acad Sci USA* 1992; **89**: 6099–103.
67 Gao L, Wagner E, Cotten M, et al. Direct in vivo gene transfer to airway epithelium employing adenovirus–polylysine–DNA complexes. *Hum Gene Ther* 1993; **4**: 17–24.

68 Wagner E, Plank C, Zatloukal K, et al. Influenza virus hemagglutinin HA-2 N-terminal fusogenic peptides augment gene transfer by transferrin–polylysine–DNA complexes: toward a synthetic virus-like gene transfer vehicle. *Proc Natl Acad Sci USA* 1992; **89**: 7934–8.

69 Isberg RR, Lelong JM. Multiple $\beta$-chain integrins are receptors for invasin, a protein that promotes bacterial penetration into mammalian cells. *Cell* 1990; **60**: 861–71.

70 Gaillard J-L, Berche P, Frehel C, et al. Entry of *L. monocytogenes* into cells is mediated by internalin, a repeat protein reminiscent of surface antigens from Gram-positive cocci. Cell 1991; **65**: 1127–41.

71 Ortega-Barria E, Pereira MEA. A novel *T. cruzi* heparin binding protein promotes fibroblast adhesion and penetration of engineered bacteria and trypanosomes into mammalian cells. *Cell* 1991; **67**: 411–21.

72 Isberg RR. Discrimination between intracellular uptake and surface adhesion of bacterial pathogens. *Science* 1991; **252**: 934–8.

73 Wickham TJ, Mathias P, Cheresh DA, et al. Integrins $\alpha v\beta 3$ and $\alpha v\beta 5$ promote adenovirus internalization but not virus attachment. *Cell* 1993; **73**: 309–19.

73a Hart SL, Knight AM, Harbottle RP, et al. Cell binding and internalization by filamentous phase displaying a cyclic RGD-containing peptide. *J Biol Chem* 1994; **269**: 12468–74.

74 Willard HF. Centromeres of mammalian chromosomes. *Trends Genet* 1990; **6**: 410–416.

75 Bloom K. The centromere frontier: kinetochore components, microtubule-based motility, and the CEN-value paradox. *Cell* 1993; **73**: 621–4.

76 Cooper KF, Fishery RB, Tyler-Smith C. Structure of sequences adjacent to the centromeric alphoid satellite DNA array on the human Y chromosome. *J Mol Biol* 1993; **230**: 787–99.

77 Itzhaski JE, Barnett MA, MacCarthy AB, et al. Targeted breakage of a human chromosome mediated by a cloned human telomeric DNA. *Nature Genet* 1992; **2**: 283–7.

78 Barnett MA, Buckle VJ, Evans EP, et al. Telomere directed fragmentation of mammalian chromosomes *Nucleic Acids Res* 1993; **21**: 27–36.

79 Featherstone T, Huxley C. Extrachromosomal maintenance and amplification of yeast artificial chromosome DNA in mouse cells. *Genomics* 1993; **17**: 267–78.

Chapter Three

# Splicing of the CFTR Gene

Garry R. Cutting
*Center for Medical Genetics, and Departments of Pediatrics and Medicine, Johns Hopkins University School of Medicine, Baltimore, Maryland, USA*

## INTRODUCTION

The coding regions of eukaryotic genes are arranged in discontinuous elements called exons. Following the transcription of a gene into heterogeneous nuclear RNA (hnRNA) the intron sequences between the exons are removed in a process called splicing. This allows the creation of mature messenger RNA (mRNA) containing only coding sequence. The splicing process is guided by DNA sequences called the splice donor at the 5′ end of the intron and the splice acceptor at the 3′ end (Figure 1). These sequences define the boundaries between exons and introns and have been highly conserved during evolution[1–4]. A third conserved sequence is the branch point consensus surrounding an adenine nucleotide that is linked by a 5′–2′ phosphodiester bond to the first nucleotide of the intron during the initial phase of intron removal[4]. The splicing of hnRNA can be altered to produce mRNAs which encode proteins with different properties (isoforms). This process, termed alternative splicing, has been observed in a variety of genes, including immunoglobulins[5,6], myelin basic protein[7] and structural proteins[8,9]. It can occur in a tissue-specific and/or developmentally regulated fashion to significantly increase the diversity of proteins produced by a single gene[10,11]. In some instances an alternatively spliced transcript may include a single exon that contributes a novel domain or regulatory region to the protein[5,12,13]. The situation can also be very

*Cystic Fibrosis—Current Topics, Volume 2.* Edited by J. A. Dodge, D. J. H. Brock and J. H. Widdicombe

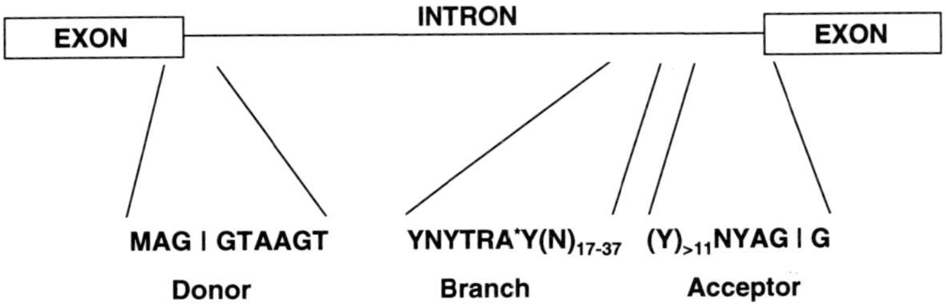


**Figure 1** Relative locations of consensus sequences that direct RNA splicing. The most common nucleotide at each position is shown[1–4]. The boundary between exon and intron sequences is indicated by a line. Asterisk indicates the adenine nucleotide of the branch site that forms a phosphodiester bond with the 5′ end of the intron. Nucleotide codes for M, Y, R and N are the same as in Table 1

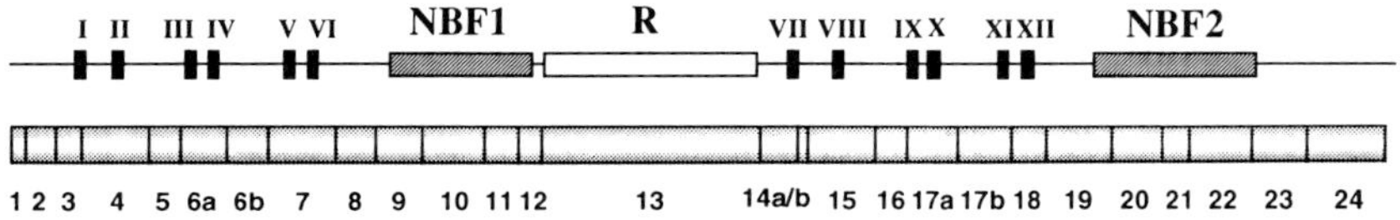


**Figure 2** Location of CFTR functional domains relative to exons in CFTR mRNA. Solid boxes indicate hydrophobic segments with roman numerals I–VI forming transmembrane domain 1 (TM 1) and numerals VII–XII forming TM 2. Hatched boxes represent the nucleotide-binding folds (NBF). Open box indicates the single regulatory (R) domain. Shaded boxes are CFTR exons with numbers shown below

complex with multiple differing splice patterns involving numerous exons, as demonstrated by the rat skeletal muscle troponin T gene, which gives rise to 64 different mRNAs[11].

Mutations in the cystic fibrosis transmembrane conductance regulator (CFTR) gene are responsible for cystic fibrosis (CF). Twenty-seven exons encompassing 250 000 nucleotides of DNA are spliced to form the CFTR protein, which functions as a cAMP-activated chloride channel[14,15]. CFTR also appears to function as a regulator of a separate chloride channel called the outward rectifier and may have additional functions[16–19]. The majority of CFTR exons are 200 nucleotides or less in length, with the notable exception of exon 13, which is 723 nucleotides long and encodes the regulatory (R) domain of the protein[20,21] (Figure 2). None of the remaining exons individually encodes entire functional or structural domains of the protein[21].

## ALTERNATIVE SPLICING AT THE 5′ END OF THE CFTR GENE

Subsequent to the cloning of the CFTR gene and determination of its genomic structure, two additional exons (1a and −1a) upstream of the 5′ most exon (exon 1) were identified[22,23]. Exons 1a and −1a are within 1000 nucleotides of exon 1 and were found spliced to exon 2 by RNA polymerase chain reaction (PCR) assays using primers located in exon −1a and exon 2[23]. Two forms of splicing were found to occur: −1a to 1a to 2 and −1a to 2. Transcripts hybridizing to a probe derived from exon −1a were detected in RNA from a human colonic epithelial adenocarcinoma cell line (Caco2) that expresses high levels of CFTR mRNA. A sequence similar to the splice acceptor consensus sequence could not be found in the exon −1a region, leading the authors to conclude that transcription initiates from exon −1a. The characterization of a cluster of transcriptional start sites in exon −1a supports this hypothesis[23].

The data presented by Koh and coworkers provide convincing evidence for alternative splicing at the 5′ end of CFTR. However, exon −1a does not contain an AUG codon in the correct frame to enable translation to initiate from this exon. Exon 1a has termination codons in all three reading frames. Therefore it is unclear whether transcripts bearing exon −1a (−1a/1a/2 or −1a/2) are translated to produce an isoform of CFTR. A non-AUG codon would have to be used for translation to begin in exon −1a. Alternatively, an AUG codon in the proper context elsewhere in the transcript could be used to translate a CFTR isoform. A similar mechanism is used to produce different versions of the myosin alkali light chain protein[24,25]. The next appropriate AUG in CFTR occurs in exon 4 at codon 150 and is preceded by and immediately followed by AUG codons (at position 82 and 152) in less suitable contexts for translation initiation. This situation is not favourable for translation initiation[26]. It is possible that these transcripts are not translated but are involved in the regulation of CFTR expression in a tissue or developmental stage-specific manner. This form of regulation has been observed for other genes[27–29].

Alternative splicing of the 5′ of CFTR was originally discovered in cDNAs from a pancreatic library and has been studied in cell lines derived from adenocarcinomas (T84, Caco2 and CFPAC)[23]. It is not known whether this process occurs at an appreciable level *in vivo* and in which tissues. Therefore further studies are necessary to define the biological role of the 5′ alternative splicing of CFTR.

## ALTERNATIVE SPLICING OF EXONS ENCODING PORTIONS OF THE FIRST TRANSMEMBRANE DOMAIN

Exons 4 and 5 encode portions of the first transmembrane domain (TM 1) of CFTR (Figure 2). Exon 4 has been found deleted in a small fraction ($\leqslant 2\%$) of CFTR transcripts from a variety of human and mouse tissues and human cell lines[30,31]. Deletion of exon 4 would leave the reading frame intact, making possible the translation of a CFTR isoform. Whether this isoform would be functional is debatable since a sequence encoding half of the first and the entire second hydrophobic segments would be missing. This would be expected to significantly alter the topology of the protein, possibly making it unstable and prone to degradation or improperly trafficked and retained in the endoplasmic reticulum similar to the situation observed for CFTR bearing the ΔF508 mutation[32]. The discovery of a disease-associated mutation (621 + 1 G → T) that causes the deletion of exon 4 supports the concept that functional isoforms of CFTR are not encoded by transcripts missing exon 4[33,34].

Exon 5 has been found to be deleted in a significant fraction (20–40%) of CFTR transcripts in expressing tissues in the mouse[31]. A smaller fraction (1–8%) of murine CFTR transcripts had exons 4 and 5 deleted[31]. RNA PCR of CFTR mRNA from rabbit and guinea-pig cardiac tissues revealed a deletion of 90 nucleotides corresponding to the boundaries of exon 5 in human CFTR. This alternative splicing occurs in a tissue-specific manner. All of the CFTR transcripts in cardiac ventricular tissue in these species were missing exon 5, while only full-length transcripts were found in the rabbit pancreas[35]. CFTR transcripts could not be detected by this method in rabbit, guinea-pig or canine atria or canine ventricles.

Deletion of exon 5 also leaves the reading frame intact, raising the possibility that CFTR isoforms may be translated from exon 5− transcripts. Although this form of alternative splicing has not been detected in human tissue[30] it is plausible that it has a biologically significant role in mice, rabbits and guinea-pigs. This hypothesis is supported by high levels of exon 5− transcripts in these species and apparent tissue specificity of this form of alternative splicing. In addition, exon 5 encodes a portion of a putative intracellular loop between hydrophobic segments 2 and 3 and contains two potential sites for phosphorylation by protein kinase C[35]. Therefore, loss of this region might not drastically alter protein topology and may provide a CFTR isoform with distinct functional properties.

Electrophysiological studies have revealed cAMP-activated chloride channels in guinea-pig ventricle but not in guinea-pig or canine atrium[35]. Only CFTR 5− transcripts were detected in the guinea-pig ventricle, suggesting that CFTR missing exon 5 encoded residues (CFTRΔ5) is functional in guinea-pigs. Expression of human CFTRΔ5, however, does not confer cAMP-activated chloride conductance when expressed in epithelial cervical carcinoma (HeLa) cells[13]. This mutant CFTR protein appears to be abnormally processed, as demonstrated by the lack of mature fully glycosylated protein on SDS–PAGE gels following radiolabelling of immunoprecipitated mutant CFTR with protein kinase A[13]. A mutation in the splice donor sequence of intron 5 (711 + 1 G → T) that causes skipping of exon 5 is invariably associated with CF[33,36]. The differences between guinea-pig and human CFTRΔ5 function may be species-specific. The lack of alternative splicing of exon 5 in human tissues is consistent with this hypothesis. Alternatively, the guinea-pig and rabbit ventricles may express very low levels of full-length CFTR that was below the detection threshold of the techniques employed by Horowitz et al.[35]. Either way, the species- and tissue-specific character of the exon 5 alternative splicing suggests a biological role that may have been modified during evolution.

## ALTERNATIVE SPLICING OF EXONS ENCODING THE FIRST NUCLEOTIDE BINDING FOLD

One of the first forms of alternative splicing discovered in CFTR was deletion of exon 9[22,37]. This exon encodes the beginning of the first nucleotide-binding fold (NBF 1), including motif A of the Walker ATP binding consensus sequence[38]. The amount of exon 9− transcript varies widely (0–92%) and can account for the majority of CFTR transcripts in airway epithelia[30,37,39]. The variability in exon 9 splicing efficiency is explained, for the most part, by a variation in the splice acceptor site in intron 8[40]. As shown in Figure 1, the splice acceptor consensus contains a polypyrimidine tract that optimally has 11 consecutive thymidine or cytosine nucleotides[4]. Sequencing of the splice acceptor site preceding exon 9 demonstrated that three variations of uninterrupted pyrimidines occur in the population; 5, 7 and 9 thymidines[37]. Semi-quantitative PCR analysis of bronchial and nasal epithelial cell RNA revealed that the amount of exon 9− CFTR transcripts correlated with the type of intron 8 polypyrimide tract variant[30,40]. The fraction of total CFTR mRNA transcripts that were missing exon 9 ranged from 0 to 50% in individuals homozygous for the 7 thymidine variant (7T) and 0% to 40% in 9 thymidine (9T) homozygotes[40]. Three individuals homozygous for the 5 thymidine (5T) variant had the vast majority (89%, 90% and 92%) of their CFTR transcripts deleted for exon 9[39,40].

The association between exon 9 splicing efficiency and the length of the polypyrimidine tract provided a genetic basis for this process and emphasized the importance of the polypyrimidine tract in splice site selection[40]. However, variation in length of the polypyrimidine tract in intron 8 does not appear to be the only factor leading to inefficient exon 9 splicing. Several other CFTR introns have splice acceptor sites with short polypyrimidine tracts (e.g. introns 6a and 17a), yet alternative splicing of the exons following these introns has not been observed[30]. Intron 8 is unique among CFTR introns in that its splice donor site has a cytosine nucleotide following the first two nucleotides of the intron (see Table 1). This position is occupied by a purine nucleotide in all other CFTR introns consistent with the donor splice site consensus sequence[3,4]. Therefore, reduced efficiency of exon 9 splicing may be the consequence of a short polypyrimidine tract in the splice acceptor and a deviation from the optimum consensus sequence in the splice donor of intron 8.

The abundance of exon 9− CFTR transcripts in epithelial tissues lead two groups of investigators to determine whether it encoded a functional isoform of CFTR. Transduction of CFPAC (pancreatic adenocarcinoma cell line from a CF patient) or HeLa cells with the CFTR cDNA missing exon 9 did not confer novel cAMP-regulated chloride conductance[31,41]. Protein analysis of transduced cells detected mutant CFTR but it was immature and incompletely glycosylated in both studies. This suggests exon 9 – CFTR mRNA transcripts are translated but the protein product is improperly processed and never reaches the cell membrane. Degradation within the endoplasmic reticulum is the probable fate of the mutant protein. Expression of the CFTR missing exon 9 encoded amino acids in *Xenopus* oocytes incubated at room temperature also failed to produce a cAMP-regulated chloride conductance. This is significant because other CFTR mutants that are improperly processed at 37 °C appear to properly fold and regain function at lower temperatures[32,42]. Therefore CFTR protein missing a crucial region of NBF 1 does not function as a chloride channel and it appears likely that it does not have any intracellular function.

Alternative splicing of exon 9 may play a role in post-transcriptional regulation of CFTR expression. Studies of the HT29 cell line, a model for differentiating intestinal epithelia indicate that CFTR transcription increases by an order of magnitude during differentiation[43]. The level of CFTR protein and magnitude of cAMP-activated chloride transcript were unchanged[44,45]. Interestingly, the amount of exon 9 – CFTR transcripts increased by 18-fold during HT29 cell differentiation[43]. This raises the possibility that this form of alternative splicing and/or its encoded isoform modulates the level of mature functional CFTR protein.

Although the biological role of alternative exon 9 splicing remains obscure it has provided important insights into the relationship between CFTR levels and disease. Individuals homozygous for the inefficient intron 8 splice variant with 5T had only 8–12% of CFTR mRNA transcripts in airway epithelia with exon 9, yet did not have progressive lung disease associated with CF[39]. The identification of healthy individuals carrying the common mutation ΔF508 and the 5T variant on the other CFTR allele suggests that only a minor fraction of CFTR transcripts needs to be full-length to produce a normal phenotype[46].

Variant exon 9 splicing of CFTR transcripts can also alter the phenotype produced by a disease-associated mutation. The missense mutation which substitutes an arginine residue at codon 117 with histidine (R117H) has been associated with the pancreatic sufficient form of CF[47]. Patients with this phenotype have chronic obstructive pulmonary disease that is indistinguishable from that observed in classic CF. However, they do not develop clinically significant pancreatic exocrine insufficiency and their sweat chloride levels are only modestly elevated[48]. The R117H mutation has also been identified in males with infertility due to congenital bilateral absence of the vas deferens (CBAVD) who do not have lung disease. Interestingly, it was discovered that the R117H mutation had occurred twice; in a CFTR gene with the inefficient splice acceptor 5T and in a gene with the common and more efficient 7T variant[46]. Individuals heterozygous for a CF mutation associated with classic CF (e.g. ΔF508 or G551D) and the R117H mutation associated with the 5T variant developed the lung disease characteristic of CF. However, the R117H mutation found in healthy males with CBAVD is exclusively associated with the more efficient splice acceptor 7T[46]. Analysis of the CFTR coding regions of the R117H alleles associated with each intron 8 splicing variant uncovered only one other difference. In addition to the intron 8 splice variant, a G to C transversion was found for nucleotides prior to the AUG initiator codon in exon 1[46]. The consequence of the latter alteration upon translation efficiency is unknown; however, the difference in intron 8 splice acceptor sites is predicted to have a profound effect upon the amount of full-length CFTR protein bearing the R117H mutation. This is important because CFTR bearing the R117H mutation is partially functional[49–51]. Taken together, these data suggest that low levels of partially functioning CFTR results in progressive lung disease whereas higher levels allow individuals to escape life-limiting lung disease. How much partially functional CFTR protein is required for a normal pulmonary phenotype is unknown.

Deletion of exon 12 has been observed in a significant fraction of CFTR transcripts from a variety of human epithelial tissues and cell lines[30,52,53]. It does not occur in a tissue-specific manner and has not been identified in murine tissues[31]. One study has reported that exon 12– transcripts constituted 5–30% of transcripts. A second study of lymphocyte RNA found a wide variability of exon 12– transcript levels ranging from 0% to 100% in 12 controls. In two of these individuals the proportion of exon 12– transcripts in epithelial cell mRNA was found to correlate with the levels found in lymphocytes[52]. The aetiology of alternative splicing of exon 12 is unclear. The splice site sequences flanking exon 12 are in good agreement with the consensus sequences for splicing. One group of investigators has suggested that the exon 12 deletion is due to the lack of a sequence that precisely matches the branch point consensus in intron 11. This situation occurs in a number of other CFTR introns where alternative splicing has not been observed (e.g. introns 6b and 17b)[30]. In addition, intron 12 has a reasonable branch point sequence (ATTTAAT) in the correct location[21].

The region of CFTR encoded by exon 12 includes the last portion of NBF1 and motif B of the Walker ATP binding consensus sequence[20,38]. Therefore, although deletion of this exon would not alter the reading frame of the mature transcript, it appears unlikely that a functional isoform would be created. Indeed, a mutation in the splice donor of intron 12 that causes deletion of exon 12 in all mRNA transcripts from this allele causes CF when paired with the ΔF508 mutation[53]. Expression of CFTR missing exon 12 encoded residues in heterologous cells has not been reported.

In the process of identifying the CFTR gene, a cDNA clone (T16-4.5) isolated from a T84 cell library was found to contain extraneous sequence between exons 10 and 11[20]. A larger than expected fragment from the same region was PCR amplified from lymphocyte and nasal epithelial cell cDNA[54]. Four of 20 individuals had this larger fragment in lymphocyte RNA which constituted 7–83% of total CFTR mRNA transcripts[54]. Sequence analysis revealed a novel fragment of 199 nucleotides inserted precisely between exons 10 and 11. Approximately 5% of CFTR mRNA in T84 cells also contain this insertion[55]. This sequence originates from intron 10, where it is flanked by splice donor and acceptor consensus sequences[54]. Based upon these characteristics, the sequence has been designated exon 10b[54]. A 120-nucleotide sequence with 74% nucleotide identity to human exon 10b occurs in intron 10 of the mouse genome[55]. However, alternative splicing of exon 10b has not been observed in murine CFTR transcripts[31]. This may be due to the fact that splice sites flanking murine exon 10b vary at a number of positions from the splice consensus sequences and the putative splice acceptor site lacks a poly-pyrimide tract[55]. Both exons contain in-frame termination codons and human exon 10b shifts the reading frame of the CFTR transcript.

The biological role of alternative splicing of exon 10b is unknown. Inclusion of exon 10b in CFTR mRNA transcripts introduces a premature termination codon that would be predicted to drastically lower transcript levels similar to the situation observed for nonsense mutations[56]. A few individuals had high levels of CFTR mRNA transcripts containing exon 10b, suggesting that a CFTR protein truncated in the NBF 1 might be present in those persons. However, it seems unlikely that a CFTR isoform truncated in the middle of a region known to be important would retain any function. One group of investigators claimed that a protein of 61 kDa, immunoprecipitated with an anti-CFTR antibody from T84 cells, was the product of an exon $10b^+$ CFTR transcript[55]. Unfortunately, additional studies were not presented that definitively identified the lower molecular weight fragment as a CFTR isoform.

The presence of exon $10b^+$ in the mouse genome suggests that this sequence may be a remnant of CFTR evolution. This exon may have been included in a primitive version of CFTR. Mutations occurring over time then excluded it from the normal pattern of CFTR splicing. This situation became permanent since loss of the region encoded by this exon produced a protein which conferred a selective advantage to its host. An intriguing observation is that human exon 10b has excellent splice donor and acceptor sequences but is not included in the normal form of CFTR mRNA. Since this exon contains an in-frame stop codon, it is tempting to speculate that mechanisms causing skipping of exons containing nonsense mutations might operate to exclude exon 10b from mature CFTR transcripts[57].

A situation similar to that observed for exon $10b^+$ has been documented in CFTR mRNA from murine testis[31,58]. In this case, insertions of 89, 90 and 108 nucleotides between exons 11 and 12 have been identified which appear to be the result of alternative splicing of a novel region in intron 11. The 89-nucleotide insertion was observed in 10–15% of CFTR transcripts in testicular mRNA[31]. Sequence analysis of mouse genomic DNA identified a sequence corresponding to the 89 nucleotides in intron 11. This region was flanked by splice acceptor and donor sequences and has been designated exon 11b[31]. The 108-nucleotide fragment contains the 89 nucleotide sequence and arises by use of an alternative splice acceptor site 19 nucleotides upstream from the start of the 89 nucleotide sequence in intron 11. The 90 nucleotide fragment is identical to the 89-nucleotide exon 11b but contains an additional adenine nucleotide in the middle of the sequence[58]. Reverse transcriptase and Taq polymerase errors have been ruled out by the characterization of multiple independent clones amplified from the exon 11 to exon 12 region of testicular CFTR cDNA. The most likely explanation for the 89- and 90-nucleotide sequences is a polymorphism in the mouse population[58].

The inclusion of the 89-nucleotide fragment causes a frame shift and subsequent introduction of a premature termination codon into the CFTR mRNA. The 90-nucleotide and 108-nucleotide insertions each contain in-frame termination codons. Therefore, it seems unlikely that a functional CFTR isoform would be encoded by transcripts containing any of these exon 11b variants. However, the tissue specificity of this splicing process suggests a possible gene-regulatory role. Indeed there are a number of examples where alternative splicing of exons containing termination codons alter the expression of a gene in a developmentally regulated or tissue-specific manner[59–63]. This form of alternative splicing is not observed in humans or rats, suggesting that if the exon 11b splicing does have a biological role, it is species specific.

## ALTERNATIVE SPLICING OF THE CARBOXYL TERMINUS OF CFTR

PCR amplification of CFTR exons 21–24 from cDNA derived from several epithelial and non-epithelial cell lines revealed a larger than expected product[64]. Sequencing of this larger fragment identified a 260-nucleotide novel sequence inserted between exons 23 and 24. The alternatively spliced product represented 3–16% of the total CFTR transcripts and could be detected in T84 and HT29 cell line mRNA by Northern blot analysis. Analysis of the intron between exons 23 and 24 revealed that the 260-nucleotide sequence was immediately 5′ of exon 24 and is preceded by a reasonable splice acceptor consensus sequence. This suggests that the insertion of the additional sequence termed exon 24a is due to use of a cryptic splice acceptor in intron 23[64].

Inclusion of exon 24a introduces a termination signal 183 nucleotides prior to the normal termination codon. CFTR translated from transcripts

**Table 1** Location of mutations reported in CFTR splice donor and acceptor site

| Intron | Nucleotide No. | Donor Exon/intron | | Acceptor Intron/exon | Refs |
|---|---|---|---|---|---|
| Consensus | | MAG/GTRAGT | ..... | YYYYYYYYYYNYAG/G | |
| 1 | 185/186 | CAG/GTGAGa | ..... | CTCTCTTTaTTTTAG/c | |
| 2 | 296/297 | AAG/GTAtGT | ..... | TTTaTTCTTTTGCAG/a | |
| 3 | 405/406 | ggG/GTAAGg | ..... | TTTCCCCTTTTGTAG/G | 81,82 |
| 4 | 621/622 | AAG/GTAAta | ..... | CaTTTTTTCTTTTAG/a | 69,33 |
| 5 | 711/712 | gAa/GTAtGT | ..... | gCTTTTaTTTTCCAG/G | |
| 6a | 875/876 | CAG/GTAgca | ..... | TTgaTTgaTTTACAG/a | |
| 6b | 1001/1002 | Aca/GTAAGT | ..... | TaTTgTTTTTTATAG/a | |
| 7 | 1248/1249 | CAG/GTAAtg | ..... | CTCTTTTaTaaATAG/G | |
| 8 | 1341/1342 | gAG/GTcAGa | ..... | gTgTTTTTTTaACAG/G | 69,84 |
| 9 | 1524/1525 | AAG/GTAGtT | ..... | gggTTTTaTTTCCAG/a | 85 |
| 10 | 1716/1717 | gAG/GTAAGa | ..... | TaTTTTTggTaATAG/G | |
| 11 | 1811/1812 | AAG/GTGAaT | ..... | CCaTTTTCTTTTTAG/a | 69 |
| 12 | 1898/1899 | AAG/GTAtGT | ..... | TTTTaTaTCTTAaAG/c | 69 |

| | | | | | |
|---|---|---|---|---|---|
| 13 | 2622/2623 | AAG/GTAgGT | ..... | aaTTCTTTTaTTCAG/G | 86 |
| 14a | 2751/2752 | CAG/GTAAGa | ..... | CTTgTTCCaTTCCAG/G | |
| 14b | 2789/2790 | aAa/GTGAGT | ..... | CTaTTTgCTTTACAG/c | 69 |
| 15 | 3040/3041 | CAG/GTActT | ..... | TCTTgTaTaTTATAG/G | |
| 16 | 3120/3121 | CAG/GTAtGT | ..... | TCTTTgaTCTTACAG/t | |
| 17a | 3271/3272 | AAG/GTAtGa | ..... | ggaaaTaTTTCACAG/G | 69 |
| 17b | 3499/3500 | CAG/GTActa | ..... | TTTgTgCaTCTATAG/G | |
| 18 | 3600/3601 | ttG/GTAAGT | ..... | TTaTTTTaTTTCAG/a | 85 |
| 19 | 3849/3850 | AgG/GTGAGa | ..... | aCTTTTaCCTTATAG/G | 69,85 |
| 20 | 4005/4006 | CAG/GTGAGc | ..... | TCTTTTTTgCTATAG/a | 69 |
| 21 | 4095/4096 | gAG/GTAAGg | ..... | CTTCTCTaaCTGCAG/G | |
| 22 | 4268/4269 | Agt/GTGAGT | ..... | TTCTTTCTTTTCTAG/a | |
| 23 | 4374/4375 | ttG/GTGAGT | ..... | CagCCaTTTCCCTAG/G | 69 |

Nucleotide numbers refer to the last nucleotide in the exon of the splice donor and the first nucleotide in the exon of the slice acceptor[21]. Splice site sequences are as published by Zielenski et al.[21]. Nucleotides in lower case differ from consensus[1,3]. Underlined bases are sites of mutations in CFTR which cause a deviation from the consensus sequence. Double underlined nucleotides have been published in the references shown at the right; single underlined nucleotides have been reported to the CF Genetic Analysis Consortium. Nucleotide codes: M can be A or C; Y can be C or T; R can be A or G and N can be A, C, G or T.

containing exon 24a would be shorter than the normal CFTR by 61 amino acids. Whether this protein would be functional is unknown. Alternative splicing that can produce proteins with different carboxyl terminal domains has been observed in several other genes[8,65].

## ABERRANT SPLICING OF CFTR

Over 350 putative mutations have been identified in CFTR genes from affected individuals and reported to the CF Genetic Analysis Consortium. Approximately 10% of these mutations are predicted to cause disease by altering splicing of CFTR RNA. The location of mutations that cause a deviation from the respective splice consensus sequence are indicated in Table 1. The effect upon RNA splicing has been reported for seven of these mutations (Table 2).

The mutation 621 + 1G → T alters the highly conserved GT in the splice donor site of exon 4[66]. PCR amplification of cDNA reverse-transcribed from nasal epithelial RNA of two patients carrying this mutation revealed skipping of exon 4 as predicted[33,34]. In addition, aberrantly spliced transcripts were identified that resulted from the use of a cryptic donor splice site within exon 4. This form of splicing occurred in 100% of CFTR transcripts from the 621 + 1G → T allele in one patient[34] and a fraction of the transcripts in a second patient who also had transcripts missing exon 4[33]. Lymphoblastoid cell RNA from the latter patient showed the same pattern of aberrant CFTR splicing. This suggests that lymphoblasts or peripheral lymphocytes can be used to analyse the consequences of putative splice mutations in the CFTR gene. This is an important observation since lymphocytes are more readily available than CFTR expressing epithelial cells. However, there is ample evidence that splicing patterns can vary by developmental stage and tissue type[11]. Caution should be exercised when evaluating the consequences of a putative splice site mutation in a tissue that is not involved in the disease. This problem is exemplified by the observation that 50% of dystrophin transcripts from peripheral lymphocyte RNA contained a novel exon that is rarely (<5%) present in dystrophin-expressing tissues such as skeletal muscle[67]. The CFTR mutation 711 + 1G → T alters the conserved GT of the splice donor site of exon 5[66]. RNA PCR analysis of nasal epithelial cells and lymphoblastoid cells from one patient and lymphoblastoid cells from a second patient revealed skipping of exon 5[33,36]

Each of the aberrantly spliced transcripts produced by mutations 621 + 1G → T and 711 + 1G → T retain the normal reading frame. CFTR protein might be translated from these transcripts but does not have normal function since individuals carrying this mutation paired with a second disease-associated mutation (e.g. ΔF508) invariably have cystic fibrosis. Neither

**Table 2** Mutations and polymorphisms in the CFTR gene shown to alter RNA splicing

| Mutation[a] | Location | Tissue studied | Effect(s) | Phenotype[b] | Refs |
|---|---|---|---|---|---|
| $621 + 1$ G → T | Intron 4 | Nasal epithelia<br>Lymphoblasts | Deletion of exon 4, use of cryptic splice donor site in exon 4 | Severe CF | 33,34 |
| $711 + 1$ G → T | Intron 5 | Nasal epithelia<br>Lymphoblasts | Deletion of exon 5 | Severe CF | 33,36 |
| 5,7 or 9 thymidines in polypyrimidine tract | Intron 8 | Nasal and bronchial epithelia, lymphocytes | Variable deletion of exon 9 | Normal | 40 |
| $1717 - 1$ G → T | Intron 10 | Nasal epithelia | Deletion of exon 11 | Severe CF | 34 |
| $1898 + 1$ G → T | Intron 12 | Nasal epithelia | Deletion of exon 12 | Severe CF | 34,53 |
| $2789 + 5$ G → A | Intron 14b | Nasal epithelia | Deletion of exon 14a | Mild CF | 69,77 |
| $3849 + 10$ Kb C → T | Intron 19 | Nasal epithelia | Insertion of 84 bp sequence | Mild CF | 69,76 |
| 4005 G → C | Exon 20 | Nasal and rectal epithelia | Use of cryptic slice donor site in intron 20 | Severe CF | 74 |

[a] For mutation nomenclature see review by Beaudet and Tsui[87]
[b] Severe and mild primarily refer to pancreatic status; the adult patients classified as mild also had minimal lung disease.

mutation is rare; the 621 + 1G → T and 711 + G → T mutations account for approximately 1.4% and 0.9%, respectively, of CF alleles worldwide[68,69]. In certain ethnic groups the frequency of 621 + 1G → T reaches 23% and 711 + 1G → T attains 9%, presumably as a result of a founder effect[70].

The mRNA splicing pattern produced by a mutation in the splice acceptor site preceding exon 11 (1717 – 1G → A) has been examined in nasal epithelial cell RNA from three patients[34]. Skipping of exon 11 was observed in all three cases. Although transcript deleted for exon 11 is present in epithelial cells it is probably not translated into a functional protein. Loss of this exon causes a shift in the reading frame of the mRNA transcript. Nasal epithelial CFTR mRNA transcripts from patients carrying the 1898 + 1G → T mutation in the splice donor site of intron 12 have been analysed[34,53]. The only aberrantly spliced product identified is deleted for exon 12. This mutation accounts for about 0.9% of CF alleles and has invariably been associated with classic pancreatic insufficient CF[53,68]. Although loss of exon 12 leaves the reading frame of CFTR transcripts intact, it appears highly unlikely that a translated product retains any function.

The mutation (4005G → C) changes the last nucleotide of exon 20 and causes an amino acid substitution (histidine for glutamine at codon 1291). The last three nucleotides of exons are reasonably well conserved and participate in splice site selection. Mutations of these nucleotides can affect splicing efficiency as reported for the human β-globin and mouse omithine transcarbamylase genes[71,72]. Therefore, the 4005G → C mutation was studied for its effect upon splicing[73]. RNA PCR analysis of rectal and nasal epithelial cells from the patient carrying the 4005G → C mutation revealed normal and aberrant splicing in the region from exons 20 to 21. The abnormal products were found to result from the use of a cryptic splice donor site in intron 20 located 30 nucleotides downstream from the normal donor site. Although the cryptic donor site did not contain the almost invariant GT dinucleotide of splice donors, it was hypothesized that the remainder of the splice site sequence matched the consensus sequence sufficiently often to compete with the mutated intron 20 splice donor site[74].

The four mutations described above that affect the almost invariant GT–AG nucleotides of splice sites are found in patients with severe forms of CF (Table 2). The likely explanation is that change of these nucleotides abolishes the normal pattern of splicing, leading to abnormal transcripts and absence of a protein product from those alleles. A similar situation has been observed in other genetic disorders, exemplified by β-thalassaemia, where a dozen different mutations that change GT or AG dinucleotides cause loss of gene product and a severe phenotype[75]. On the other hand, mutations of other positions in the β-globin gene splice sites were associated with reduced but not absent of β-globin, producing a mild phenotype[75]. Mutations causing aberrant splicing have been reported in patients with 'mild' CF by Highsmith, Knowles and colleagues[76,77]. One mutation (2789 + 5G → A) changes the conserved guanine in the donor splice site of intron 14b five nucleotides from the splice junction. One adult patient homozygous for this mutation had exon 14b deleted from all CFTR mRNA transcripts in nasal epithelia[77]. This patient and two affected adult members of the same consanguineous family had mild CF[78,79]. Loss of this exon would cause a frameshift and introduction of a premature termination codon to the transcript.

The mild phenotype might be explained if a functional truncated protein is translated from the aberrantly spliced allele. Alternatively, since the mutation occurs at a less critical position in the splice donor site, some level of normally spliced transcript may be present in epithelial tissue. This is the likely explanation for the second mutation, a C to T transition which activates a cryptic splice acceptor 10 kb from the normal splice junction in intron 19[76]. The result is an insertion of a novel 84-nucleotide exon that retains reading frame. A small fraction of transcripts from this allele were reported to retain the normal splicing pattern. Patients carrying one or two genes with this mutation have a variable but generally mild course of disease[80]. The presence of a very reduced quantity of the normally functioning protein or partial function of the protein containing residues encoded by the novel 84 nucleotide exon may explain the milder phenotype.

In summary, several patterns of alternative RNA splicing have been identified for the CFTR gene. The biological significance of these events is unclear and some may be the consequence of evolution or random DNA variation. At the present time, alternate patterns of splicing have not given rise to a functional CFTR isoform. Tissue specificity suggests a regulatory role for alternate splicing in CFTR expression. The analysis of a select group of splicing mutations has provided valuable insight into the significance of alternatively spliced exons. Additional insight is likely to be gained by further study of the tissue specificity and developmental regulation of the splicing variants and by identification and characterization of disease-associated mutations within the intron splice donor or acceptor sequences.

## ACKNOWLEDGEMENTS

The author wishes to thank Ada Hamosh, Haig H. Kazazian and Iain McIntosh for helpful discussions, Janice Staton for excellent secretarial support and the members of the CF Genetic Analysis Consortium for mutation data prior to publication. This work is supported by grants from the Cystic Fibrosis Foundation and the NIDDK.

## REFERENCES

1 Mount SM. A catalogue of splice junction sequences. *Nucleic Acids Res* 1982; **10**: 459–72.

2 Jackson IJ. A reappraisal of non-consensus mRNA splice sites. *Nucleic Acids Res* 1991; **19**: 3795–8.
3 Padgett RA, Grabowski PJ, Konarska MM. Splicing of messenger RNA precursors. *Annu Rev Biochem* 1986; **55**: 1119–50.
4 Krainer AR, Maniatis T. RNA splicing. In: *Transcription and Translation*. (eds BD Hames, DM Glover) IRL Press, Eynsham, Oxford, 1988, pp 131–206.
5 Early P, Rogers J, Davis M, et al. Two mRNAs can be produced from a single immunoglobulin μ gene by alternative RNA processing pathways. *Cell* 1980; **20**: 313–19.
6 Moore KW, Rogers J, Hunkapillar T, et al. Expression of IgD may use both DNA rearrangement and RNA splicing mechanisms. *Proc Natl Acad Sci USA* 1981; **78**: 1800–4.
7 de Ferra F, Engh H, Hudson L, et al. Alternative splicing accounts for the four forms of myelin basic protein. *Cell* 1985; **43**: 721–7.
8 Feeney CA, Koenig M, Kunkel LM. Alternative splicing of human dystrophin mRNA generates isoforms at the carboxy terminus. *Nature* 1989; **338**: 509–11.
9 Helfman DM, Cheley S, Kuismanen E, et al. Nonmuscle and muscle tropomyosin isoforms are expressed from a single gene by alternative RNA splicing and polyadenylation. *Mol Cell Biol* 1986; **6**: 3582–95.
10 Leff SE, Rosenfeld MG, Evans RM. Complex transcriptional units: diversity in gene expression by alternative RNA processing. *Annu Rev Biochem* 1986; **55**: 1091–117.
11 Breitbart RE, Andreadis A, Nadal Ginard B. Alternative splicing: a ubiquitous mechanism for the generation of multiple protein isoforms from single genes. *Annu Rev Biochem* 1987; **56**: 467–95.
12 Günthert U, Hofmann M, Rudy W, et al. A new variant of glycoprotein CD44 confers metastatic potential to rat carcinoma cells. *Cell*; 1991; **65**: 13–24.
13 Whiting P, McKernan RM, Iversen LL. Another mechanism for creating diversity in gamma-aminobutyric type A receptors: RNA splicing directs expression of two forms of gamma2 subunit, one of which contains a protein kinase C phosphorylation site. *Proc Natl Acad Sci USA* 1990; **87**: 9966–70.
14 Anderson MP, Rich DP, Gregory RJ, et al. Generation of cAMP-activated chloride currents by expression of CFTR. *Science* 1991; **251**: 679–82.
15 Bear CE, Li C, Kartner N, et al. Purification and functional reconstitution of the cystic fibrosis transmembrane conductance regulator (CFTR). *Cell* 1992; **68**: 809–18.
16 Egan M, Flotte T, Afione S, et al. Defective regulation of outwardly rectify Cl– channels by protein kinase A corrected by insertion of CFTR. *Nature* 1992; **358**: 581–4.
17 Gabriel SE, Clarke LL, Boucher RC, Stutts MJ. CFTR and outward rectifying chloride channels are distinct proteins with a regulatory relationship. *Nature* 1993; **363**: 263–6.
18 Hasegawa H, Skach W, Baker O, et al. A multifunctional aqueous channel formed by CFTR. *Science* 1992; **258**: 1477–9.
19 Quinton PM, Reddy MM. Control of CFTR chloride conductance by ATP levels through non-hydrolytic binding. *Nature* 1992; **360**: 79–81.
20 Riordan JR, Rommens JM, Kerem B, et al. Identification of the cystic fibrosis gene: cloning and characterization of complementary DNA. *Science* 1989; **245**: 1066–73.
21 Zielenski J, Rozmahel R, Bozon D, et al. Genomic DNA sequence of the cystic fibrosis transmembrane conductance regulator (CFTR) gene. *Genomics* 1991; **10**: 214–28.

22 Strong TV, Koh J, Tsui L-C, Collins FS. Analysis of CFTR transcription. *Pediat Pulmonol* 1991; (Suppl 5) 195.
23 Koh J, Sferra TJ, Collins FS. Characterization of the cystic fibrosis transmembrane conductance regulator promoter region. *J Biol Chem* 1993; **268**: 15912–21.
24 Nabeshima Y, Fujii-Kuriyama Y, Muramatsu M, Ogata K. Alternative transcription and two modes of splicing result in two myosin light chains from one gene. *Nature* 1984; **308**: 333–8.
25 Robert B, Daubas P, Akimenko M-A, et al. A single locus in the mouse encodes both myosin light chains 1 and 3, a second locus corresponds to a related pseudogene. *Cell* 1984; **39**: 129–40.
26 Kozak M. The scanning model for translation: an update. *J Cell Biol* 1989; **108**: 229–41.
27 Foo N-C, Carter D, Murphy D, Ivell R. Vasopressin and oxytocin gene expression in rat testis. *Endocrinology* 1991; **128**: 2118–28.
28 Nudel U, Zuk D, Einat P, et al. Duchenne muscular dystrophy gene product is not identical in muscle and brain. *Nature* 1989; **337**: 76–8.
29 Young RA, Hagenbüchle O, Schibler U. A single mouse $\alpha$-amylase gene specifies two different tissue-specific mRNAs. *Cell* 1981; **23**: 451–8.
30 Bremer S, Hoof T, Wilke M, et al. Quantitative expression patterns of multidrug-resistance P-glycoprotein (MDR1) and differentially spliced cystic-fibrosis transmembrane-conductance regulator mRNA transcripts in human epithelia. *Eur J Biochem* 1992; **206**: 137–49.
31 Delaney SJ, Rich DP, Thomson SA, et al. Cystic fibrosis transmembrane conductance regulator splice variants are not conserved and fail to produce chloride channels. *Nature Genet* 1993; **4**: 426–30.
32 Denning GM, Anderson MP, Amara JF, et al. Processing of mutant cystic fibrosis transmembrane conductance regulator is temperature-sensitive. *Nature* 1992; **358**: 761–4.
33 Zielenski J, Bozon D, Markiewicz D, et al. Analysis of CFTR transcripts in nasal epithelial cells and lymphoblasts of a cystic fibrosis patient with 621 + 1G → T and 711 + 1G → T mutations. *Hum Mol Genet* 1993; **2**: 683–7.
34 Hull J, Shackleton S, Harris A. Abnormal mRNA splicing resulting from three different mutations in the CFTR gene. *Hum Mol Genet* 1993; **2**: 689–692.
35 Horowitz B, Tsung SS, Hart P, et al. Alternative splicing of CFTR $Cl^-$ channels in the heart. *Am J Physiol* 1993; **264**: H2214–20.
36 Fonknechten N, Chomel J-C, Kitzis A, et al. Skipping of exon 5 as a consequence of the 711 + 1G → T mutation in the CFTR gene. *Hum Mol Genet* 1992; **1**: 281–2.
37 Chu C-S, Trapnell BC, Murtagh JJ, et al. Variable deletion of exon 9 coding sequences in cystic fibrosis transmembrane conductance regulator gene mRNA transcripts in normal bronchial epithelium. *EMBO J* 1991; **10**: 1355–63.
38 Walker JE, Saraste M, Runswick MJ, Gay NJ. Distantly related sequences in the alpha and beta subunits of ATP synthase, myosin, kinases and other ATP-requiring enzymes and a common nucleotide binding fold. *EMBO J* 1982; **1**: 945–51.
39 Chu C-S, Trapnell BC, Curristin SM, et al. Extensive post-translational deletion of the coding sequences for part of nucleotide-binding fold 1 in respiratory epithelial mRNA transcripts of the cystic fibrosis transmembrane conductance regulator gene is not associated with the clinical manifestations of cystic fibrosis. *J Clin Invest* 1992; **90**: 785–90.
40 Chu C-S, Trapnell BC, Curristin S, et al. Genetic basis of variable exon 9 skipping in cystic fibrosis transmembrane conductance regulator mRNA. *Nature Genet* 1993; **3**: 151–6.

41 Strong TV, Wilkinson DJ, Mansoura MK, et al. Expression of an abundantly alternatively spliced form of the cystic fibrosis transmembrane conductance regulator (CFTR) gene is not associated with a cAMP-activated chloride conductance. *Hum Mol Genet* 1993; **2**: 225–30.
42 Drumm ML, Wilkinson DJ, Smit LS, et al. Chloride conductance expressed by deltaF508 and other mutant CFTRs in *Xenopus* oocytes. *Science* 1991; **254**: 1797–9.
43 Montrose-Rafizadeh C, Blackmon DL, Hamosh A, et al. Regulation of cystic fibrosis transmembrane conductance regulator (CFTR) gene transcription and alternative RNA splicing in a model of developing intestinal epithelium. *J Biol Chem* 1992; **267**: 19299–305.
44 Sood R, Bear C, Auerbach W, et al. Regulation of CFTR expression and function during differentiation of intestinal epithelial cells. *EMBO J* 1992; **11**: 2487–94.
45 Montrose-Rafizadeh C, Guggino WB, Montrose MH. Cellular differentiation regulates expression of $Cl^-$ transport and cystic fibrosis transmembrane conductance regulator mRNA in human intestinal cells. *J Biol Chem* 1991; **266**: 4495–9.
46 Kiesewetter S, Macek M,Jr, Davis C, et al. A mutation in the cystic fibrosis transmembrane conductance regulator gene produces different phenotypes depending on chromosomal background. *Nature Genet* 1993; **5**: 274–8.
47 Kristidis P, Bozon D, Corey M, et al. Genetic determination of exocrine pancreatic function in cystic fibrosis. *Am J Hum Genet* 1992; **50**: 1178–84.
48 Hamosh A, Corey M, Cystic fibrosis genotype/phenotype consortium: correlation between genotype and phenotype in cystic fibrosis. *N Engl J Med* 1993; **329**: 1308–13.
49 McIntosh I, Carroll TP, Zeitlin PL, et al. Cystic fibrosis (CF) transmembrane conductance regulator bearing a mild CF mutation, R117H, is partially functional when expressed in *Xenopus* oocytes. *Am J Hum Genet* 1992; **51** (Suppl): A37.
50 Carroll TP, McIntosh I, Egan ME, et al. Transmembrane mutations alter the channels characterisitics of the cystic fibrosis transmembrane conductance regulator expressed in *Xenopus* oocytes. *Cell Physiol Biochem* 1994; **4**: 10–18.
51 Sheppard DN, Rich DP, Ostedgaard LS, et al. Mutations in CFTR associated with mild-disease-form $Cl^-$ channels with altered pore properties. *Nature* 1993; **362**: 160–4.
52 Slomski R, Schloesser M, Berg LP, et al. Omission of exon 12 in cystic fibrosis transmembrane conductance regulator (CFTR) gene transcripts. *Hum Genet* 1992; **89**: 615–19.
53 Strong TV, Smit LS, Nasr S, et al. Characterization of an intron 12 splice donor mutation in the cystic fibrosis transmembrane conductance regulator (CFTR) gene. *Hum Mutat* 1992; **1**: 380–7.
54 Will K, Stuhrmann M, Dean M, Schmidtke J. Alternative splicing in the first nucleotide binding fold of CFTR. *Hum Mol Genet* 1993; **2**: 231–5.
55 Melo CA, Serra C, Stoyanova V, et al. Alternative splicing of a previously unidentified CFTR exon introduces an in-frame stop codon 5′ of the R region. *FEBS Lett* 1993; **329**: 159–62.
56 Hamosh A, Trapnell BC, Zeitlin PL, et al. Severe deficiency of CFTR mRNA carrying nonsense mutations R553X and W1316X in respiratory epithelial cells of patients with cystic fibrosis. *J Clin Invest* 1991; **88**: 1880–5.
57 Dietz HC, Francomano CA, Kendzior RJ Jr, et al. The skipping of constitutive exons in vivo induced by nonsense mutations. *Science* 1993; **259**: 680–3.
58 Trezise AEO, Buchwald M, Higgins CF. Testis-specific, alternative splicing of rodent CFTR mRNA. *Hum Mol Genet* 1993: **2**: 801–2.

59 Petch LA, Harris J, Raymond VW, et al. A truncated, secreted form of the epidermal growth factor receptor is encoded by an alternatively spliced transcript in normal rat tissue. *Mol Cell Biol* 1990; **10**: 2973–82.
60 Bond RW, Wyborski RJ, Gottlieb DI. Developmentally regulated expression of an exon containing a stop codon in the gene for glutamic acid decarboxylase. *Proc Natl Acad Sci USA* 1990; **87**: 8771–5.
61 Waeber G, Habener JF. Nuclear translocation and DNA recognition signals co-localized within the bZIP domain of cyclic adenosine 3′,5′-monophosphate response element-binding protein CREB. *Mol Endocrinol* 1991; **5**: 1431–8.
62 Bell LR, Maine EM, Schedl P, Cline TW. Sex-lethal, a drosophila sex determination switch gene, exhibits sex-specific RNA splicing and sequence similarity to RNA binding proteins. *Cell* 1998; **55**: 1037–46.
63 Gower HJ, Barton CH, Elsom VL, et al. Alternative splicing generates a secreted form of N-CAM in muscle and brain. *Cell* 1988; **955**: 964.
64 Yoshimura K, Chu CS, Crystal RG. Alternative splicing of intron 23 of the human cystic fibrosis transmembrane conductance regulator gene resulting in a novel exon and transcript coding for a shortened intracytoplasmic C terminus. *J Biol Chem* 1993; **268**: 686–90.
65 Kress M, Glaros D, Khoury G, Jay G. Alternative RNA splicing in expression of the H-2K gene. *Nature* 1983; **306**: 602–4.
66 Zielenski J, Bozon D, Kerem B-S, et al. Identification of mutations in exons 1 through 8 of the cystic fibrosis transmembrane conductance regulator (CFTR) gene. *Genomics* 1991; **10**: 229–35.
67 Roberts RG, Bentley DR, Bobrow M. Infidelity in the structure of ectopic transcripts: a novel exon in lymphocyte dystrophin transcripts. *Hum Mutat* 1993; **2**: 293–9.
68 Tsui L-C. The spectrum of cystic fibrosis mutations. *Trends Genet* 1992; **8**: 392–8.
69 Tsui L-C. Mutations and sequence variations detected in the cystic fibrosis transmembrane conductance regulator (CFTR) gene: a report from the Cystic Fibrosis Genetic Analysis Consortium. *Hum Mutat* 1992; **1**: 197–203.
70 Rozen R, De Braekeleer M, Daigneault J, et al. Cystic fibrosis mutations in French Canadians: three CFTR mutations are relatively frequent in a Quebec population with an elevated incidence of cystic fibrosis. *Am J Med Genet* 1992; **42**: 360–4.
71 Vidaud M, Gattoni R, Stevenin J. et al. A 5′ splice-region G → C mutation in exon 1 of the human beta-globin gene inhibits pre-mRNA splicing: a mechanism for beta + -thalassemia. *Proc Natl Acad Sci USA* 1989; **86**: 1041–5.
72 Hodges PE, Rosenberg LE. The $spf^{ash}$ mouse: a missense mutation in the ornithine transcarbamylase gene also causes aberrant mRNA splicing. *Proc Natl Acad USA* 1989; **86**: 4142–6
73 Chow J-L, Rozmahel R, Tsui L-C. Characterization of the promoter region of the cystic fibrosis transmembrane conductance regulator gene. *J Biol Chem* 1991; **266**: 24471–6.
74 Jones CT, McIntosh I, Keston M, et al. Three novel mutations in the cystic fibrosis gene detected by chemical cleavage: analysis of variant splicing and a nonsense mutation. *Hum Mol Genet* 1992; **1**: 11–17
75 Kazazian HH Jr. The thalassemia syndromes: molecular basis and prenatal diagnosis in 1990. *Semin Hematol* 1990; **27**: 209–28.
76 Highsmith WE Jr, Burch LH, Boat TF, et al. Identification of a homozygous point mutation in intron 19 in an inbred CF patient with mild disease and normal sweat chloride: creation of an alternative splice site resulting in base-sequence insertion in CFTR coding region between exons 19 and 20. *Pediatr Pulmonol* 1991 (Suppl 6) 22A.

77 Highsmith WE Jr, Strong T, Burch N, et al. Identification of a splicing error of exon 14b giving rise to a frameshift mutation in a consanguineous family with mild cystic fibrosis. *Pediatr Pulmonol* 1990 (Suppl 5): 11A.
78 McConkie-Rosell A, Chen Y-T, Harris D, et al. Mild cystic fibrosis linked to chromosome 7q22 markers with an uncommon haplotype. *Ann Intern Med* 1989; **111**: 797–801.
79 Knowles MR, Barnett TB, McConkie-Rosell A, et al. Mild cystic fibrosis in a consanguineous family. *Ann Intern Med* 1989; **110**: 599–605.
80 Augarten A, Kerem B-S, Yahav Y, et al. Mild cystic fibrosis and normal or borderline sweat test in patients with the 3849 + 10 kb C → T mutation. *Lancet* 1993; **342**: 25–6.
81 Bonizzato A, Nicolis E, Gasparini P. Identification of a new splicing mutation (406-1 G-C) in the CFTR gene. *Hum Mutat* 1992; **1**: 432–3.
82 Nunes V, Chillon M, Dörk T, et al. A new missense mutation (E92K) in the first transmembrane domain of the CFTR gene causes a benign cystic fibrosis phenotype. *Hum Mol Genet* 1993; **2**: 79–80.
83 Claustres M, Maguelone L, Desgeorges M, et al. Analysis of the 27 exons and flanking regions of the cystic fibrosis gene: 40 different mutations account for 91.2% of the mutant alleles in Southern France. *Hum Mol Genet* 1993; **2**: 1209–13.
84 Dörk T, Fislage R, Rappen U, Tümmler B. Severe splice site mutation preceding exon 9 of the CFTR gene. *Hum Mol Genet* 1993; **2**: 1313–14.
85 Dörk T, Wulbrand B, Tümmler B. Four novel cystic fibrosis mutations in splice junction sequences affecting the CFTR nucleotide binding folds. *Genomics* 1993; **15**: 688–91.
86 Audrezet MP, Mercier B, Guillermit H, et al. Identification of 12 novel mutations in the CFTR gene. *Hum Mol Genet* 1993; **2** 51–4.
87 Beaudet AL, Tsui L-C. A suggested nomenclature for designating mutations. *Hum Mutat* 1993; **2**: 245–8.

Chapter Four

# Hypotheses of Postnatal and Prenatal Selection in Cystic Fibrosis

Giovanni Romeo, Olga Zegarra-Moran and
Luis Juan Vicente Galietta
*Servizio di Genetica Molecolare e Laboratorio di Citogenetica, Istituto Giannina Gaslini, Genoa, Italy*

## INTRODUCTION

The high frequency of the cystic fibrosis (CF) gene in Caucasian populations has always puzzled geneticists. The usual hypotheses put forward to explain such frequency vary from heterozygote advantage to random genetic drift[1]. Strong evidence against the drift hypothesis represented by the southeast to northwest gradient of ΔF508, the main CF mutation in Europe, was collected soon after the cloning of the gene[2]. This gradient is not compatible with random independent events which, according to the drift hypothesis, should have occurred in small populations. In addition the analysis of intragenic haplotypes associated with ΔF508 in different European populations indicates a unifocal origin of this mutation[3]. The most obvious explanation in selective terms for the frequency of CF is the hypothesis of heterozygote advantage. However, in view of recent data which cannot be reconciled with postnatal selection of CF carriers, we shall also discuss additional hypotheses dealing with prenatal selection.

*Cystic Fibrosis—Current Topics, Volume 2.* Edited by J. A. Dodge, D. J. H. Brock and J. H. Widdicombe

The CF gene was cloned in 1989 through a positional cloning approach[4–6]. The product of the gene, named CFTR (cystic fibrosis transmembrane conductance regulator), is a plasma membrane $Cl^-$ channel activated by cAMP-dependent phosphorylation and direct binding of ATP to nucleotide-binding domains[7,8]. CFTR was localized in the apical membrane of many epithelial cells, among which are intestinal crypt cells[9]. This localization is consistent with previous models for $Cl^-$ secretion which postulated that $Cl^-$ exits at the apical membrane following the favourable electrochemical gradient created by the combined action of $Na^+/K^+$-ATPase, the $Na^+/K^+/Cl^-$ cotransporter and $K^+$ channels in the basolateral membrane (Figure 1).

The impairment of CFTR function in CF is responsible for the abnormalities in fluid secretion which cause airways obstruction and chronic respiratory infections. In the pancreas, the reduced ability to secrete ions and water affects the flushing of mucous secretions produced by the acinar portion. This results in pancreatic duct obstruction and thus pancreatic insufficiency in 85% of patients.

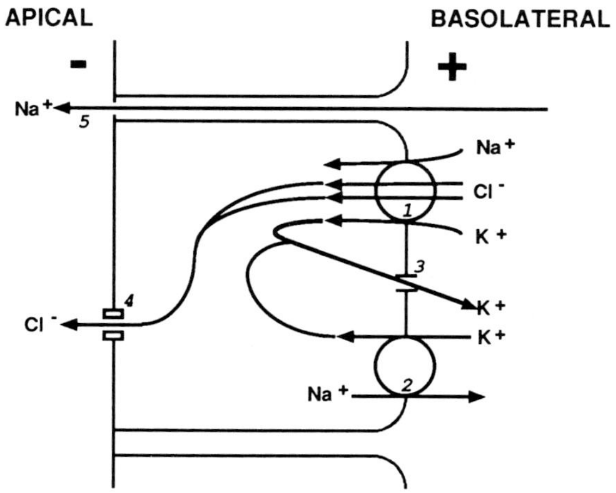


**Figure 1** Model for intestinal $Cl^-$ secretion. The $Cl^-$ entry at the basolateral membrane is coupled with that of $K^+$ and $Na^+$ by a cotransporter (*1*). $Na^+$ ions are then pumped outside through the $Na^+/K^+$ ATPase (*2*), whereas $K^+$ ions which have entered the cell by the combined action of the cotransporter and the pump can exit through specific ion channels (*3*) placed in the basolateral membrane. The accumulation of $Cl^-$ inside the cell by the cotransporter and the negative membrane potential produced by the $K^+$ exit favours the subsequent $Cl^-$ efflux (*4*) at the apical membrane. This results in a transepithelial potential difference, negative at the apical side, that drives $Na^+$ through the paracellular pathway (*5*) which is actually permeable to cations. The net NaCl secretion is osmotically followed by water. According to this model, the $Cl^-$ secretion process is possible only if $Cl^-$ channels are active in the apical membrane

The most frequent CF mutation, ΔF508 consists of deletion of a phenylalanine codon in the first nucleotide-binding domain[6]. This mutation is classified as 'severe' since it is associated with pancreatic insufficiency. In contrast with other mutations which give a mild phenotype[10], ΔF508 does not seem to affect the channel activity of CFTR[11], but rather is responsible for the arrest of correct protein processing[10]. Indeed, no channel activity is observed when the mutated CFTR is expressed in human or rodent cells[12,13]. Nevertheless, CFTR with the ΔF508 mutation is able to produce $Cl^-$ currents when expressed in non-mammalian cells which are cultured at low temperatures[11,14]. This discrepancy was recently explained as ΔF508 being a temperature-sensitive mutation. At 37 °C the correct processing and maturation of the synthesized protein[15] is blocked, whereas at lower temperatures the mutated CFTR can reach the cell membrane. Accordingly, the absence of CFTR in the apical membrane of epithelial cells was demonstrated in patients homozygous for ΔF508[16,17].

The frequencies of ΔF508 in European populations range from 30% to 88%[2]. The other mutations (at present more than 300) are much less frequent[18]. As already anticipated, the analysis of intragenic haplotypes associated with ΔF508 suggests that a single mutational event occurred in the past[3]. To explain the spreading of the mutation in the original European populations, the hypothesis of heterozygote advantage has been postulated. This advantage might consist of a higher resistance (and therefore survival) of CF carriers to intestinal infectious diseases causing profuse diarrhoeas. In the following pages this hypothesis will be reviewed in light of the present knowledge on the stimulation of intestinal secretion by physiological and pathological agents.

## $Cl^-$ CHANNELS IN THE INTESTINE OF CYSTIC FIBROSIS PATIENTS

Several *in vivo* and *in vitro* studies demonstrate that the intestine of CF patients is unresponsive to agents that stimulate ion secretion in normal individuals (Table 1). In particular, cAMP-elevating agonists such as theophylline, forskolin and prostaglandin $E_2$ fail to stimulate $Cl^-$ secretion in the small intestine, the colon and rectum of CF patients[19–23] in accordance with CFTR being a cAMP-activated channel. Nevertheless, in contrast to airway epithelia, the CF intestine is also unresponsive to agents that elevate cytosolic $Ca^{2+}$-like cholinergic agonists and $Ca^{2+}$ ionophores[19–25]. This is a notable difference since patch-clamp studies have demonstrated that $Ca^{2+}$-activated $Cl^-$ channels are normal in CF cells[26]. This puzzling behaviour may be explained by the observation made by Anderson and Welsh[27] that polarized intestinal T84 cells lack $Ca^{2+}$-dependent $Cl^-$ channels in the apical membrane (Figure 2). If this

**Table 1** Agents that fail to stimulate chloride secretion in the intestine of CF patients

| Stimulating agent | Second messenger |
|---|---|
| Theophylline | cAMP |
| Prostaglandin $E_2$ | cAMP |
| Forskolin | cAMP |
| A23187 | $Ca^{2+}$ |
| Betanechol | $Ca^{2+}$ |
| Carbachol | $Ca^{2+}$ |
| Histamine | $Ca^{2+}$ |
| Acetylcholine | $Ca^{2+}$ |
| Cholera toxin | cAMP |
| *E. coli* heat-stable toxin | cGMP |

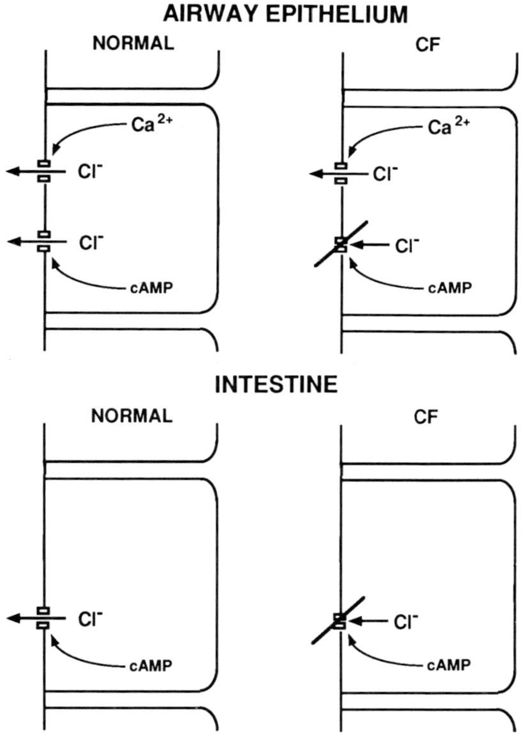


**Figure 2** $Cl^-$ secretion in airway and intestinal epithelial cells. Airway cells possess cAMP- and $Ca^{2+}$-activated $Cl^-$ channels in the apical membrane. Consequently, these two second messengers are able to separately induce $Cl^-$ secretion in airway epithelial cells of normal individuals. In contrast, CF airway cells display only the $Ca^{2+}$-activated pathway. According to recent findings obtained on T84 cultured cells, intestinal epithelia would express only cAMP-activated $Cl^-$ channels in the apical membrane. The defect of such channels in CF cells accounts for the impaired $Cl^-$ secretion in the CF intestine

is also true in the intestinal epithelium *in vivo*, it would explain why CF intestine does not respond to cytosolic $Ca^{2+}$ increases. However, it still remains to be explained how the normal intestine can display $Ca^{2+}$-mediated $Cl^-$ secretion if the $Ca^{2+}$-activated $Cl^-$ channels are absent. A plausible explanation postulated by Anderson and Welsh[27] assumes that the cytosolic $Ca^{2+}$ increase stimulates basolateral $Ca^{2+}$-dependent $K^+$ channels. The resulting hyperpolarization would provide the driving force for $Cl^-$ exit through apical channels. This model requires some apical CFTR channels to be open in resting conditions (Figure 2) since a direct activation of CFTR by cytosolic $Ca^{2+}$ has not been demonstrated so far. CF cells would lack these functioning channels and thus would not respond to $Ca^{2+}$-elevating agents.

In addition to pharmacological agents, bacterial toxins have also been tested. Choleragen does not stimulate $Cl^-$ secretion in the CF intestine[28] (Table 1), as expected by the fact that the toxin action is mediated by the cAMP pathway. *Escherichia coli* heat-stable enterotoxin ($ST_A$) also fails to produce a response[28,29]. Since this toxin is known to increase cGMP, it appears that the CF intestine is also insensitive to this second messenger. Actually recent experiments demonstrate that CFTR can be phosphorylated *in vitro* by the cGMP-dependent protein kinase[30], and a $Cl^-$ channel similar to CFTR has been activated in T84 cells by this nucleotide[31].

Besides choleragen and *E. coli* $ST_A$, other bacterial toxins listed in Table 2 are able to affect the intestinal $Cl^-$ secretion[32–36]. All these toxins act by

**Table 2** Modes of action of different infectious agents causing diarrhoea

| Diarrhoea-causing agent | Toxin | Pathway | Mechanism |
|---|---|---|---|
| *Vibrio cholerae* | Choleragen (CT) | cAMP | Chloride secretion increased |
| Enterotoxigenic *E. coli* | Heat-stable toxin (STA)<br>Heat-labile toxin | cGMP<br>cAMP | |
| *Yersinia enterocolitica*<br>*Klebsiella pneumoniae*<br>*Enterobacter* | STA-like enterotoxin | cGMP | |
| *Salmonella* (some)<br>*Campylobacter*<br>*Pseudomonas aeruginosa* | CT-like enterotoxin | cAMP | |
| *Clostridium difficile* | Toxin A | $Ca^{2+}$, cGMP | |
| *Shigella* | Shiga toxin<br>(also invasive) | – | Sodium absorption impaired |
| *Salmonella* (other strains) | No toxin (invasive) | – | |
| Rotavirus | No toxin (invasive) | – | |

increasing cAMP, cGMP or $Ca^{2+}$. Although only the first two have been tested on CF intestine[28,29], it is presumed that the other toxins also fail to stimulate $Cl^-$ secretion since CFTR in intestinal cells seems to be the $Cl^-$ channel where many stimulatory signals (cAMP, $Ca^{2+}$, cGMP) converge to induce $Cl^-$ secretion. In contrast, other infectious agents like shigella, some strains of salmonella and rotaviruses cause diarrhoea by impairing $Na^+$ absorption without affecting $Cl^-$ secretion[33,35,36] (Table 2).

## HETEROZYGOTE ADVANTAGE AND ACUTE GASTROENTERITIS

The hypothesis, of a selective advantage of CF carriers against acute gastroenteritis must be in agreement with at least one of the following assumptions:

(1) Acute gastroenteritis was endemic and, to a significant degree, lethal in European populations, thus representing a constant selective pressure.
(2) Acute gastroenteritis was epidemic (or pandemic) in Europe and mortality was extremely high, in such a way that although the events were of relatively short duration, the pressure was sufficient for the selection of CF carriers in the same populations.

In this context one could accept the hypothesis that cholera epidemics were the main selective factor in favour of the CF gene[37] and in particular of ΔF508, which is the most frequent mutation in Europe[2]. However, the first pandemic of cholera in Europe is recorded in the nineteenth century as documented by the *Annals of Epidemics in Italy*, which mentions 'asiatic cholera' for the first time in 1835[38]. According to different estimates, the age of ΔF508 is between 3000 and 6000 years[39] or between 65 000 and 215 000[3]. It is very unlikely, therefore, that cholera represented a selective factor for CF in Europe.

Acute gastroenteritis is among the major causes of childhood morbidity and mortality throughout the world. In developing countries there are between 3 and 5 billion cases of acute infectious diarrhoea per year, from which 5–10 millions die[36]. It is estimated that in Third World countries up to 15% of children die of acute diarrhoeal disease before the age of three. Although in industrialized nations most cases of diarrhoea are due to viral agents (rotaviruses and others), in developing countries the incidence of bacterial intestinal infections is much higher, accounting for near 50% of the total cases. Most of these bacterial infections produce secretory diarrhoeas, which are characterized by large losses of water and electrolytes from the gastrointestinal tract. The secretory stimuli for active $Cl^-$ secretion from intestinal crypts are cAMP, cGMP and $Ca^{2+}$ stimulated by bacterial enterotoxins

(Table 2). Diarrhoea in small children is particularly likely to lead to serious fluid and electrolyte imbalance. The water losses could be massive, thus leading rapidly to dehydration and acid–base imbalances, which, if not adequately treated, may lead to serious central nervous system complications and death. Socioeconomic factors play a major role in the frequency of bacterial gastrointestinal infections. Lack of clean water, crowding, lack of minimal hygienic conditions, major nutritional deficiencies and poor sanitation are the most relevant risk factors for these diarrhoeal diseases.

All these conditions, still present in some regions of Third World countries, were common in Europe up to the last century. It is not unreasonable to assume that the incidence of diarrhoea in Europe 100 years ago was similar to that of developing countries of the present time or even higher.

The hypothesis of a selective advantage against infectious disease causing profuse diarrhoea, first proposed by Quinton[40], requires that CF heterozygotes have an intestinal secretory response to bacterial toxins equal to 50% of that present in normal individuals[41]. Actually, a significantly reduced secretion induced by cholinergic agents has been revealed not only in the intestine of CF patients[24] but also in carriers[42]. Although the latter study does not include stimulation with bacterial toxins, it is reasonable to expect that CF heterozygotes show a phenotype intermediate between normal individuals and CF patients. Analogous observations were made on sweat glands, where a decreased secretory response has been found in heterozygotes with respect to normal individuals after $\beta$-adrenergic stimulation[43,44].

In conclusion, a decreased $Cl^-$ secretion in response to some bacterial toxins is highly likely in CF carriers with respect to normal controls, suggesting that the former individuals might have had a significant advantage in surviving acute gastroenteritis. Genetic evidence in support of this hypothesis might only come from the observation of distorted segregation ratios in favour of CF carriers in sibships which have been exposed to acute bacterial gastroenteritis during early childhood. A study of the segregation of CF mutations in such sibships (e.g. uncles and aunts of CF patients) might yield information on this particular question, but the amount of data to be collected would be enormous. If we assume a selective advantage of 2% in favour of carriers, we estimate that, in order to detect a significant segregation distortion among uncles and aunts of CF patients, a sample of more than 10 000 of these relatives would be needed. In addition, since an advantage of 2% could be blurred by non-paternity, only the offspring of female CF carriers should be taken into account. The effort to collect the appropriate genetic information to test the hypothesis of heterozygote advantage therefore seems overwhelming. However, other hypotheses which will be described in the following pages justify the collection, even on a smaller scale, of segregation data in CF nuclear families and extended pedigrees.

## EVIDENCE SUGGESTING PRENATAL SELECTION

Prenatal selection can occur either at the prezygotic or postzygotic level. The former type of selection, named meiotic drive, is documented when an allele is recovered in more than 50% of the gametes from heterozygous individuals. In genetics there are several well-documented examples of meiotic drive[45], which has been invoked to account for the results obtained in a preliminary study of gametes segregated by a CF carrier[46]. When sperm from a single carrier of the F508 mutation were individually genotyped, a small but statistically significant difference was detected between the proportion carrying the ΔF508 mutation (44%) and that carrying the normal allele (56%). If confirmed, these data might have considerable bearing on the topics dealt with in this review.

A puzzling piece of evidence yet to be confirmed, pointing towards prenatal selection associated with CF genotypes, was published before the cloning of the CF gene[47]. In a sample of 1003 sibs of patients, typed as carriers or homozygous normals by haplotype reconstruction of closely linked restriction fragment length polymorphisms (RFLP), a significant distortion in the expected sex ratio was observed in both groups. An excess of girls was noticed among normal homozygotes together with a reciprocal excess of carrier boys inheriting the CF gene from either their father or their mother. These data would point to an underlying mechanism giving a selective advantage to the association between the CF gene and the Y chromosome, either before fertilization, or at the time of fertilization, or after fertilization. Data from a larger sample of CF families, different from those used by Kitzis et al.[47], typed on the basis of mutations (not of haplotypes) are now being collected at the European level to confirm this finding. According to a different hypothesis, the dissemination of CF mutations might have taken place through the higher size and the decreased sex ratio supposedly observed in sibships of carrier mothers with respect to those of carrier fathers[48]. That the high frequency of CF is simply due to a fertility advantage in CF carriers is not supported by comparative data on the progeny of grandparents of patients and matched controls[49].

A more recent indication of the possible role of prenatal selection comes from the difference observed in the frequencies of the W1281X and ΔF508 mutations between Ashkenazi patients and carriers[50]. A sample of 295 patients from Israel and the USA showed that the frequency of the major mutation among Ashkenazi Jews (W1282X) is almost twice (51%) the frequency of the ΔF508 mutation (27%). In contrast, among 1946 Ashkenazi Jews screened for carrier status, an essentially equal number of ΔF508 and W1282X chromosomes was found. The difference in the proportions was statistically significant ($p = 0.025$). A possible postzygotic mechanism that might explain the observed difference is prenatal selection against homozygotes for a disadvantageous recessive allele preferentially associated with ΔF508 in the Jewish Ashkenazi population.

On the contrary, the hypothesis of genes closely linked to CF, which might have a selective advantage through a hitch-hiking effect, was proposed in the attempt to explain the high frequency of CF[51]. Along the same lines, the presence in the surroundings of the CF gene of an imprinted region which might be critical for growth has been postulated to account for short stature in two CF children who showed uniparental isodisomy of maternal origin[52,53]. Further support for the presence of gene(s) acting on development and closely linked to CF comes from data collected in German patients which indicate an association between CF marker haplotypes and the patient's height, weight and percentage of weight for height[54].

Association between haplotype B, as defined by extragenic polymorphisms (XV2C, KM19) and the severity of the disease in non-ΔF508 chromosomes, was originally noticed in the EWGCFG report[2]. A similar effect of the B haplotype was hypothesized to account for its noteworthy increase among non-ΔF508 chromosomes from patients with meconium ileus (MI) with respect to non-MI patients[2]. According to a previous report[55], published before the identification of the ΔF508 mutation, the association of MI in all CF chromosomes was particularly strong with allele 1 of the RFLP revealed by probe J3.11 , while allele 2 appeared strongly associated with CF without MI. In the same paper[55] an unexplained segregation distortion was reported from the prospective study of 282 CF couples. While the recurrence of CF among children of those couples who had given birth to a previous CF child without MI was 25% (as expected in a prospective study for an autosomal recessive disorder), the recurrence observed for the couples with a previous CF child with MI was 45%. To the best of our knowledge there is no record of any further data confirming or disproving this finding.

## CONCLUSIONS

The evidence presented in this review indicates the existence of selective factors which might have favoured in the past the spreading of some CF mutations. This conclusion is supported, among others, by the study of RFLPs closely linked to the CF gene. A recent report points out that, while the majority of the CF mutations (called private, demic or local) are randomly associated with RFLP markers, those observed in most populations (called general mutation) are more likely to be associated with a specific RFLP marker[56]. The unifocal origin of each of these mutations might be a sufficient explanation for the linkage disequilibrium observed in the latter and in other studies[2,3]. However, when different mutations of independent origin are associated with the same haplotype, as reported by Sereth et al.[56], there arises again the question of a

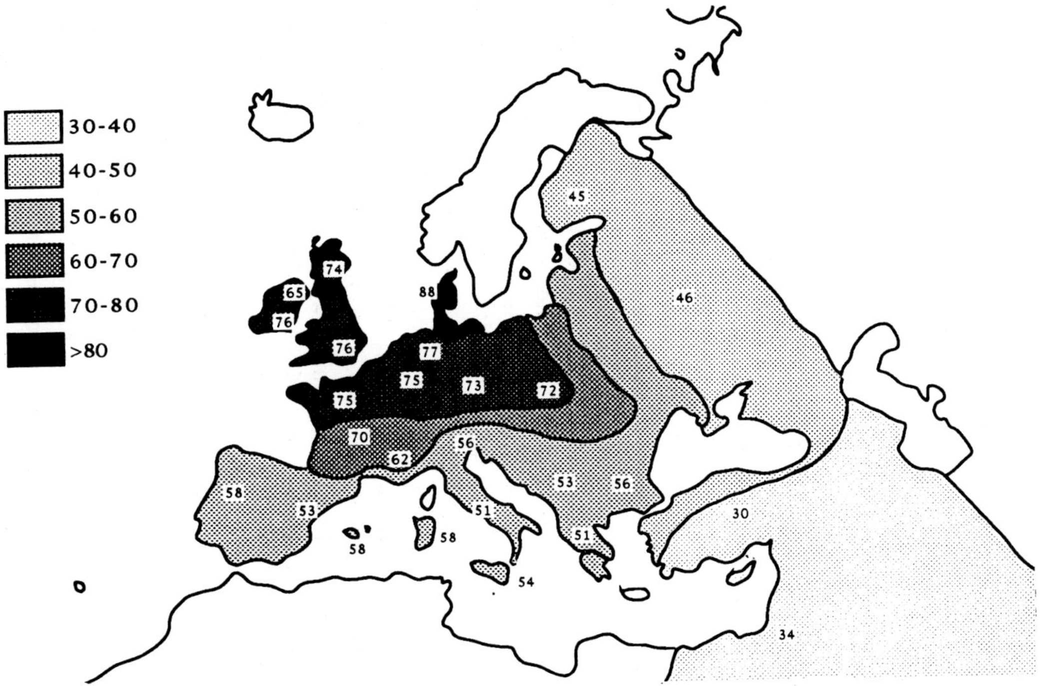


**Figure 3** Southeast to northwest gradient of the ΔF508 mutation in Europe. The numbers indicate the relative frequency of ΔF508 among mutations causing CF. This map, kindly provided by Prof. A. Piazza (Turin), was constructed using data of the EWGCFG (European Working Group on CF Genetics)

selectively advantageous and closely-linked gene (or genes) present on that haplotype which might hitch-hike with different mutations. Unfortunately this hypothesis has not been tested sufficiently because the typing for extragenic polymorphic markers has been replaced more and more in the last years by direct identification of mutations.

The southeast–northwest gradient of ΔF508 in Europe[2] (Figure 3) was interpreted as an effect of the neolithic demic expansion associated with the spreading of agriculture. However, it is impossible to reconcile the upward gradient (30–88%) with migration from the southeast towards the northwest. The current interpretation is therefore that ΔF508 was present in Europe before the neolithic period, and that its frequency was diluted by the introduction of other mutations, brought in by the neolithic farmers. This hypothesis implies that the latter mutations, more recent than ΔF508, confer a similar selective advantage and that they had more time to expand in the southeast rather than in the northwest of Europe, where they arrived more recently.

The preneolithic origin of ΔF508 is in agreement with its relatively high frequency among Basques[57], in contrast with the frequency observed in the surrounding populations, and with the dating attempted through the use of intragenic microsatellites[3]. While the arguments in favour of the presence of ΔF508 in the preneolithic European populations are quite strong, its approximate dating is dependent on the stability of the mutation rate of the intragenic microsatellites used in the calculations which led to the estimated age of 65 000–215 000 years[3]. If so, ΔF508 might have the same age as *Homo sapiens*, or might even predate its appearance. It would therefore be interesting to investigate in primates the haplotypes used in man for the dating of ΔF508[3].

Two main hypotheses have been invoked to account for the observations made, and they can be identified under the general terms of postnatal and prenatal selection. These are not mutually exclusive hypotheses and actually the high frequency of CF might be the result of an interplay between developmental (or prenatal) causes and postnatal advantage of heterozygotes. In other words, it might well be that the answer to the high frequency of CF is not simple and unequivocal but, more interestingly, contains several different and even contrasting reasons. This line of thought tends to give a biological significance to most of the data and discrepancies summarized in the previous pages, especially to the haplotype data obtained with extragenic RFLPs. We should be aware, however, that simple explanations (like bias of ascertainment) might account for some of the discrepancies reported in segregation and population studies. This, as an example, seems to be the explanation for a recent report in which the frequency of the R117H mutation among carriers was found to be higher than expected on the basis of its relative frequency among CF patients[58]. This latter discrepancy is probably due to the milder expression of CF in patients who are compound heterozygotes carrying this mutation[59], and who might go in part undiagnosed or show a different disease, namely congenital bilateral absence of the vas deferens. Even this interpretation is only apparently in contrast with that previously mentioned regarding the possible prenatal selection against ΔF508 homozygotes (see above under 'Evidence suggesting prenatal selection'). The common hypothesis underlying these interpretations is the existence of genes closely linked and interacting with CFTR that cause the phenotypic variability which in turn might lead to the apparent distortion of segregation ratios in families and/or of the Hardy–Weinberg equilibrium in populations. The search for such modifier genes needs, however, a rationale that should be stronger than the one presently available, based on the study of extragenic RFLPs.

It is surprising that, in spite of the number of tools which molecular genetics has made available during the past years for research on CF, so many questions regarding the formal genetic analysis of this disorder (namely segregation distortion, meiotic drive, etc.) have been left unanswered. Future work along the different lines of research reviewed in this chapter may contribute to some of the questions raised and, at the same time, will help in setting up the methodology by which the spreading of mutations should be approached, not only for CF but also for other relatively common disorders, like phenylketonuria, whose genes might have been subjected to selection.

## REFERENCES

1 Romeo G, Devoto M, Galietta LJV. Why is the cystic fibrosis gene so frequent? *Hum Genet* 1989; **84**: 1–5.
2 EWGCFG (European Working Group on CF Genetics). Gradient of distribution in Europe of the major CF mutation and of its associated haplotype. *Hum Genet* 1990; **85**: 436–41.
3 Morral N, Bertranpetit J, Estivill X, et al. Tracing the origin of the major cystic fibrosis mutation (F508) in European populations. *Nature Genet* 1994; **7**: 169–75.
4 Rommens JM, Iannuzzi MC, Kerem B, et al. Identification of the cystic fibrosis gene: chromosome walking and jumping. *Science* 1989; **245**: 1059–65.
5 Riordan JR, Rommens JM, Kerem B, et al. Identification of the cystic fibrosis gene: clonic and characterization of complementary DNA. *Science* 1989; **245**: 1066–73.
6 Kerem B, Rommens JM, Buchanan JA, et al. Identification of the cystic fibrosis gene: genetic analysis. *Science* 1989; **245**: 1073–80.
7 Drumm ML, Pope HA, Cliff WH, et al. Correction of the cystic fibrosis defect *in vitro* by retrovirus mediated gene transfer. *Cell* 1990; **62**: 1227–33.
8 Anderson MP, Berger HA, Rich DP, et al. Nucleoside triphosphates are required to open the CFTR chloride channel. *Cell* 1991; **67**: 775–84.
9 Trezise AEO, Buchwald M. *In vivo* cell-specific expression of the cystic fibrosis transmembrane conductance regulator. *Nature* 1991; **353**: 436–7.
10 Sheppard DN, Rich DP, Ostedgaard LS, et al. Mutations in CFTR associated with mild-disease-form $Cl^-$ channels with altered pore properties. *Nature* 1993; **362**: 160–4.

11 Li C, Ramjeesingh M, Reyes E, et al. The cystic fibrosis mutation (ΔF508) does not influence the chloride channel activity of CFTR. *Nature Genet* 1993; **3**: 311–16.
12 Rich DP, Anderson MP, Gregory RJ, et al. Expression of cystic fibrosis transmembrane conductance regulator corrects defective chloride channel regulation in cystic fibrosis airway epithelial cells. *Nature* 1990; **347**: 358–63.
13 Anderson MP, Rich DP, Gregory RJ, et al. Generation of cAMP-activated chloride currents by expression of CFTR. *Science* 1991; **251**: 679–82.
14 Drumm ML, Wilkinson DJ, Smit LS, et al. Chloride conductance expressed by ΔF508 and other mutant CFTRs in *Xenopus* oocytes. *Science* 1991; **254**: 1797–9.
15 Denning GM, Anderson MP, Amara JF, et al. Processing of mutant cystic fibrosis transmembrane conductance regulator is temperature-sensitive. *Nature* 1992; **358**: 761–4.
16 Engelhardt JF, Yankaskas JR, Ernst SA, et al. Submucosal glands are the predominant site of CFTR expression in the human bronchus. *Nature Genet* 1992; **2**: 240–7.
17 Denning GM, Ostedgaard LS, Welsh MJ. Abnormal localization of cystic fibrosis transmembrane conductance regulator in primary cultures of cystic fibrosis airway epithelia. *J Cell Biol* 1992; **118**: 551–9.
18 Tsui L-C, Markiewicz D, Zielenski J, et al. Mutation analysis in cystic fibrosis. In: *Cystic Fibrosis: Current Topics*, vol 1 (eds JA Dodge, DJH Brock, JH Widdicombe) Wiley, Chichester, 1993, pp 27–44.
19 Taylor CJ, Baxter PS, Hardcastle J, Hardcastle PT. Absence of secretory response in jejunal biopsy samples from children with cystic fibrosis. *Lancet* 1987; **ii**: 107–8.
20 Baxter PS, Wilson AJ, Read NW, et al. Abnormal jejunal potential difference in cystic fibrosis. *Lancet* 1989; **i**: 464–6.
21 Berschneider HM, Knowles MR, Azizkhan RG, et al. Altered chloride transport in cystic fibrosis. *FASEB J* 1988; **2**: 2625–9.
22 Goldstein JL, Shapiro AB, Rao MC, Layden TJ. *In vivo* evidence of altered chloride but not potassium secretion in cystic fibrosis rectal mucosa. *Gastroenterology* 1991; **101**: 1012–19.
23 Veeze HJ, Sinaasappel M, Bijman J, et al. Ion transport abnormalities in rectal suction biopsies from children with cystic fibrosis. *Gastroenterology* 1991; **101**: 398–403.
24 Taylor CJ, Hughes H, Hardcastle PT, Hardcastle J. Genotype and secretory response in cystic fibrosis. *Lancet* 1992; **339**: 67–8.
25 Hardcastle J, Hardcastle PT, Taylor CJ, Goldhill J. Failure of cholinergic stimulation to induce a secretory response from the rectal mucosa in cystic fibrosis. *Gut* 1991; **32**: 1035–9.
26 Wagner JA, Cozens AL, Schulman H, et al. Activation of chloride channels in normal and cystic fibrosis airway epithelial cells by multifunctional calcium/calmodulin-dependent protein kinase. *Nature* 1991; **349**: 793–6.
27 Anderson MP, Welsh MJ. Calcium and cAMP activate different chloride channels in the apical membrane of normal and cystic fibrosis epithelia. *Proc Natl Acad Sci USA* 1991; **88**: 6003–7.
28 Baxter PS, Goldhill J, Hardcastle J, et al. Accounting for cystic fibrosis. *Nature* 1988; **335**: 211.
29 Goldstein JL, Bhuva MB, Layden TJ, Rao MC. *E. coli* heat stable enterotoxin stimulated chloride secretion is abnormal in cystic fibrosis (CF) rectal mucosa *in vivo*. *Pediatr Pulmonol Suppl* 1991; **6**: 260 (Abstract).

30 Berger HA, Travis SM, Welsh MJ. Regulation of the cystic fibrosis transmembrane conductance regulator $Cl^-$ channel by specific protein kinases and protein phosphatases. *J Biol Chem* 1993; **268**: 2037–47.
31 Meiqiu L, Nairn AC, Guggino SE. cGMP-dependent protein kinase regulation of a chloride channel in T84 cells. *Am J Physiol* 1992; **262**: C1304–12.
32 Ghishan FK. The transport of electrolytes in the gut and the use of oral rehydration solutions. *Pediatr Clin North Am* 1988; **35**: 35–51.
33 Keusch GT, Jacewicz M, Mobassaleh M, Donohue-Rolfe A. Shiga toxin: intestinal cell receptors and pathophysiology of enterotoxic effects. *Rev Infect Dis* 1991; **13** (Suppl 4): S304–10.
34 Field M, Rao MC, Chang EB. Intestinal electrolyte transport and diarrheal disease. *N Engl J Med* 1989; **321**: 879–83.
35 Hamilton JR. Viral enteritis. *Pediatr Clin North Am* 1988; **35**: 89–101.
36 Bishop WP, Ulshen MH. Bacterial gastroenteritis. *Pediatr Clin North Am* 1988; **35**: 69–87.
37 Rodman DM, Zamucho S. The CF heterozygote-advantage in surviving cholera? *Med Hypothesis* 1991; **36**: 253–8.
38 Corradi A. *Annali delle epidemic occorse in Italia*. Vol 6 parte VI. *Indice cronologico e topografico*. Memorie della Società Medico chirurgica di Bologna. Tipografia Gamberini e Parmeggiani, Bologna, 1876.
39 Serre JL, Simon-Bouy B, Mornet E, et al. Studies of RFLP closely linked to the cystic fibrosis locus throughout Europe lead to new considerations in population genetics. *Hum Genet* 1990; **84**: 449–54.
40 Quinton PM. Abnormalities in electrolyte secretion in cystic fibrosis sweat glands due to decreased anion permeability. In: Quinton PM, Martinez RJ, Hopfer U (eds). *Fluid and Electrolyte Abnormalities in Exocrine Glands in Cystic Fibrosis* (eds PM Quinton, RJ Martinez, U Hopfer) San Francisco Press, San Francisco, 1982, pp. 53–76.
41 Hansson GC. Cystic fibrosis and chloride secreting diarrhoea. *Nature* 1988; **333**: 711.
42 Baxter PS. MD thesis, Cambridge University, 1991.
43 Behm JK, Hagiwara G, Lewiston NJ, et al. Hyposecretion of β-adrenergically induced sweating in cystic fibrosis heterozygotes. *Pediatr Res* 1987; **22**: 271–6.
44 Sato K, Sato F. Variable reduction in β-adrenergic sweat secretion in cystic fibrosis heterozygotes. *J Lab Clin Med* 1988; **111**: 511–18.
45 Little TW. Cheaters sometimes prosper: distortion of mendelian segregation by meiotic drive. *Trends Genet* 1993; **9**: 205–10.
46 Williams C, Davies D, Williamson R. Segregation of DF508 and normal CFTR alleles in human sperm. *Hum Mol Genet* 1993; **2**: 445–8.
47 Kitzis E, Chomel JC, Haliassos A. et al. Unusual segregation of CF alleles. *Nature* 1988; **336**: 316.
48 Pritchard DJ. Cystic fibrosis allele frequency, sex ratio anomalies and fertility: a new theory for the dissemination of mutant alleles. *Hum Genet* 1991; **87**: 671–6.
49 Jorde LB, Lathrop GM. A test of the heterozygote-advantage hypothesis in cystic fibrosis carriers. *Am J Hum Genet* 1988; **42**: 808–15.
50 Kalman YM, Kerem B. Inference of CF carrier frequency from CF patients' data: is it justified'? *Am J Hum Genet* 1993; **53**: 1492A.
51 Wagner DK, Cavalli Sforza LL. Ethnic variation and genetic disease: possible roles of hitch-hiking and epistasis. *Am J Hum Genet* 1975; **27**: 348–64.

52 Spence JE, Perciaccante RG, Greig GM, et al. Uniparental disomy as a mechanism for human genetic disease. *Am J Hum Genet* 1988; **42**: 217–26.
53 Voss R, Ben-Simon E, Avital A, et al. Isodisomy of chromosome 7 in a patient with cystic fibrosis: could uniparental disomy be common in humans? *Am J Hum Genet* 1989; **45**: 373–80.
54 Tummler B, Aschendorff A, Darnedde T, et al. Marker haplotype association with growth in German cystic fibrosis patients. *Hum Genet* 1990; **84**: 267–73.
55 Mornet E, Simon-Bouy B, Serre JL, et al. Genetic heterogeneity between two clinical forms of cystic fibrosis evidenced by familial analysis and linked DNA probes. *Clin Genet* 1989; **35**: 81–7.
56 Sereth H, Shoshani T, Bashan N, Kerem BS. CF extended haplotype analysis and implication to the selective advantage hypothesis. *Hum Genet* 1993; **92**: 289–95.
57 Casals T, Vazquez C, Lazaro C, et al. Cystic fibrosis in the Basque Country: high frequency of mutation ΔF508 in patients of basque origin. *Am J Hum Genet* 1992; **50**: 404–10.
58 Lee R, Nezmer L, Witt DR. Identification of previously undiagnosed cystic fibrosis patients: an unexpected outcome of prenatal carrier screening. *Am J Hum Genet* 1992; **51**: A32.
59 The Cystic Fibrosis Genotype–Phenotype Consortium. Correlation between genotype and phenotype in patients with cystic fibrosis *N Engl J Med* 1993; **329**: 1308–13.

Chapter Five

# Heterozygote Screening

David J. H. Brock
*Human Genetics Unit, University of Edinburgh, Edinburgh, UK*

## INTRODUCTION

Soon after the cystic fibrosis (CF) gene was cloned in 1989, an active debate began about the merits of population screening for heterozygotes. Substantial screening programmes for three other autosomal recessive disorders, Tay-Sachs disease[1], β-thalassaemia[2] and sickle cell anaemia[3], had already been carried out with varying degrees of success. Although none of these disorders is particularly common in populations of highest CF frequency, there was a feeling that adequate lessons had been learned about how to apply genetic screening to a comprehensive population group.

There was, however, one major difference. In Tay-Sachs disease, β-thalassaemia and sickle cell anaemia the test for heterozygosity is simple, sensitive and specific. Because tests were based on analysis of the products of mutant genes, there was no need to worry about molecular heterogeneity. CF was quite different. From the first reports of the gene cloning two factors were apparent. There was no chance of carrying out tests of CF heterozygosity through measurement of the gene product, the CF transmembrane conductance regulator, since it was not expressed in accessible tissues. Furthermore, the CF gene was heterogeneous. In the original study only 70% of CF chromosomes could be accounted for by the predominant mutant allele, ΔF508, and it was expected that there would be at least 7–10 other mutations responsible for the disorder[4]. As laboratories moved into action in the search

*Cystic Fibrosis—Current Topics, Volume 2.* Edited by J. A. Dodge, D. J. H. Brock and J. H. Widdicombe

for mutations to be found in their respective populations, it became apparent that the CF gene was characterized by a quite remarkable degree of heterogeneity.

## THE PROBLEM OF HETEROGENEITY

In virtually every major population group analysed to date, the CF gene is heterogeneous. Amongst Caucasian populations, where CF prevalence is highest, the major ΔF508 allele ranges from a high of about 90% to a low of below 50%[5]. Any genetics centre contemplating a programme of CF screening must survey its local population for the nature and frequency of CF alleles, and then calculate how many of these it is practical to cover in laboratory analyses. This in turn is determined by the size of the population to be screened. It is comparatively easy to assay for 20 or 30 mutant alleles if the only subjects are a small group of high-risk individuals. It is relatively difficult to assay for more than 10 CF alleles if any substantial through-put of samples is to be achieved.

For most centres contemplating population screening, the realistic expectation was that between 85% and 90% of CF alleles would be analysed. Inevitably this would create a problem for couples where one partner was found to carry a mutant allele while the other did not. Such 'positive–negative' couples would have a residual risk of carrying a CF child which would depend on the proportion of CF alleles detectable (Table 1). For most of these couples the residual risk would be higher than the starting risk. In a population where the birth incidence is one in 2500, the residual risk for a positive–negative couple would only fall below the starting risk when over 96% of CF alleles were analysed.

**Table 1** Residual risk of a CF child if one partner tests positive and the other negative (CF incidence one in 2500) against proportion detectable alleles

| Residual risk | Proportion of all alleles detectable (%) |
|---|---|
| 1 in 311 | 70 |
| 1 in 388 | 75 |
| 1 in 484 | 80 |
| 1 in 644 | 85 |
| 1 in 964 | 90 |
| 1 in 1924 | 95 |
| 1 in 2404 | 96 |
| 1 in 3204 | 97 |

The problem of the positive–negative couple loomed large in the minds of many commentators[6,7] It was suggested that the figure of 96% for detectable alleles should be a minimum one before population screening was contemplated in a population with a one in 2500 birth incidence[8]. This was the attitude taken by the American Society of Human Genetics in its 1990 statement[9]. However, others were not persuaded that this was a legitimate point of view and pointed to the success of other prenatal screening programmes at substantially lower sensitivities[10]. It was felt that even at a 75% heterozygote detection rate, half of all high-risk couples would be able to make an informed decision about child bearing. It was pointed out that several commentators were too concerned about their own legal and moral position and had lost sight of the needs of their patients[11,12].

In a number of countries, and in particular in Britain, it was decided to launch pilot trials of population heterozygote testing for CF. By the time that the trials commenced it was already clear that it would only be practical to detect about 85% of CF alleles. These programmes were therefore launched in the full knowledge that CF screening was likely to start and to remain as an incomplete process. It was clearly important that information provided to the participating population and the counselling of those found to be at risk should take this fully into account.

## TARGET GROUPS

Four main target groups have been identified as possibly appropriate for heterozygote testing (Table 2). However, there has been little enthusiasm for neonatal testing, despite the ease with which this might be grafted onto existing screening programmes that used Guthrie cards. Problems of consent might prove vexatious, and the information gathered would have no practical use until the screened person reached reproductive age. It was noted that some of the new programmes of neonatal testing for CF homozygosity were inadvertently detecting CF heterozygotes[13]. The problem of how to deal with these had yet to be addressed.

There were several theoretical advantages in screening children of high-school age. Scriver et al. had demonstrated that this worked well for

**Table 2** Potential target groups for CF heterozygote testing

| |
|---|
| Neonates |
| High-school children |
| Young adults, alone or as couples |
| Pregnant women or couples |

Tay-Sachs and β-thalassaemia screening in Montreal schools[14,15]. The whole concept of genetic risk could be tied into an imaginative programme of biology teaching. In a pilot study of CF heterozygosity screening they showed a take-up rate of 42% in four public high schools in 1991[16]. Nonetheless, in the UK there are unresolved problems of parental consent for those under 16. There is also some information suggesting that knowledge of carrier status may not be retained by school children until the appropriate age at which to use it[14].

Largely for these reasons, the major pilot programmes of CF heterozygosity testing which have been reported have been concerned with the two last groups in Table 2.

## HETEROZYGOSITY SCREENING IN PRIMARY CARE

In many respects screening through primary health care services, such as general practitioner surgeries or family planning clinics, and at or near reproductive age, is the ideal programme. It is most compatible with the principle of individual autonomy. An identified carrier can, if he or she wishes, ignore the information, change marriage partners, have artificial insemination by a screened donor, forgo reproduction or choose to have a pregnancy monitored by prenatal diagnosis. In practice, however, experience from the Tay-Sachs[1] and β-thalassaemia[2] screening programmes has shown that the only option seriously considered by carriers identified in this way is prenatal diagnosis and selective termination of pregnancy. Thus the main advantage of screening in primary care is that it allows individuals the opportunity for considered reflection before they make the choice as to how to handle their carrier status.

Two pilot trials of carrier screening through primary health care services have shown that the method of approach to potential participants is critical

**Table 3** Take-up rates of CF heterozygote testing in primary care

| Ref. | Approach to identified target group | Take-up | (%) |
|---|---|---|---|
| 17 | Opportunistic screening, general practice | 340/513 | (66) |
| 17 | Opportunistic screening, family planning clinics | 371/431 | (87) |
| 17 | Invitation letter, general practice | 87/852 | (10) |
| 18 | Letter at beginning of trial in one general practice | 59/502 | (12) |
| 18 | Letter and booklet | 47/496 | (9) |
| 18 | Passive opportunistic | 81/471 | (17) |
| 18 | Active opportunistic—test now | 453/649 | (70) |
| 18 | Active opportunistic—test at return visit | 22/88 | (25) |
| 18 | Letter at end of trial | 128/2953 | (4) |

in determining the take-up rate (Table 3). Watson et al.[17] found that when the offer of screening was made opportunistically and in person by a member of the research team, between 66% and 87% of those approached agreed to be tested. In contrast, when screening was presented by an invitation letter, the take-up rate was only 10%. Bekker et al.[18] reached similar conclusions. When there was active opportunistic contact and immediate testing the acceptance rate was 70%. For other methods of presentation participation was meagre. Bekker et al.[18] concluded that the most important variable determining participation rates in screening was the personal approach by a professional and the offer of immediate carrier testing.

## PREGNANCY SCREENING IN ANTENATAL CLINICS

In Britain a very high proportion of women attend the antenatal clinics of maternity hospitals during pregnancy. Such clinics therefore represent a 'turnstile' where the offer of heterozygote testing for CF may be efficiently made. Furthermore, following successful trials of $\alpha$-fetoprotein (AFP) screening, initially for the detection of neural tube defects but more recently for segregating out those at high risk of bearing an infant with Down's syndrome, pregnancy screening has become a relatively routine aspect of antenatal care. Heterozygote screening may therefore be added to existing programmes with a relatively small input of additional staff.

Two types of antenatal CF screening have been proposed: 'two-step'[19] and 'couple'[20]. Although they are not mutually exclusive, the two-step model tests women first and then moves on to the male partner only when the woman is shown to be a carrier. There is a delay between the phases of testing and it is possible in principle for a woman to be tested while her partner refuses to participate. In contrast, in the couple model both partners must agree to participate before testing begins. In most cases only one of the partners need be tested, since a negative result means that the couple is not at high risk.

A large trial of two-step screening in the antenatal clinics of a major Edinburgh maternity hospital has recently been completed[21]. The offer of testing was made by a specially designed leaflet[22] sent with a booking clinic appointment at an early stage of pregnancy. Women agreeing to participate were tested for six mutant CF alleles, representing 85% of CF chromosomes. If a woman was found to be positive, her partner was also tested. No further action was taken when a woman was negative, or if she was positive and her partner negative. An offer of prenatal diagnosis was made to couples with a one in four risk of bearing an affected child. The full results of this trial are presented in Table 4. The take-up rate of screening was 83% when related to eligible women, and 71% when set against all women to whom the offer was

**Table 4** Two-step antenatal screening in Edinburgh

| | | | | |
|---|---|---|---|---|
| Women offered screening | | 7011 | | (100%) |
| Not eligible for screening | | 981 | | (14%) |
| Late gestation | 701 | | | |
| Abnormal pregnancy | 125 | | | |
| Partner unavailable | 124 | | | |
| Other | 31 | | | |
| Eligible | | 6030 | (100%) | (86%) |
| Declined screening | | 1052 | (17%) | (15%) |
| Women screened | | 4978 | (83%) | (71%) |
| Carriers | | 190 | (1/26) | |
| Carrier partners screened | | 189 | | |
| Heterozygous couples | | 7 | | |
| Affected fetuses | | 2 | | |

made. All but one of the 190 carriers identified were able to persuade their male partners to undergo testing. All seven couples where each partner was a CF heterozygote elected to undergo prenatal diagnosis. One couple had two successive pregnancies with an affected fetus, and in each case the pregnancy was terminated and the diagnosis confirmed. Similar results have been reported by Schwartz et al.[23] in a Danish population where 80% of 3000 women accepted the offer of screening.

Two-step screening of the type outlined in Table 4 does generate some anxiety amongst women found to be positive for CF alleles while they await their partner's test result. A way round this problem was suggested by Wald[20]. He proposed that the screening unit should be the couple; positive couples were those where each partner carried a CF allele, while negative couples were those where only one partner was tested or where both partners were tested and only one found to be a carrier. Whereas two-step screening generates two types of screen-negative couple—a large group with a low risk and a smaller group with an intermediate risk—couple screening generates a single class of screen-negative couple, whose composite risk is satisfactorily low (Figure 1). Because, in a majority of cases it is only necessary to test one sample from a couple, the number of assays performed is no different from that in two-step screening.

Couple screening has not hitherto been tested in clinical practice. Initially, there were doubts as to whether the take-up rate would be satisfactory, since the decision to participate must be a joint one between the pregnant woman and her partner. Data from the Edinburgh two-step screening trial suggest that up to 40% of women make the decision to be tested without reference to their partner[22]. Fears have also been expressed that denying information about individual carrier status to those participating in the trials would lead to low acceptance rates.

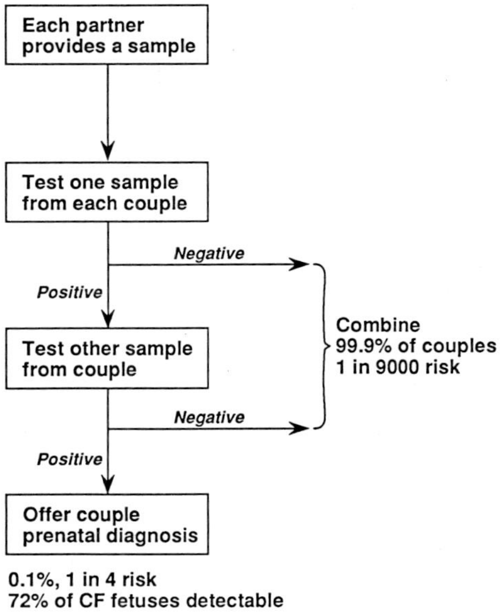


**Figure 1** Flow chart of couple screening

An extended trial of couple screening in the antenatal clinics of two Edinburgh maternity hositals shows that the take-up rates are little different from those encountered in two-step screening (Table 5)[24,25]. Some 76% of eligible couples participated, while the figure for the overall group was 69%. There was little sign that participants wished to know their individual carrier status. The data were freely available either in the obstetric notes or on application to the screening coordinator; only 3% of participants sought this

**Table 5** Couple screening in Edinburgh

| | | | | |
|---|---|---|---|---|
| Women offered screening | | 6932 | | (100%) |
| Not eligible for screening | | 632 | | (9%) |
| Late gestation | 358 | | | |
| Abnormal pregnancy | 37 | | | |
| Partner unavailable | 212 | | | |
| Other | 25 | | | |
| Eligible | | 6300 | (100%) | (91%) |
| Declined screening | | 1519 | (24%) | (22%) |
| Women screened | | 4781 | (76%) | (69%) |
| Carriers | | 184 | (1/26) | |
| Heterozygous couples | | 3 | | |
| Affected fetuses | | 2 | | |

information. Couple screening is a remarkably easy and trouble-free mode of delivery of carrier testing, and has become the method of choice in Edinburgh maternity hospitals. Wald et al.[26] have also reported a satisfactory 68% take-up of couple screening.

## PREGNANCY SCREENING IN PRIMARY CARE

One of the problems of screening in antenatal clinics is that the time of first booking may be too late to allow necessary action to be taken in the first trimester of pregnancy. Harris et al.[27] have suggested that this problem can be circumvented if general practitioners offer heterozygote testing to women at the time of a positive pregnancy test. A pilot trial claimed that this was a viable option, although no data on take-up rates were provided. However, it was pointed out that there are 33 839 general practitioners in the UK, and the chance of persuading a reasonable number of these to participate in CF screening seems improbable. At best, such screening must be seen as a useful adjunct to more generally applicable programmes.

## OPPORTUNISTIC TESTING

It has been argued that if a woman undergoes an invasive and potentially hazardous investigation such as amniocentesis or chorionic villus biopsy, she is entitled to obtain maximum information from the process[28]. Schwartz et al.[23] offered CF heterozygote testing to 3545 women about to undergo first-trimester prenatal diagnosis usually because of advanced maternal age, and recorded an acceptance rate of 98%.

Instead of screening mothers and fathers for heterozygosity, Brambati et al.[29] chose to test the fetal sample in 780 pregnancies undergoing first and early second-trimester transabdominal chorionic villus sampling. The acceptance rate was 98%. One affected fetus was detected as well as 12 who were apparently heterozygous for the ΔF508 allele. However, in two of the latter cases termination of pregnancy was requested. A worrying aspect of this type of opportunistic testing is that women at a heightened state of anxiety may not be able to accept CF heterozygosity in their fetus as normal[30].

## CASCADE TESTING

Most genetic centres now offer testing for CF heterozygosity to first-degree relatives of affected individuals. In general such programmes are reactive, and respond to consultand's requests. Super et al.[31] suggest a more pro-active approach, taking screening out into the population by focusing on the relatives of index cases. They argue that the ratio of carriers detected to people tested will be higher this way, that only one or two mutant alleles need be screened for and that less anxiety would be generated among the screened population.

There is no doubt that cascade testing could be a very effective way of identifying large numbers of carriers and carrier couples with a great deal less effort than in any standard population screening. However, it is not screening in the conventional sense of the word. Access to the test is not equal, and the probability of being offered screening is a function of relatedness to the index case. Most people have difficulty remembering the names of first cousins once removed or second cousins. Cascade testing would need to reach to the fourth cousin level (Figure 2) to attempt the same cover as population screening (Table 6)[32]. Even at that level it would detect a relatively small proportion of carriers. There is also the chance that the aggressive features involved in contacting distant relatives, which are necessary if cascade screening is to be effective, will rebound on the concept of community genetics.

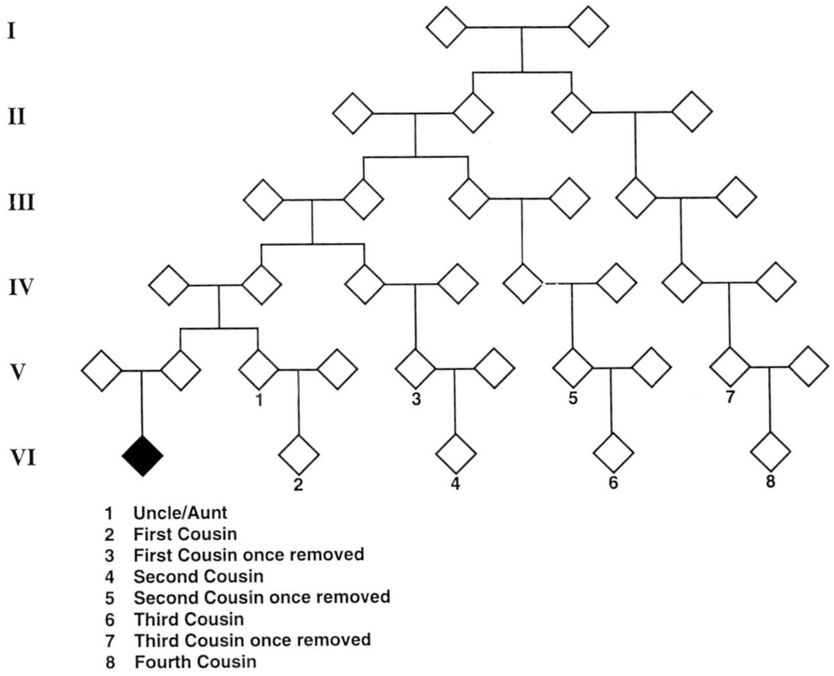


**Figure 2** Hypothetical pedigree showing fourth cousin level in cascade testing

**Table 6** Cascade testing: numbers of different categories of relative for sibships of size 2 and 3, probabilities of being a carrier and numbers positive on testing

| Relative | Probability of being a carrier | Probability of having same allele as proband | Probability positive on testing | Sibship size 2 | | Sibship size 3 | |
|---|---|---|---|---|---|---|---|
| | | | | Total relatives | Number positive | Total relatives | Number positive |
| Aunt/uncle | 0.50251 | 0.50000 | 0.50213 | 2 | 1.00426 | 4 | 2.00852 |
| First cousin | 0.26230 | 0.25000 | 0.26046 | 4 | 1.04184 | 12 | 3.12552 |
| First cousin once removed | 0.14631 | 0.12500 | 0.14311 | 8 | 1.14488 | 24 | 3.43464 |
| Second cousin | 0.09002 | 0.06250 | 0.08589 | 16 | 1.37424 | 72 | 6.18408 |
| Second cousin once removed | 0.06296 | 0.03125 | 0.05820 | 32 | 1.86240 | 144 | 8.38080 |
| Third cousin | 0.04988 | 0.01563 | 0.04474 | 64 | 2.86336 | 432 | 19.32768 |
| Third cousin once removed | 0.04361 | 0.00781 | 0.03824 | 128 | 4.89472 | 864 | 33.03936 |
| Fourth cousin | 0.04057 | 0.00391 | 0.03507 | 256 | 8.97792 | 2592 | 90.90144 |
| Total | – | – | – | 510 | 23.16362 | 4144 | 166.40204 |

## PSYCHOSOCIAL ASPECTS OF SCREENING

It is sometimes suggested that screening does more harm than good[33]. Although a negative test result is usually reassuring[34], a positive result may lead to loss of self-esteem and worries about future health. Considerable experience has been gained from Tay-Sachs disease screening programmes amongst Jewish communities in North America. McQueen[35] found that 45% of participants stated that it would matter a great deal if they were found to be gene carriers, despite the recessive nature of the disease. Zeesman et al.[14] found that some eight years after a screening programme 19% of carriers were anxious about their status. Marteau et al.[36] reported similar data; Tay-Sachs disease carriers were in general less optimistic about their future health than control groups. It was thought that the root of the problem lay in a poor level of understanding of what it really meant to be a carrier of a recessive disease.

These issues are relevant to potential programmes of CF heterozygote screening. Added to this is the fact that individuals who test negative for CF alleles still have a substantial residual risk of carrier status—at an 85% detection rate the chance of being a carrier declines from one in 25 to one in 167. The lack of sensitivity in CF testing was a prime factor in leading the NIH workshop on population screening for the CF gene to advocate in 1990 that no mass programmes of heterozygote testing should be carried out until carefully conducted pilot studies were complete[9]. This advice was repeated in a statement of the American Society of Human Genetics as recently as June 1992[37].

Caution in North American circles to some extent reflects different patterns of health care provision in that continent as well as worries about medico-legal action. In the UK a more forward-looking approach to screening has been adopted, with the Cystic Fibrosis Trust soliciting bids for pilot trials. One factor behind this decision has been an awareness that studies on population attitudes to CF heterozygote screening have been somewhat ahead of the medical profession. Before the gene was cloned, Williamson et al.[38] found that 84% of a mixed London population answered yes to the question ‘Given that cystic fibrosis is an inherited disease and that a healthy person may unknowingly carry it and pass it on to his/her children, would you want to know if you were a carrier?’ In a later study, Williamson[39] states that when several hundred students between 16 and 20 were asked whether they wished to be screened for CF carrier status, 90% said the test should be available to those who request it and 70% stated that they wished to be tested themselves. Similar attitudes amongst the general public have been recorded in Holland[40] and in Belgium[41]. Even amongst CF families, where a more ambivalent attitude to screening might be anticipated, opinion has been strongly in favour of population screening[42–44].

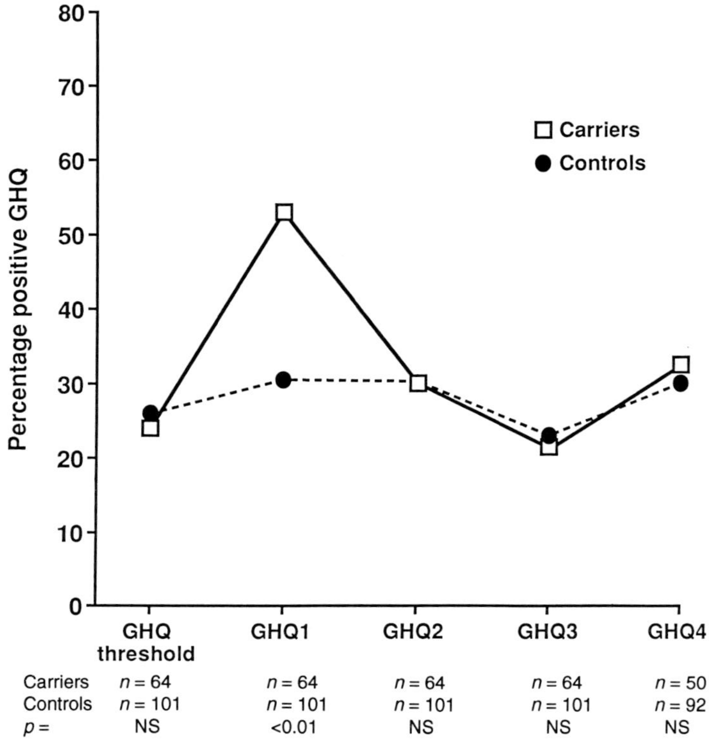


**Figure 3** Two-step screening. Stress as measured by the general health questionnaire (GHQ) is apparent amongst carriers only while awaiting partner's test result (GHQ1)

**Table 7** Attitudes to antenatal CF screening (percentages)

(A) 'I am glad that I had a CF carrier test'

| | Yes | No/don't know |
|---|---|---|
| Female carriers | 80 | 20 |
| Female controls | 97 | 3 |
| Male partners | 90 | 10 |
| Male controls | 98 | 2 |

(B) 'The CF carrier test should routinely be offered to all pregnant women'

| | Yes | No |
|---|---|---|
| Female carriers | 88 | 12 |
| Female controls | 96 | 4 |
| Male partners | 90 | 10 |
| Male controls | 98 | 2 |

**Table 8** Reasons for declining CF screening

| | | |
|---|---|---|
| Against termination of pregnancy | 111 | (43%) |
| Against termination for CF | 29 | (11%) |
| Partner opposed | 26 | (10%) |
| Risk of CF child too low | 19 | (7%) |
| Error rate unacceptable | 15 | (6%) |
| Test causes anxiety | 13 | (5%) |
| Don't want test during pregnancy | 11 | (4%) |
| Not enough information | 11 | (4%) |
| Decision too difficult if positive | 10 | (4%) |
| Don't want to know | 9 | (3%) |
| No reason | 5 | (2%) |
| Advances in treatment probable | 1 | (1%) |
| | 260 | (100%) |

Pilot programmes of CF testing now make it possible to ascertain whether screening has had harmful consequences. In a programme carried out in primary care, Watson et al.[45] found that 81% of carriers were glad that they had been tested, and although varying degrees of anxiety were found to be initially associated with a positive result, most of this was allayed by genetic counselling with no adverse long-term psychological consequences. At six months after the test 55% of carriers reported that they were not worried. A large proportion of partners (87%) of carriers were also tested. In this group it was difficult to ascertain attitudes to future reproduction; however, significantly fewer individuals in 'at-risk' partnerships felt that they would refrain from having children after testing and counselling than before. This may be the consequence of an increased awareness of the availability of prenatal diagnosis or simply that carriers now give more concerted thought to potential risks in future pregnancies.

Carrier testing during pregnancy, particularly using the two-step mode of delivery, might be expected to generate some anxiety. Mennie et al.[21,46] showed that this was of comparatively short duration, with a reversion to the normal state by the time that the partner was tested (Figure 3). Partners of identified female carriers also showed some stress, but again this was of short duration[46]. Most of the participants in this study reported that they were glad that they had taken the carrier test and asserted that it should be offered routinely to all pregnant women (Table 7)[47]. Amongst those who declined the offer of the CF carrier test, a majority (54%) did so because they were against termination of pregnancy (Table 8)[48].

## COSTS OF SCREENING

One of the problems in assessing the costs of screening is that the levels of royalty payments on patented CF alleles and the licensing fee for the use of the polymerase chain reaction have yet to be determined. It is likely that these, together with laboratory overheads and staff salaries, will represent a major component of the total. However, it is possible to compare the relative costs of different types of programme delivery, using data available from pilot screening trials.

Beech and colleagues[49] have made an economic evaluation of the alternative population screening programmes in the UK. The tangible outcomes were the number of individuals informed of their carrier status, the number of actual CF carriers identified, the number of CF carrier couples found and the number of CF fetuses detected. The lowest unit cost for each of the above-named outcomes was found in the antenatal screening programmes, though there was little difference between two-step and couple-orientated deliveries.

## REFERENCES

1 Kaback MM, Nathan TJ, Greenwald S. Tay-Sachs disease: heterozygote screening and prenatal diagnosis—US experience and world perspective. In: *Tay-Sachs disease: Screening and Prevention* (ed MM Kaback). Liss, New York, 1977, pp 13–36.
2 Modell B, Berdoukas V. *The Clinical Approach to Thalassaemia*, Grune & Stratten, London, 1984, pp 354–378.
3 Bowman JE. Invited editorial: prenatal screening for haemoglobinopathies. *Am J Hum Genet* 1991; **48**: 433–438.
4 Riordan JR, Rommens JM, Kerem B, et al. Identification of the cystic fibrosis gene: cloning and characterization of complementary DNA. *Science* 1989; **245**: 1066–73.
5 The Cystic Fibrosis Genetic Analysis Consortium. Worldwide survey of the ΔF508 mutation. *Am J Hum Genet* 1990; **47**: 354–9.
6 Wilfond BS, Fost N. The cystic fibrosis gene: medical and social implications for heterozygote detection. *JAMA* 1990; **263**: 2778–83.
7 Gilbert F. Is population screening for cystic fibrosis appropriate now? *Am J Hum Genet* 1990; **46**: 394–5.
8 Ten Kate LP. Carrier screening in CF. *Nature* 1989; **342**: 131.
9 Workshop on population screening for the cystic fibrosis gene. Statement from the National Institutes of Health workshop on population screening for the cystic fibrosis gene. *N Engl J Med* 1990; **323**: 70–71.
10 Super M, Schwartz MJ, Sardhawalla IB. CF screening. *Nature* 1990; **344**: 113–14.
11 Brock DJH. Population screening for cystic fibrosis. *Am J Hum Genet* 1990; **47**: 164–5.
12 Schulman JD, Maddalena A, Black SH, Bick DP. Screening for cystic fibrosis carriers. *Am J Hum Genet* 1990; **47**: 740.
13 Ranieri E, Ryall RG, Morris CP, et al. Neonatal screening strategy for cystic fibrosis using immunoreactive trypsinogen and direct gene analysis. *Br Med J* 1991; **302**: 1237–40.
14 Zeesman S, Clow CL, Cartier L, Scriver CR. A private view of heterozygosity: eight year follow-up study of carriers of the Tay-Sachs gene detected by high-school screening in Montreal. *Am J Med Genet* 1984; **18**: 769–78.

15 Scriver CR, Bardanis M, Cartier L, et al. $\beta$-Thalassaemia disease prevention: genetic medicine applied. *Am J Hum Genet* 1984; **35**: 1024–38.
16 Kaplin F, Clow C, Scriver CR. Cystic fibrosis carrier screening by DNA analysis: a pilot study of attitudes among participants. *Am J Hum Genet* 1991; **49**: 240–2.
17 Watson EK, Mayall E, Chappell J, et al. Screening for carriers of cystic fibrosis through primary health care services. *Br Med J* 1991; **303**: 504–7.
18 Bekker H, Modell M, Denniss G, et al. Uptake of cystic fibrosis testing in primary care: supply push or demand pull? *Br Med J* 1993; **306**: 1584–6.
19 Brock DJH, Shrimpton AE, Jones C, McIntosh I. Cystic fibrosis: the new genetics. *J R Soc Med* 1991; **84** (Suppl 18) 2–9.
20 Wald NJ. Couple screening for cystic fibrosis. *Lancet* 1991; **338**: 1318–19.
21 Mennie ME, Gilfillan A, Compton M, et al. Prenatal screening for cystic fibrosis. *Lancet* 1992; **340**: 214–16.
22 Mennie ME, Liston WA, Brock DJH. Prenatal cystic fibrosis carrier testing: designing an information leaflet to meet the specific needs of the target population. *J Med Genet* 1992; **29**: 308–12.
23 Schwartz M, Brandt NJ, Skovby F. Screening for carriers of cystic fibrosis among pregnant women: a pilot study. *Eur J Hum Genet* 1993: 239–44.
24 Livingstone J, Axton RA, Mennie M, et al. A preliminary trial of couple screening for cystic fibrosis: designing an appropriate information leaflet. *Clin Genet* 1993; **43**: 57–62.
25 Livingstone J, Axton RA, Gilfillan A, et al. Antenatal screening for cystic fibrosis: a trial of the couple model. *Br Med J* 1994; **308**: 1459–62.
26 Wald NJ, George LM, Wald NM, MacKenzie IZ. Couple screening for cystic fibrosis. *Lancet* 1993; **342**: 1307–8.
27 Harris H, Scotcher D, Hartlie N, et al. Cystic fibrosis carrier testing in early pregnancy by general practitioners. *Br Med J* 1993; **306**: 1580–3.
28 Young ID. Pregnancy screening for cystic fibrosis. *Lancet* 1993, **342**: 569–70.
29 Brambati B, Tului L, Fattore S, Ferec C. First-trimester fetal screening of cystic fibrosis in low risk population. *Lancet* 1993; **342**: 624.
30 Black SH, Bick DB, Maddalena A, et al. Pregnancy screening for cystic fibrosis. *Lancet* 1993; **342**: 1112–13.
31 Super M, Schwarz MJ, Malone G. Screening for cystic fibrosis carriers. *Lancet* 1992; **340**: 490–1.
32 Holloway S, Brock DJH. Cascade testing for the identification of carriers of cystic fibrosis. *J Med Screening*. In press.
33 Marteau TM. Psychological costs of screening. *Br Med J* 1989; **299**: 527.
34 Marteau TM, Johnstone M, Shore RW, et al. The impact of prenatal screening and diagnostic tests upon the cognitions, emotions and behaviour of pregnant women. *J Psychosom Res* 1989; **33**: 7–16.
35 McQueen DV. Social aspects of genetic screening for Tay-Sachs disease: the pilot community screening programme in Baltimore and Washington. *Soc Biol* 1975; **22**: 125–33.
36 Marteau TM, van Duijn M, Ellis I. Effects of genetic screening on perceptions of health: a pilot study. *J Med Genet* 1992; **29**: 24–6.
37 Statement of the American Society of Human Genetics on cystic fibrosis carrier screening. *Am J Hum Genet* 1992; **51**: 1443–4.
38 Williamson R, Allison MED, Bentley TJ, et al. Community attitudes to cystic fibrosis carrier testing in England: a pilot study. *Prenat Diagn* 1989; **9**: 727–34.
39 Williamson R. Universal community carrier screening for cystic fibrosis? *Nature Genet* 1993; **3**: 195–201.

40 Ten Kate LP, Tijmstra TJ. Carrier screening for cystic fibrosis. *Lancet* 1989; **ii**: 973–4.
41 Decruyenaere M, Evers-Kiebooms G, Denayer L, Van Den Berghe H. Cystic fibrosis: community knowledge and attitudes towards carrier screening and prenatal diagnosis. *Clin Genet* 1992; **41**: 189–96.
42 Turner G, Wilcken B, Griffiths H. Cystic fibrosis screening and community genetics. *J Med Genet* 1991; **28**: 575–6.
43 Watson EK, Marchant J, Bush A, Williamson B. Attitudes towards prenatal diagnosis and carrier screening for cystic fibrosis among the parents of patients in a paediatric cystic fibrosis clinic. *J Med Genet* 1992; **29**: 490–1.
44 Green JM. Principles and practicalities of carrier screening: attitudes of recent parents. *J Med Genet* 1992; **29**: 313–19.
45 Watson EK, Mayall ES, Lamb J, et al. Psychological and social consequences of community carrier screening programme for cystic fibrosis. *Lancet* 1992; **340**: 217–20.
46 Mennie ME, Compton ME, Gilfillan A, et al. Prenatal screening for cystic fibrosis: psychological effects on carriers and their partners. *J Med Genet* 1993; **30**: 543–8.
47 Mennie M, Gilfillan A, Compton ME, et al. Prenatal cystic fibrosis carrier screening: factors in a woman's decision to decline testing. *Prenat Diagn* 1993; **13**: 807–14.
48 Mennie ME, Cornpton ME, Gilfillan A, et al. Prenatal screening for cystic fibrosis: attitudes and responses of participants. *Clin Genet* 1993; **44**: 102–6.
49 Beech R, Bekker H. The costs and outcomes of population carrier screening for cystic fibrosis. *J Med Screening* (in press).

# Part II

## Cell Biology

## Chapter Six

# Altered Regulation of Airway Fluid Content in Cystic Fibrosis

J. H. Widdicombe[a,b] S. S. Miller[c] and W. E. Finkbeiner[a,d]

*[a]Cardiovascular Research Institute, Departments of [b]Physiology and [d]Pathology, University of California—San Francisco, and [c]School of Optometry and Department of Molecular and Cell Biology, University of California—Berkeley, USA*

## THE EPITHELIAL LINING FLUID

The airways are lined with a film of fluid from 5 to 100 μm in depth. This fluid is a complex mixture of secretions from cells of both the surface and glandular epithelia. Its components include plasma proteins, surfactant, DNA, antibacterial substances (such as lysozyme, lactoferrin and proteases), and mucins[1]. Mucins are high molecular weight glycoproteins, which bind together in a number of ways[2] to create a gel which entraps inhaled particulate matter. The peculiar viscoelastic properties of the mucous gel[3] allow it, together with entrapped particles, to be propelled by ciliary motion at ~5 mm/min towards the mouth[4,5], where it is swallowed or expectorated. Thus, it is this process of 'mucociliary clearance' which keeps the surface of the airways clean. The mucous gel may be absent in healthy, uninflamed airways[6] but becomes thicker in bronchitis, asthma and cystic fibrosis, where defective mucociliary clearance results in obstruction and plugging of the airways with mucous secretions.

*Cystic Fibrosis—Current Topics, Volume 2.* Edited by J. A. Dodge, D. J. H. Brock and J. H. Widdicombe

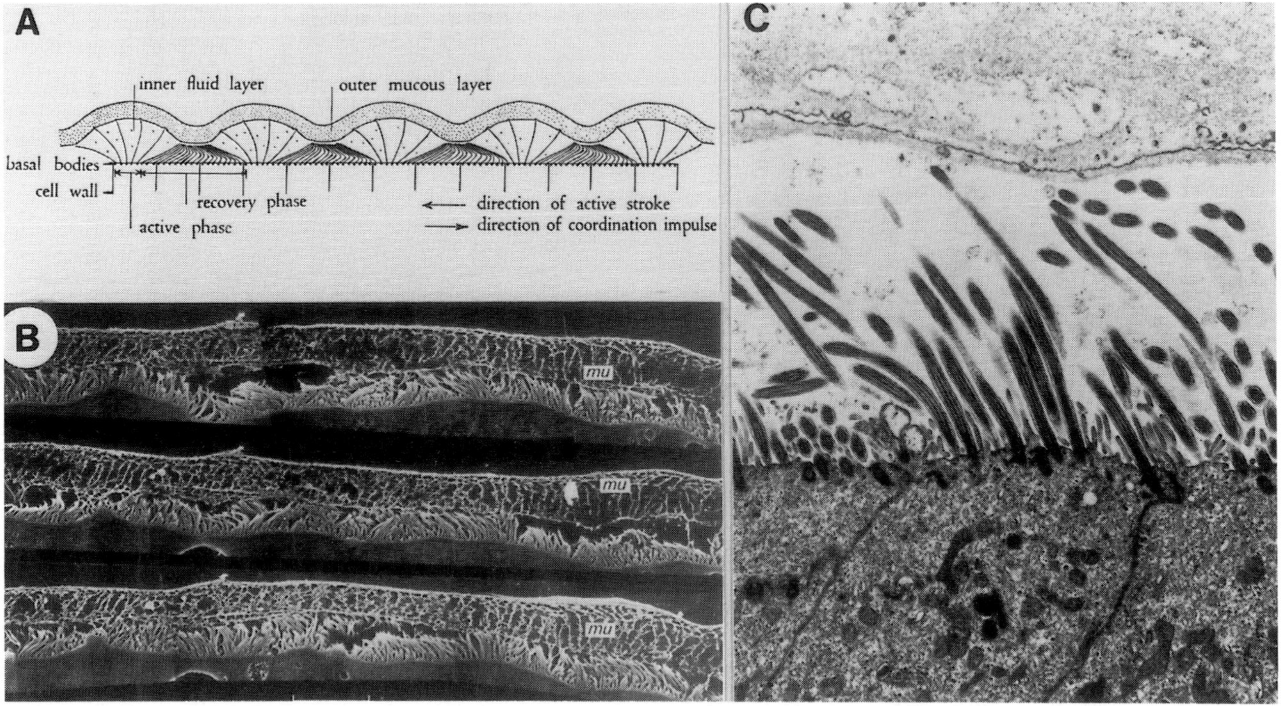


**Figure 1** The two-layer hypothesis for airway secretions. (A) As originally proposed by Lucas and Douglas. (Reproduced from Lucas and Douglas[7], with permission.) (B) Two layers as revealed by electron microscopy of rat trachea. (Reproduced from Yoneda[9], with permission.) (C) Two layers seen in rapidly frozen preparations from rabbit tracheal cultures. (Reproduced from Sanderson and Sleigh[10], with permission)

Visual inspection of the surface of monkey nasal mucosa led Lucas and Douglas[7] to propose that the airway lining fluid consisted of two layers, with a mucous blanket lying on top of a watery sol bathing the cilia (see Figure 1A). They suggested that the periciliary fluid was of low viscosity and almost exactly the same depth as the length of the cilia. The cilia were able to beat in this layer, and during their effective strokes their tips contacted the underside of the mucous blanket and propelled it forward. Later, two layers were clearly demonstrated in several electron microscopical studies[8,9] (see Figure 1B). However, perhaps the most convincing evidence for a periciliary sol layer comes from studies in which explant cultures of rabbit trachea were fixed by rapid freezing[10] (Figure 1C). As fixation occurred within a few milliseconds, it seems unlikely that the periciliary sol layer was an artifact of the fixation procedure.

## ACTIVE TRANSPORT OF IONS AND WATER ACROSS SURFACE EPITHELIUM OF HUMAN AIRWAYS

Active fluid transport across epithelia is secondary to active transepithelial transport of solutes, which creates local concentration gradients across the epithelium and results in fluid movement by osmosis[11]. Such directional solute transport is believed to play a critical role in mucociliary clearance by altering the depth of the periciliary sol layer and/or the hydration of the mucous gel.

The major active ion transport process of surface epithelia from the nose[12], trachea[13] and bronchi[14] of humans is amiloride-sensitive absorption of Na. This makes the airway lumen electrically negative (by 10–30 mV), inducing net passive movement of Cl towards the submucosa, probably via the paracellular pathway. The resulting transfer of salt is believed to create an osmotic gradient locally across the epithelium which results in fluid absorption. In human airways, Cl secretion can be transiently induced by mediators such as isoproterenol, bradykinin, UTP and ATP[13,15,16]. Active secretion of Cl is expected to promote secretion of fluid into the airway lumen.

We have developed cultures of surface epithelium from human trachea, which show ion transport and ultrastructure similar to those of the original tissues[13]. Active transport of fluid across these cultures has recently been measured[17] by a double-sided capacitance probe technique that has an accuracy of ±1 nl/min[18,19]. In this technique, a sheet of epithelium is mounted between two lucite half-chambers. Probes detect the capacitance between their tips and the menisci of the fluid in both the mucosal and serosal reservoirs. Movement of fluid across the epithelium is registered as equal and opposite changes in the capacitance sensed by the serosal and mucosal probes. Transepithelial potential difference (PD) is recorded continuously, and estimates of transepithelial resistance are made at regular intervals from the voltage deflections caused by transepithelial current pulses of known magnitude.

With this apparatus, we[17] found a baseline fluid absorption of 2.3 ± 0.3 (20 cultured cell sheets from 11 tracheae) and 4.4 ± 0.6 μl/cm$^2$ per hour (eight cell sheets from four tracheae) across non-CF nasal and tracheal epithelial cultures, respectively. These rates of absorption are reasonably close to those predicted from open-circuit fluxes across human nasal and bronchial epithelia. In the bronchus, the rates of absorption of Na and Cl under open-circuit conditions (i.e. with the tissue at its spontaneous transepithelial PD) are 1.2 ± 0.31 and 0.46 ± 0.25 μl/cm$^2$ per hour, respectively[14]. These values are

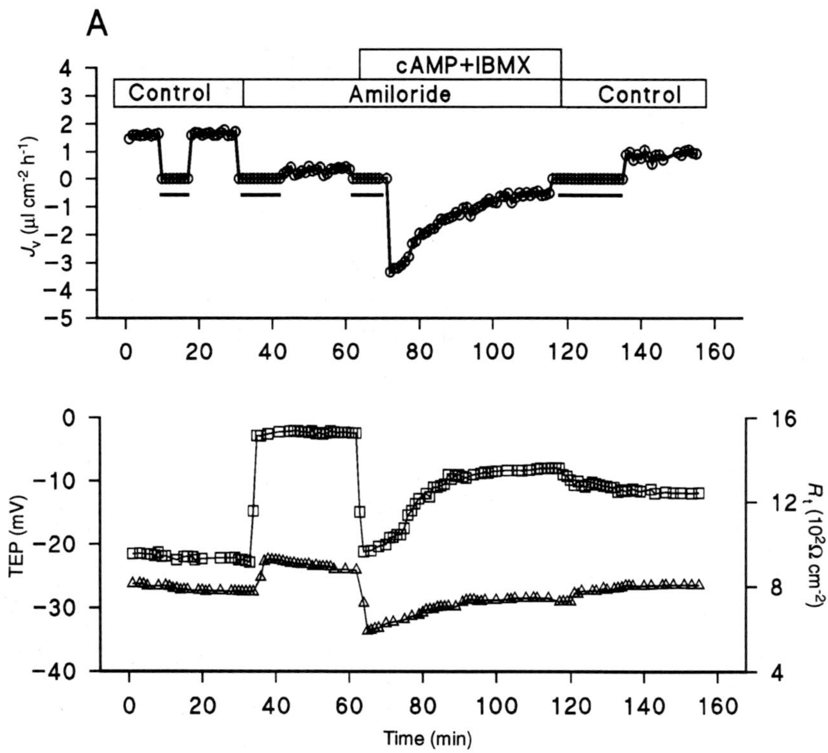


**Figure 2** Effects of amiloride, cAMP-elevating agents (CPT–cAMP and IBMX) and ATP on transepithelial volume flow ($J_v$), transepithelial resistance ($R_t$) and transepithelial potential difference (TEP) across human nasal epithelial cultures from non-CF subjects. (A) In the control period $J_v$ was from the luminal to serosal side of the cell sheet at 1.6 μl/cm$^2$ per hour. During the control period, the capacitance probes were removed (horizontal bar) and old medium replaced with fresh. This caused no changes in $J_v$, $R_t$ or TEP. At 30 min, the probes were removed again in order to allow

not statistically different, and assuming that they reflect absorption of isotonic NaCl solution, then they predict fluid absorption of 3–8 μl/cm² per hour. Smith and Welsh[20] reported rates of fluid absorption across cultures of human tracheal epithelium which were 1/10 to 1/50 those obtained by us. In their experiments, 100 μl of culture medium was added to the mucosal side of a monolayer; it was covered with mineral oil to prevent evaporation, and the volume of fluid remaining after 24 h was measured. During this period, large pH and electrolyte gradients developed that could have altered active ion and fluid transport. In our experiments, volume flow and biolectric properties are continuously measured in mucosal and serosal solutions of identical composition with a time resolution of ⩽1 min.

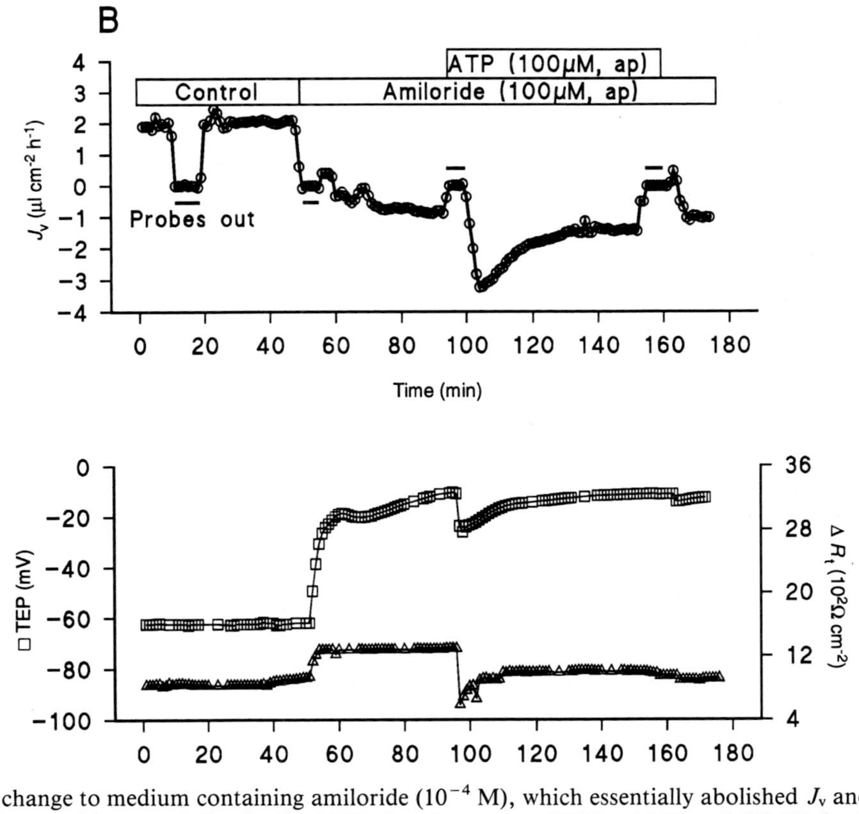


a change to medium containing amiloride ($10^{-4}$ M), which essentially abolished $J_v$ and TEP, and increased $R_t$. Cyclic AMP-elevating agents (CPT–cAMP and IBMX, both at $10^{-4}$ M in the luminal bath) induced secretion, increased TEP and reduced $R_t$, all changes consistent with stimulation of Cl secretion. On returning to drug-free medium, $J_v$ returned to 1 μl/cm² per hour. (B) In a culture from another individual, amiloride again reduced $J_v$ to zero, and ATP ($10^{-4}$ M, mucosal bath) produced a steady-state secretion of −2.2 μl/cm² per hour. (Reproduced from Jiang et al.[17], with permission)

We found that baseline fluid absorption was reduced by 90% (nasal) or 85% (tracheal) by mucosal amiloride. In both nasal and tracheal cultures, UTP, ATP or elevation of intracellular cAMP by addition of 8-(4-chlorophenylthio)cAMP(CPT-cAMP) and isobutyl-methylxanthine (IBMX) all led to transient induction of fluid secretion (~1–2 μl/cm$^2$ per hour. Representative tracings for nasal cultures are shown in Figure 2. Exactly similar results were obtained with tracheal cultures.

In the absence of other pathways for fluid movement, fluid absorption of 3–5 μl/cm$^2$ per hour will decrease the depth of the mucus layers at ~1 μm/min.

## GLAND FLUID SECRETION

Submucosal glands are the major source of the mucus needed for effective mucociliary clearance of inhaled particles. In human trachea, the combined volume of mucus-secreting cells in the glands has been estimated as 40 times that of the combined volume of surface goblet cells[21]. The glands consist of two or three orders of tubules, branching from a main duct and ending in secretory acini. Acini are lined with serous cells, characterized by electro-opaque granules, whereas the proximal ducts are lined with mucous cells, containing larger, electron-lucent secretory granules[22]. A typical gland, reconstructed from serial light microscopic sections[23], is illustrated in Figure 3. Glands are found only in the cartilaginous airways (i.e. trachea and bronchi), where they lie between neighbouring cartilaginous rings and between the rings and the epithelium[24,25]. They are found on both the luminal and serosal side of airway smooth muscle. By 25–28 weeks of gestation, the maximal number of between 3500 and 6000 glands are present in the trachea[26]. At birth, this corresponds to a gland density of ~10/mm$^2$, which with growth declines to an adult density of ~1/mm$^2$. Glands are essentially completely differentiated at birth, are evenly distributed along and around the trachea, and are found in approximately equal numbers in men and women[26].

The major secretory cells of the gland acini are the mucous and serous cells. The distal location of serous relative to mucous cells suggests that the former secrete fluid which helps to 'flush-out' mucus secreted by the latter There is other indirect evidence for a role of serous cells in fluid secretion. First, though glands exist which contain only serous acini[27,28], no glands consist entirely of mucous acini; acini consisting predominantly of mucous cells also show a terminal cluster or 'demilune' of associated serous cells[28]. Second, in the cat, gland secretions collected following stimulation with $\alpha$-adrenergic agents are more watery than baseline or cholinergically stimulated secretions, having lower protein content and viscosity[29,30]. Morphometric studies on airway glands in the ferret (an animal in the same taxonomic order as the cat) have shown that $\alpha$-adrenergic agents selectively degranulate serous cells[31]. Third,

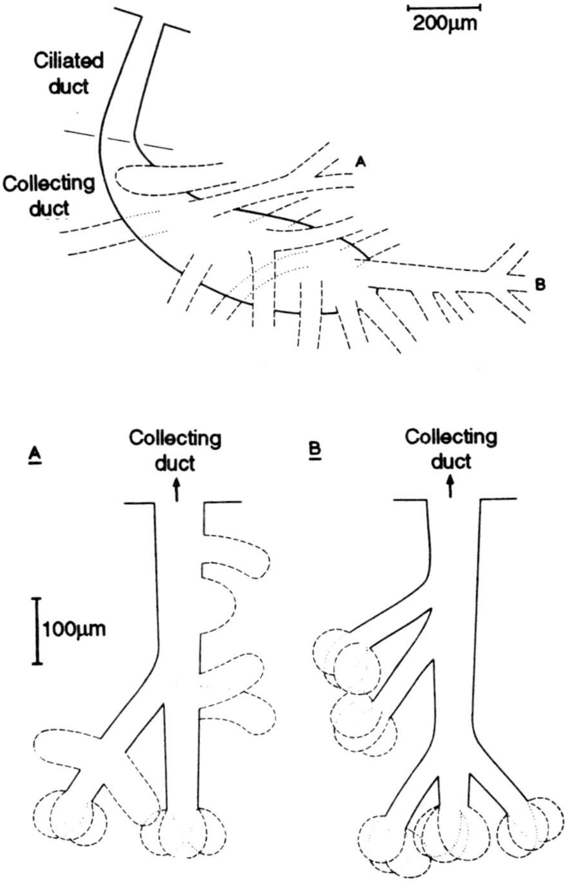


**Figure 3** Reconstruction of human submucosal gland from serial cross sections. Top: the collecting duct and its major branches. The gland opened onto the surface epithelium via a ciliated duct which joined a 'collecting duct'. This latter contained no ciliated cells and was of larger diameter than the ciliated duct. The collecting duct received 13 major secretory tubules. Bottom: secretory tubules. Each tubule branched two to three times. Areas lined by mucous cells are shown by solid lines; dashed lines denote serous cells. The location of the secretory tubules in relation to the collecting duct is indicated by 'A' and 'B'. (Reproduced from Meyrick et al.[23], with permission)

serous gland cells have the highest levels of the cystic fibrosis conductance regulator (CFTR) of any airway cell type[32]. CFTR is a cAMP-activated apical membrane Cl channel[33] believed to underlie transepithelial Cl and fluid secretion. Finally, a prominent feature of the serous cells is their intercellular canaliculi[22,34,35]. These tubes of about 1 μm diameter are extensions of the acinar lumen which pass between the lateral aspects of the cells. Apical membrane, containing abundant microvilli, lines these canaliculi, and is separated from the cells' basolateral membranes by typical tight junctions. By increasing the apical membrane surface area they may contribute to serous cell fluid secretion.

Serous cells are a source of endogenous antibiotics, and secrete in addition a number of compounds which protect the airway surface from the harmful effects of bacterial and neutrophil proteases[36]. In fact, most non-mucin proteins in airway secretions probably originate from the serous cells. Based on cytochemical[37] and immunocytochemical[38,39] data, the major secretory component of mucous gland cells is mucins. Mucins have not been conclusively demonstrated in serous cells[39,40].

Light microscopical autoradiography has shown that acetylcholine induces secretion from both mucous and serous cells of human tracheal submucosal glands[41]. Measurements of release of high molecular weight, $^{35}SO_4$-labelled material have also shown that cholinergic agents stimulate gland secretion, but that $\alpha$- and $\beta$-adrenergic agents are somewhat less potent secretagogues[42–44]. Other agents known to stimulate gland mucous secretion in human airways include arachidonic acid, prostaglandin $A_2$ ($PGA_2$), $PGD_2$, $PGF_{2\alpha}$, mono-HETE, leukotrienes $LTC_4$ and $LTD_4$, PGF-A histamine and neutrophil elastase[45,46].

Little is known about the mechanism of fluid secretion by submucosal glands. Yang et al.[47] showed that isolated swine gland cells actively accumulate Cl and that this process is inhibited by loop diuretics—inhibitors of Na-linked Cl entry across the basolateral membrane[48]. These results suggest that fluid transport by gland acini is due to the same Na-dependent Cl secretion as present in the airway surface epithelium and other mammalian Cl-secreting epithelia[49].

Quantitative estimates of human gland secretory rates have not been made. However, Quinton[50] covered the surface of cat trachea with mineral oil and then collected the droplets that formed at the duct openings. Though fluid output was essentially zero in the resting state ($<1$ nl/min), cholinergic and $\alpha$-adrenergic agents induced fluid secretion of $\sim 10$ nl/min. The $\beta$-adrenergic agent isoproterenol was a less effective secretagogue. Similar flow rates were obtained by Ueki et al.[51], who placed the fire-polished tips of glass microcapillaries directly over the duct openings of cat tracheal glands and collected secretions. Assuming similar flow rates in human glands and a gland density of $1/mm^2$ [26], then maximal gland secretion in human airways amounts to 60 $\mu l/cm^2$ per hour. In the absence of other routes of fluid movement across the airway wall, gland secretion would increase the depth of the mucous layers at $\sim 10$ $\mu m/min$.

## PASSIVE FLUID FLOWS

Active transport of solutes is not the only factor regulating fluid movement across airway epithelium. In addition to the local osmotic gradients set up by active solute transport, fluid will flow in response to bulk differences in osmotic pressure between the interstitial and luminal fluids. Transepithelial hydrostatic pressure gradients may also contribute to fluid flow. Finally, the dense packing of the cilia themselves may generate significant forces of capillarity tending to hold fluid in the airway lumen.

However visualized, the depth of the periciliary sol layer has always been about the same as the length of the cilia. Attempts were not made in these experiments to alter ion transport across the surface epithelium, but this constant depth of the periciliary sol phase suggests that forces other than active fluid transport may be controlling its depth. One possibility is that ciliary motion has a thixotropic or liquefying action on mucus[52]. However, the sol layer does not react with dyes that stain the mucous gel[7]. Another more likely possibility[53] is that the sol layer is produced by capillary (surface tension) forces generated by the presence of the cilia. There are about eight cilia per $\mu m^2$ of apical membrane[54]. The diameter of the ciliary shaft is ~200 nm. In a cross-section through the ciliary bed at right angles to the ciliary shafts, there will therefore be 600 m of ciliary plasma membrane per square centimetre of apical surface area. Assuming a zero contact angle, and a surface tension of 25 mN/m, J. G. Widdicombe[55] has calculated that the forces of capillarity between the cilia generate a pressure holding fluid in place equivalent to a transepithelial concentration gradient of ~40 mOsm (assuming a reflection coefficient of one). This is probably considerably greater than the local osmotic gradient generated by active absorption of Na[11], and suggests that as long as there are cilia there will be a periciliary sol.

The submucosal hydrostatic pressure in airways is not known. However, at least during inflammation[56] and asthma[57], the widespread dilation of the lateral intercellular spaces (LIS) suggests that it is positive[58], and should drive fluid into the lumen. Even small pressure gradients (<5 $cmH_2O$) directed towards the lumen will dilate the LIS and disrupt tight junctions of airway and other epithelia causing radical increases in the hydraulic conductivity (the ratio of fluid flow to hydrostatic pressure)[59–61]. In gallbladder, for instance, a 10 $cmH_2O$ pressure gradient directed towards the lumen caused volume flows some 100-fold greater than the same pressure gradient directed towards the submucosa[60]. LIS are generally collapsed in healthy airways, suggesting that in the absence of inflammatory exudates the interstitial pressure in the submucosa may be negative (in other tissues it averages ~ −2 mmHg[62]), tending to produce small flows of fluid towards the submucosa.

Transepithelial osmotic pressures gradients are hard to estimate; sampling and measurement of the ion contents of airway lining fluid are made difficult by the small volume of this fluid. Airway lining fluid has been sampled *in vivo* by placing filter paper[63,64] or glass-fibre screens[65] on the airway surface, or *in vitro* by allowing secretions to run out of the bottom of the trachea under the influence of gravity[66]. In experimental animals, samples so collected have generally been hyperosmotic (by ~10–15%) to plasma. K levels in secretions collected from dog trachea with filter paper were ~7.5–10-fold greater than plasma[67]. As active K secretion by airway epithelia is negligible[45], K should distribute passively according to the transepithelial PD. For the 30 mV lumen negative PD of dog tracheal epithelium, a three-fold increase above plasma levels is expected for the K content of airway lining fluid. Thus, the unexpectedly high K levels suggest that the filter paper used for sample collection had damaged the epithelium[68], a not surprising conclusion given that the thickness of the filter papers used (160 or 220 μm) is considerably greater than the depth of respiratory tract fluid. Using small filter papers delivered by bronchoscopy, Joris and Quinton[63,69] reported that Na and Cl levels of human airway lining fluid were both 80–90 mM (i.e. considerably less than plasma). Interestingly, in CF, the same authors found Na and Cl levels not significantly different from those of plasma[69].

The forces, both active and passive, regulating fluid movement into and out of the airways are summarized in Figure 4. In healthy airways, active Na absorption, the transepithelial hydrostatic pressure gradient and the bulk

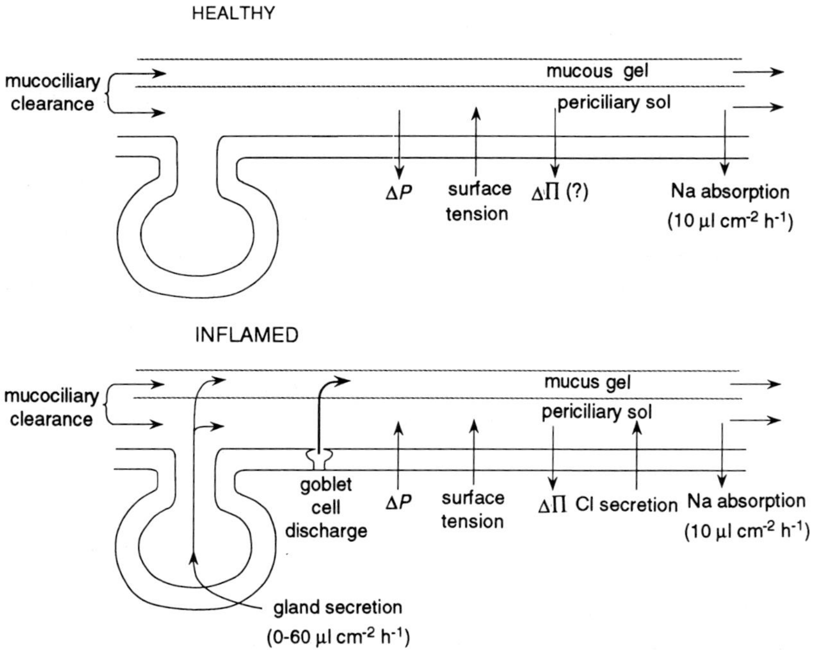


**Figure 4** Routes of fluid movement across airway epithelium. Where they can be made, estimates of fluid flow by the different routes are given

osmotic pressure difference between luminal and interstitial fluid may all favour fluid absorption. The only identifiable force retaining fluid in the airways would seem to be forces of capillarity generated by the closely packed cilia. In asthma and other inflammatory airway diseases, fluid flows in response to elevated submucosal hydrostatic pressure may play the dominant role in airway fluid balance. In addition, inflammatory mediators will induce gland secretion, Cl secretion by the surface epithelium and goblet cell discharge. We speculate that active fluid secretion, by glands or the surface epithelium, is induced focally by inflammatory mediator release in response to irritation, and serves to 'flush out' particles landing on the airways. Constitutive Na absorption in neighbouring regions of the airway then serves to reabsorb the excess fluid secreted.

## CHANGES IN AIRWAY ION AND FLUID TRANSPORT IN CYSTIC FIBROSIS

Elevation of cAMP by $\beta$-adrenergic and other agents is not altered in surface epithelia from CF airways[70-72]. However, whereas these agents induce Cl secretion across non-CF tracheal epithelium, they have essentially no effect on ion transport across CF tissues[13,73]. In addition to this change in Cl transport, amiloride-sensitive absorption of Na is elevated approximately two-fold across both nasal and tracheal cultures in CF[13,17,71].

These changes in ion transport by CF epithelia produce the expected alterations in transepithelial fluid flows[17]. Thus, fluid absorption is elevated in CF, and its inhibition by amiloride is increased (Figure 5). In addition, cAMP-dependent fluid secretion is abolished, whereas ATP- or UTP-induced fluid secretion is unaltered (see Figure 6). The combination of decreased cAMP-dependent fluid Cl secretion and increased Na absorption in CF should remove fluid from the lumen of the airways, and impair mucociliary clearance by reducing the depth of the periciliary sol, and by condensing the mucous blanket.

Involvement of airway glands in CF is suggested by the finding that the earliest detectable structural change in the airways of patients with CF is a dilation of the gland lumina[74], which becomes marked as the disease progresses. More recently, Dwyer and Farley[75] have presented indirect evidence, obtained with the Cl-sensitive fluorescent probe, SPQ[76], that the Cl permeability of human gland cells from patients with CF is less than normal.

We have investigated the possible involvement of glands in CF using cultures of airway submucosal glands[77]. The glandular origin of these cultures was demonstrated by immunocytochemical localization of antibodies to gland cells of native epithelium, as well as to lysosome and lactoferrin—known secretory products of serous gland cells[78,79]. They also contain proteins, e.g.

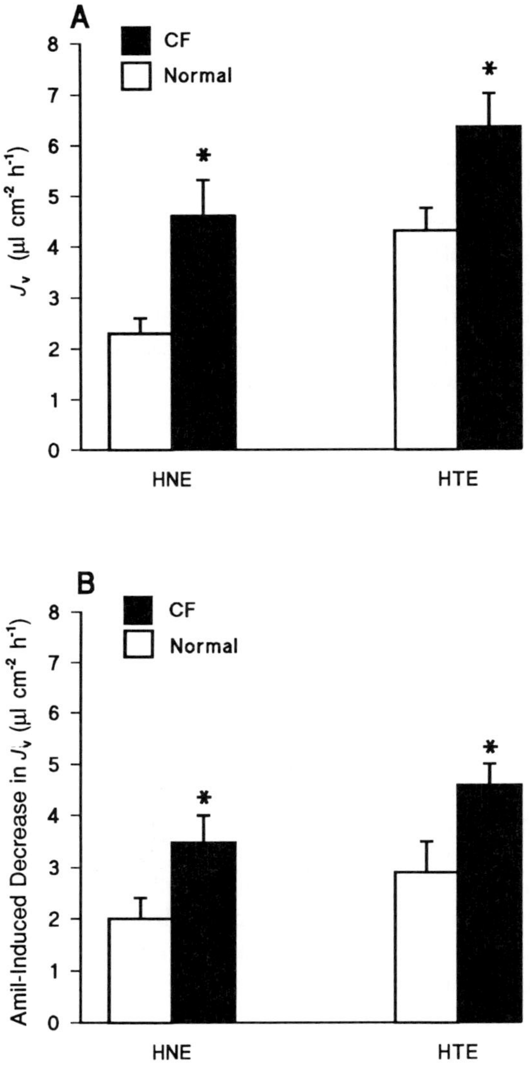


**Figure 5** (A) Comparison of baseline unstimulated $J_v$ for nasal (HNE) and tracheal (HTE) cultures from individuals with and without CF. For HNE: six cultures from four CF patients and 20 cultures from 11 individuals without CF. For HTE: six cultures from three CF patients and eight cultures from four individuals without CF. Mean values for $R_t$ and TEP were: −42 mV and 1140 Ω cm$^2$ (HNE, CF), −25 mV and 1072 Ω cm$^2$ (HNE, non-CF), −53 mV and 1240 Ω cm$^2$ (HTE, CF), −31 mV and 1123 Ω cm$^2$ (HTE, non-CF). For both HNE and HTE the mean values for TEP were significantly increased in the CF cultures (Student's $t$ test). (B) Comparison of the amiloride-induced decrease in $J_v$ in CF and non-CF cultures. (Data are presented as mean ± s.e.m. and asterisks indicate $P < 0.05$ between CF and non-CF, Student's $t$ test). (Reproduced from Jiang et al.[17], with permission)

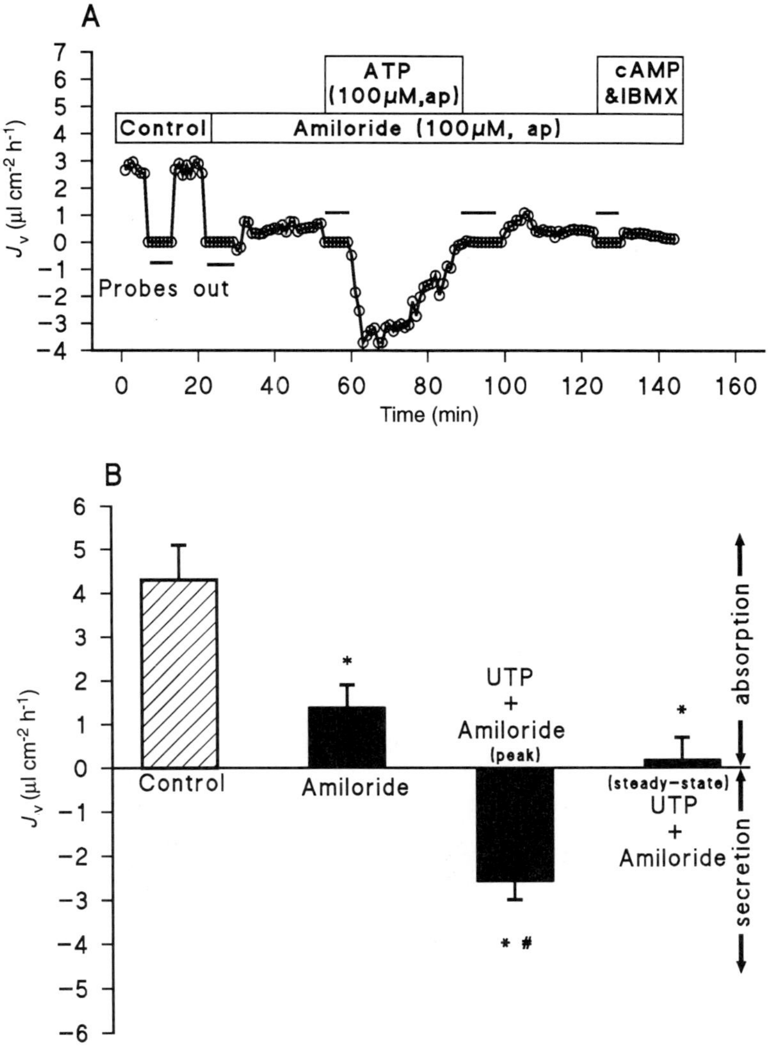


**Figure 6** Effects of amiloride, ATP (or UTP) and the combination of CPT–cAMP and IBMX on $J_v$ in CF nasal cultures. (A) Typical record. The starting $J_v$, TEP and $R_t$ were ~ 3 μl/cm$^2$ per hour, 10 mV and 1000 Ω cm$^2$. Addition of amiloride reduced $J_v$ to 0.5 μl/cm$^2$ per hour. ATP caused secretion of similar magnitude (3 μl/cm$^2$ per hour) and duration as in non-CF cultures (see Figure 2). However cAMP-elevating agents had no effect on $J_v$, $R_t$ or TEP. Changes in electrical properties in response to amiloride and ATP were similar to those observed in non-CF cultures (see Figure 2). (B) Summary of six experiments with nasal cultures from four CF patients. Cultures were treated sequentially with amiloride and UTP. ($^*P < 0.01$ compared with control; $^{\#}P < 0.01$ compared with value with amiloride alone, ANOVA). Mean control levels of TEP and $R_t$ were $-39$ mV and 1210 Ω cm$^2$. (Reproduced from Jiang et al.[17], with permission)

mucins, characteristic of mucous gland cells. These 'seromucous' gland cultures contain levels of CFTR approximately equal to those of $T_{84}$ cells as determined by immunocytochemistry[80], and by immunoprecipitation with an antibody to the C-terminal of CFTR (Genzyme) followed by phosphorylation with the catalytic subunit of protein kinase A (see Figure 7). When grown on porous supports, and studied in Ussing chambers, non-CF cultures had baseline transepithelial resistance ($R_{te}$) and short-circuit current ($I_{sc}$, a measure of total transepithelial active ion transport) of 600 Ω $cm^2$ and 12 $\mu A/cm^2$ [81]. $I_{sc}$ was transiently increased by methacholine, bradykinin, isoproterenol and histamine. As illustrated in Figure 8, amiloride (an Na transport blocker) decreased baseline $I_{sc}$ by 48 ± 8% ($n = 5$), but had little effect on the $I_{sc}$ response to mediators. Diphenylamine-2-carboxylic acid (a blocker of Cl

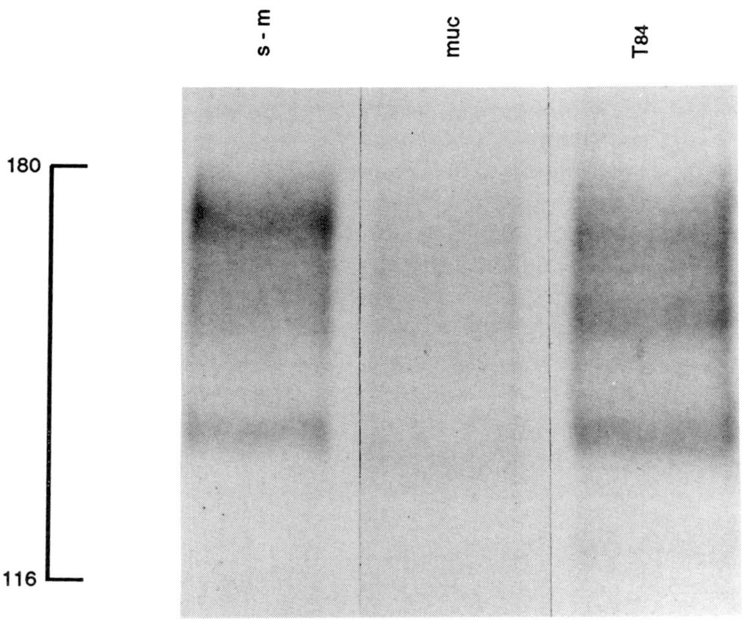


**Figure 7** Levels of CFTR in gland cultures. A mouse monoclonal to the final four amino acids of the C-terminal (Genzyme, Cambridge, MA) was added to lysate (600 μg of protein), and the immunoprecipitate labelled with $^{32}PO_4$ using the catalytic subunit of protein kinase A, run out on an SDS–PAGE gel, and CFTR was detected by autoradiography. Vertical scale gives molecular weight in kilodaltons. s-m = seromucous gland cell cultures; muc = mucous gland cell cultures—these are primary cultures of human gland cells that contain typical mucous granules, do not stain immunocytochemically for serous cell markers, and show much lower levels of Cl secretion than seromucous cells.[88]. T84 = $T_{84}$ cells—a human colonic carcinoma cell line which secretes Cl. Seromucous and mucous cell cultures were derived from the same tracheas

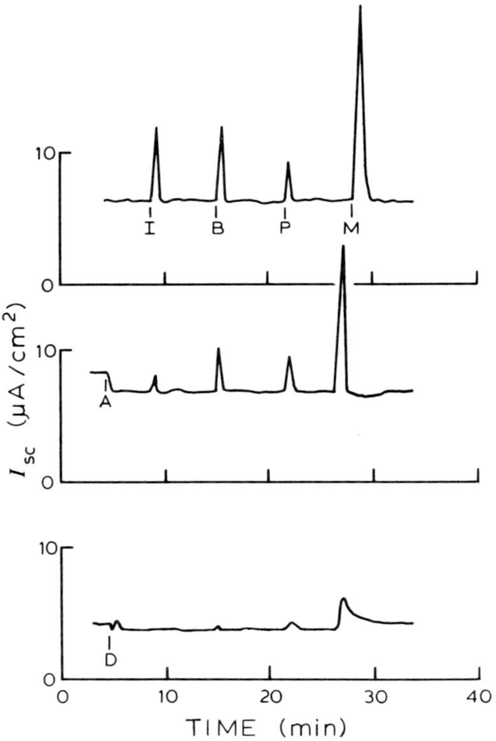


**Figure 8** Mediator-induced Cl secretion across cultures of human submucosal glands. Top: short-circuit current responses in absence of inhibitor. Middle: effects of amiloride. Bottom: effects of DPAC. Tissues from the same culture. Key: A, $10^{-5}$ M amiloride; D, $10^{-3}$ M diphenylamine-2-carboxylate; I, $10^{-5}$ M isoproterenol; B, $10^{-6}$ M bradykinin; P, $10^{-5}$ M phenylephrine; M, $10^{-5}$ M methacholine. Mediators were added in the same sequence and at approximately the same times in all three traces. (Reproduced from Yamaya et al.[81], with permission)

transport), however, had no effect on baseline $I_{sc}$ but markedly inhibited the responses to all mediators. These results suggest that the mediator-induced increases in $I_{sc}$ are due to Cl secretion.

CF submucosal gland cell cultures had $R_{te}$ and baseline $I_{sc}$ similar to those of non-CF. However, we found that the $I_{sc}$ responses to mediators of cultured cell sheets from two CF tracheas were $\leqslant 5\%$ those of non-CF cultures[82]. Experiments of this type have now been performed on cultures from several additional CF tracheas (all homo- or heterozygous for ΔF508) and the results, which essentially confirm our earlier findings, are summarized in Figure 9. That loss of mediator-induced Cl secretion is only partial in CF may reflect the fact that all agents tested elevate Ca in tracheal cultures[83], and that this

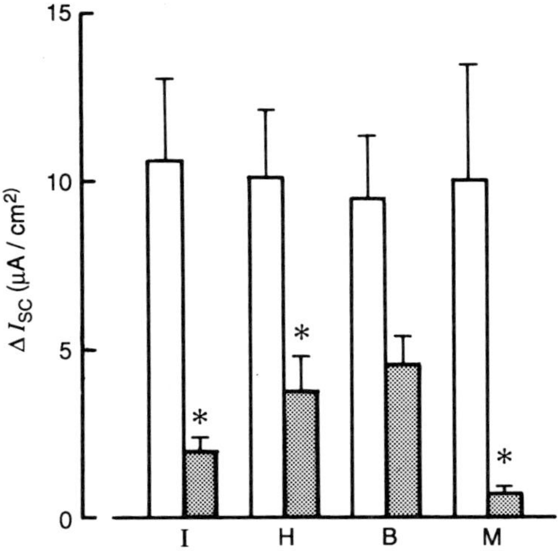


**Figure 9** Pooled data on maximal increases in $I_{sc}$ induced by mediators across seromucous gland cell cultures. Open columns: non-CF cultures (22 cell sheets from seven tracheas). Shaded columns: CF cultures (11 cell sheets from five tracheas). I, isoproterenol ($10^{-5}$ M); H, histamine ($10^{-5}$ M); B, bradykinin ($10^{-7}$ M); M, methacholine ($10^{-5}$ M). Means ± SEM, $^{*}P < 0.05$, Student's $t$ test

elevation of $[Ca^{2+}]_i$ is unaltered in CF (Shen and Widdicombe, unpublished data). Thus, the increases in $I_{sc}$ in CF cultures may reflect activation of apical membrane Ca-dependent anion channels.

In preliminary experiments[84], we have measured fluid flows across these gland cultures using the double-sided capacitance probe technique. CF cultures differed from non-CF in that the secretory response to cAMP-elevating agents was absent. By contrast, UTP stimulated secretion across both CF and non-CF cultures.

The absence of cAMP-mediated gland Cl secretion in CF will result in reduced hydration of gland mucins, which may be inadequately flushed out from the glands. They may therefore build up slowly, leading to the dilation of the gland lumina previously reported[74]. On reaching the surface, the gland mucins may fail to detach completely from the duct openings, or their dehydration may lead to inefficient mucociliary clearance[3]. Thus, the initial build-up of mucus in CF may reflect an abnormality in ion transport by the glands rather than the surface epithelium (see Figure 10).

Recently, transgenic mice have been developed in which the mouse CF gene has been disrupted by insertion of DNA[85–87]. Mouse airways differ from those of humans in many ways, of which one of the most noticeable is the lack of submucosal glands. Interestingly, 'CF mice' show relatively minor airway pathology, dying instead of gastrointestinal malfunction. This result supports

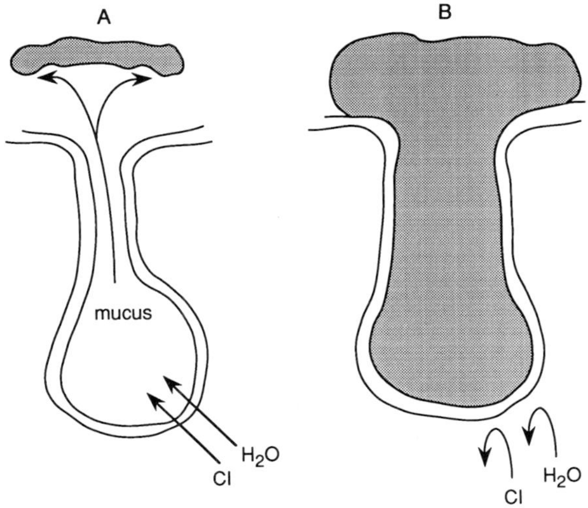


**Figure 10** Model for failure of mucociliary clearance in CF. (A) Normal gland. Chloride secretion mediates acinar fluid secretion which flushes mucins from the gland. (B) CF. Failure of acini to secrete Cl and fluid leads to build-up of dehydrated mucus in gland lumen, which distends. The dehydrated mucus may fail to detach from the duct opening or may be inefficiently cleared by the cilia, leading to its progressive build-up.

our hypothesis that submucosal glands are major contributors to the airway pathology of humans. However, it should be pointed out that the CF mice have not been studied beyond 40 days after birth, and in two out of three studies were reared in pathogen-free conditions.

## REFERENCES


1 Braga PC, Allegra L (eds). *Methods in Bronchial Mucology*. Raven Press, New York, 1988.
2 Silberberg A. Models of mucus structure. In: *Methods in Bronchial Mucology* (eds PC Braga, L Allegra) Raven Press, New York. 1988, pp 51–61;
3 King M. Mucus and mucociliary clearance. *Basics of RD* 1982; **11**: 1–7.
4 Yeates DB, Aspin N, Levison H, et al. Mucociliary tracheal transport rates in man. *J Appl Physiol* 1975; **39**: 487–95.
5 Wanner A. Mucociliary clearance in the trachea. *Clin Chest Med* 1986; **7**: 247–58.
6 Bhaskar KR, O'Sullivan DD, Seltzer J et al. Density gradient study of bronchial mucus aspirates from healthy volunteers (smokers and nonsmokers) and from patients with tracheostomy. *Exp Lung Res* 1985; **9**: 289–308.
7 Lucas AM, Douglas LC. Principles underlying ciliary activity in the respiratory tract. II. A comparison of nasal clearance in man, monkey and other mammals. *Arch Otolaryngol* 1934; **20**: 518–41.

8 Reissig M, Bang BG, Bang FB. Ultrastructure of the mucociliary interface in the nasal mucosa of chicken. *Am Rev Respir Dis* 1978; **117**: 327–41.
9 Yoneda K. Mucous blanket of rat bronchus: ultrastructural study. *Am Rev Respir Dis* 1976; **114**: 837–42.
10 Sanderson MJ, Sleigh MA. Ciliary activity of cultured rabbit tracheal epithelium: beat pattern and metachrony. *J Cell Sci* 1981; **47**: 331–47.
11 Diamond JM. Osmotic water flow in leaky epithelia. *J Membr Biol* 1979; **51**: 195–216.
12 Knowles M, Stutts MJ, Spock A, et al. Abnormal ion permeation through cystic fibrosis respiratory epithelium. *Science* 1983; **221**: 1067–70.
13 Yamaya M, Finkbeiner WE, Chun SY, Widdicombe JH. Differentiated structure and function of cultures from human tracheal epithelium. *Am J Physiol* 1992; **262**: L713–24.
14 Knowles MR, Murray GF, Shallal JA, et al. Bioelectric properties and ion flow across excised human bronchi. *J Appl Physiol* 1984; **56**: 868–77.
15 Stutts MJ, Chinet TC, Mason SJ, et al. Regulation of $Cl^-$ channels in normal and cystic fibrosis airway epithelial cells by extracellular ATP. *Proc Natl Acad Sci USA* 1992; **89**: 1621–5.
16 Boucher RC, Cheng EH, Paradiso AM, et al. Chloride secretory response of cystic fibrosis human airway epithelia: preservation of calcium but not protein kinase C- and A-dependent mechanisms. *J Clin Invest* 1989; 1424–31.
17 Jiang C, Finkbeiner WE, Widdicombe JH, et al. Altered fluid transport across airway epithelium in cystic fibrosis. *Science* 1993; **262**: 424–7.
18 Hughes BA, Miller SS, Machen TE. Effects of cyclic AMP on fluid absorption and ion transport across frog retinal pigment epithelium. *J Gen Physiol* 1984; **83**: 875–99.
19 Edelman JL, Miller SS. Epinephrine stimulates fluid absorption across bovine retinal pigment epithelium. *Invest Ophthalmol Vis Sci* 1991; **32**: 3033–40.
20 Smith J, Welsh M. Fluid and electrolyte transport by cultured human airway epithelia. *J Clin Invest* 1992; **91**: 1590–7.
21 Reid L. Measurement of the bronchial mucous gland layer: a diagnostic yardstick in chronic bronchitis. *Thorax* 1960; **15**: 132–41.
22 Meyrick B, Reid L. Ultrastructure of cells in human bronchial submucosal glands. *J Anat* 1970; **107**: 291–9.
23 Meyrick B, Sturgess JM, Reid L. A reconstruction of the duct system and secretory tubules of the human bronchial submucosal gland. *Thorax* 1969; **24**: 729–36.
24 Goco RV, Kress MB, Brantigan OC. Comparison of mucus glands in the tracheobronchial tree of man and animals. *Ann NY Acad Sci* 1963; **106**: 555–71.
25 Korhonen LK, Holopainen E, Paavolainen M. Some histochemical characteristics of tracheobronchial tree and pulmonary neoplasms. *Acta Histochem* 1969; **32**: 57–73.
26 Tos M. Development of the tracheal glands in man. *Acta Pathol Microbiol Scand* 1966 (Suppl 185): 1–130.
27 Wells U, Widdicombe JG. Lateral nasal gland secretion in the anaesthetized dog. *J Physiol* 1986; **374**: 359–74.
28 Leeson CR. Structure of salivary glands. In: *Handbook of Physiology, Section 6: Alimentary Canal* (ed CF Code) American Physiological Society, Washington, DC, 1967, pp 463–95.
29 Leikauf GD, Ueki IF, Nadel JA. Selective autonomic regulation of the viscoelastic properties of submucosal gland secretions from cat trachea. *J Appl Physiol* 1984; **56**: 426–30.

30 Ueki I, Nadel JA. Differences in total protein concentration in submucosal gland fluid: α-adrenergic vs cholinergic. *Fed Proc* 1981; **40**: 622.
31 Basbaum CB, Ueki I, Brezina L, Nadel JA. Tracheal submucosal gland serous cells stimulated in vitro with adrenergic and cholinergic agonists: a morphometric study. *Cell Tissue Res* 1981; **220**: 481–98.
32 Engelhardt JF, Yankaskas JR, Ernst SA, et al. Submucosal glands are the predominant site of CFTR expression in the human bronchus. *Nature Genet* 1992; **2**: 240–7.
33 Widdicombe JH, Wine JJ. The basic defect in cystic fibrosis. *TIBS* 1991; **16**: 474–77.
34 Sorokin SP. On the cytology and cytochemistry of the opossum's bronchial glands. *Am J Anat* 1965; **117**: 311–38.
35 Tandler B. Ultrastructure of the human submaxillary glands. I. Architecture and histological relationships of the secretory cell. *Am J Anat* 1962; **111**: 287–307.
36 Basbaum CB, Jany B, Finkbeiner WE. The serous cell. *Annu Rev Physiol* 1990; **52**: 97–113.
37 Spicer SS, Schulte BA, Chakrin LW. Ultrastructural and histochemical observations of respiratory epithelium and gland. *Exp Lung Res* 1983; **4**: 137–56.
38 Jany BH, Gallup WM, Yan PS, et al. Human bronchus and intestine express the same mucin gene. *J Clin Invest* 1991; **87**: 77–82.
39 Perini JM, Marianne T, Lafitte JJ, et al. Use of an antiserum against deglycosylated human mucins for cellular localization of their peptide precursors: antigenic similarities between bronchial and intestinal mucins. *J Histochem Cytochem* 1989; **37**: 869–75.
40 Audie JP, Janin A, Porchet N, et al. Expression of mucin genes in respiratory, digestive, and reproductive tracts ascertained by *in situ* hybridization. *J Histochem Cytochem* 1993; **41**: 1479–85.
41 Sturgess J, Reid L. An organ culture study of the effect of drugs on the secretory activity of the human submucosal gland. *Clin Sci* 1972; **43**: 533–43.
42 Phipps RJ, Richardson PS, Pack RJ, Wright N. Sympathomimetic drugs stimulate the output of secretory glycoproteins from human bronchi *in vitro*. *Clin Sci* 1982; **63**: 23–8.
43 Shelhamer JH, Marom Z, Kaliner M. Immunologic and neuropharmacologic stimulation of mucous glycoprotein release from human airways *in vitro*. *J Clin Invest* 1980; **66**: 1400–8.
44 Baker B, Peatfield AC, Richardson PS. Nervous control of mucin secretion into human bronchi. *J Physiol* 1985; **365**: 297–305.
45 Finkbeiner WE, Widdicombe JH. Control of nasal airway secretions, ion transport, and water movement. In: *Treatise on Pulmonary Toxicology. Vol 1. Comparative Biology of the Normal Lung* (ed RA Parent) CRC Press, Boca Raton, FL, 1992, pp 633–57.
46 Schuster A, Ueki I, Nadel JA. Neutrophil elastase stimulates tracheal submucosal gland secretion that is inhibited by ICI 200,355. *Am J Physiol* 1992; **262**: L86–91.
47 Yang CM, Farley JM, Dwyer TM. Acetylcholine-stimulated chloride flux in tracheal submucosal gland cells. *J Appl Physiol* 1988; **65**: 1891–4.
48 O'Grady SM, Palfrey HC, Field M. Characteristics and functions of Na–K–Cl cotransport in epithelial tissues. *Am J Physiol* 1987; **253**: C177–92.
49 Frizzell RA, Field M, Schultz SG. Sodium-coupled chloride transport by epithelial tissues. *Am J Physiol* 1979; **236**: F1–8.
50 Quinton PM. Composition and control of secretions from tracheal bronchial submucosal glands. *Nature* 1979; **279**: 551–2.

51 Ueki I, German VF, Nadel J. Micropipette measurement of airway submucosal gland secretion: autonomic effects. *Am Rev Respir Dis* 1980; **121**: 351–7.
52 Negus VE. Functions of mucus. *Acta Otolaryngol* 1963; **56**: 204–14.
53 Meyer F, Silberberg A. The rheology and molecular organization of epithelial mucus. *Biorheology* 1980; **17**: 163–8.
54 Sleigh MA. The nature and action of respiratory tract cilia. In: *Respiratory Defense Mechanisms* (eds JD Brain, DF Proctor, LM Reid) Marcel Dekker, New York, 1977, pp 247–88.
55 Widdicombe JG. Force of capillarity tending to prevent drying of ciliary mucosa. In: *The Airways* (eds MA Kaliner, PJ Barnes) Marcel Dekker, New York, 1988, p 597.
56 McDonald DM. Neurogenic inflammation in rat trachea. I. Changes in venules, leukocytes, and epithelial cells. *J Neurocytol* 1988; **17**: 583–603.
57 Laitinen LA, Heino M, Laitinen A, et al. Damage of the airway epithelium and bronchial reactivity in patients with asthma. *Am Rev Respir Dis* 1985; **131**: 599–606.
58 Spring KR, Hope A. Dimensions of cells and lateral intercellular spaces in living *Necturus* gallbladder. *Fed Proc* 1979; **38**: 128–33.
59 House CR. *Water Transport in Cells and Tissues*. Edward Arnold, London, 1974.
60 van Os CH, Wiedner G, Wright EM. Volume flows across gallbladder epithelium induced by small hydrostatic and osmotic gradients. *J Membrane Biol* 1979; **49**: 1–20.
61 Kondo M, Finkbeiner WE, Widdicombe JH. Changes in permeability of dog tracheal epithelium in response to hydrostatic pressure. *Am J Physiol* 1992; **262**: L176–82.
62 Wiig H. Evaluation of methodologies for measurement of interstitial fluid pressure (Pi): physiological implications of recent Pi data. *Crit Rev Biomed Eng* 1990; **18**: 27–54.
63 Joris L, Quinton PM. Concentration of elements in airway surface fluid. *Med Sci Res* 1987; **15**: 855–6.
64 Boucher RC, Stutts MF, Bromberg PA, Gatzy JT. Regional differences in airway surface liquid composition. *J Appl Physiol* 1981; **50**: 613–20.
65 Man SFP, Adams GK III, Proctor DF. Effects of temperature, relative humidity, and mode of breathing on canine airway secretions. *J Appl Physiol* 1979; **46**: 205–10.
66 Robinson NP, Kyle H, Webber SE, Widdicombe JG. Electrolyte and other chemical concentrations in tracheal airway surface liquid and mucus. *J Appl Physiol* 1989; **66**: 2129–35.
67 Boucher RC, Bromberg PA, Gatzy JT. Airway transepithelial electric potential in vivo: species and regional differences. *J Appl Physiol* 1980; **48**: 169–76.
68 Erjefaldt I, Persson CGA. On the use of absorbing discs to sample mucosal surface liquids. *Clin Exp Allergy* 1990; **20**: 193–7.
69 Joris L, Dab I, Quinton PM. Elemental composition of human airway surface fluid in healthy and diseased airways *Am Rev Respir Dis* 1993; **148**: 1633–7.
70 Widdicombe JH. Cystic fibrosis and $\beta$-adrenergic response of airway epithelial cell cultures. *Am J Physiol* 1986; **251**: R818–22.
71 Boucher RC, Stutts MF, Knowles RC, et al. Na transport in cystic fibrosis respiratory epithelia: abnormal basal rate and response to adenylate cyclase activation. *J Clin Invest* 1986; **78**: 1245–52.
72 Welsh MJ, Liedtke CM. Chloride and potassium channels in cystic fibrosis airway epithelia. *Nature* 1986; **322**: 467–70.
73 Widdicombe JH, Welsh MJ, Finkbeiner WE. Cystic fibrosis decreases the apical

membrane chloride permeability of monolayers cultured from cells of tracheal epithelium. *Proc Natl Acad Sci USA* 1985; **82**: 6167–71.
74 Sturgess J, Imrie J. Quantitative evaluation of the development of tracheal submucosal glands in infants with cystic fibrosis and control infants. *Am J Pathol* 1982; **106**: 303–11.
75 Dwyer TM, Farley JM. Intracellular chloride in submucosal gland cells. *Life Sci* 1991; **48**: 2119–27.
76 Illsley NP, Verkman AS. Membrane chloride transport measured using a chloride-sensitive fluorescent probe. *Biochemistry* 1987; **26**: 1215–19.
77 Sommerhoff CP, Finkbeiner, WE. Human tracheobronchial submucosal gland cells in culture. *Am J Respir Cell Mol Biol* 1990; **2**: 41–50.
78 Bowes D, Corrin B. Ultrastructural immunocytochemical localization of lysozyme in human bronchial glands. *Thorax* 1977; **32**: 163–70.
79 Bowes D, Clark AE, Corrin B. Ultrastructural localization of lactoferrin and glycoprotein in human bronchial glands. *Thorax* 1981; **36**: 108–15.
80 Finkbeiner WE, Carrier SD, Teresi CE. Reverse transcriptions–polymerase chain reaction (RT–PCR) phenotypic analysis of cell cultures of human tracheal epithelium, tracheobronchial glands and lung carcinomas. *Am J Respir Cell Mol Biol* 1993; **9**: 547–56.
81 Yamaya M, Finkbeiner WE, Widdicombe JH. Ion transport by cultures of human tracheobronchial submucosal glands. *Am J Physiol* 1991; **261**: L485–90.
82 Yamaya M, Finkbeiner WE, Widdicombe JH. Altered ion transport by tracheal glands in cystic fibrosis. *Am J Physiol* 1991; **261**: L491–4.
83 Yamaya M, Ohrui T, Finkbeiner WE, Widdicombe JH. Calcium-dependent Cl secretion across cultures of human tracheal surface epithelium and glands. *Am J Physiol* 1993; **265**: L170–7.
84 Jiang CW, Finkbeiner WE, Widdicombe JH, Miller SS. Active fluid transport across cultures of human tracheobronchial glands (HTG) in cystic fibrosis. *Pediatr Pulmonol* 1993 (Suppl 9): 208.
85 Colledge WH, Ratcliff R, Foster D, et al. Cystic fibrosis mouse with intestinal obstruction [letter]. *Lancet* 1992; **340**: 680.
86 Snouwaert JN, Brigman KK, Latour AM, et al. An animal model for cystic fibrosis made by gene targeting. *Science* 1992; **257**: 1083–8.
87 Dorin JR, Dickinson P, Alton EW, et al. Cystic fibrosis in the mouse by targeted insertional mutagenesis. *Nature* 1992; **359**: 211–15.
88 Finkbeiner WE, Shen B-Q, Widdicombe JH. Chloride secretion and function of serous and mucous gland cells of human airways. *Am J Physiol: Lung* (in press).

## Chapter Seven

# Reconstitution of CFTR

Neil A. Bradbury, Charles J. Venglarik and Robert J. Bridges
*Department of Physiology and Biophysics, and Gregory Fleming James Cystic Fibrosis Research Center, University of Alabama at Birmingham, Birmingham, Alabama, USA*

## INTRODUCTION

Gene expression in both epithelial and non-epithelial cells, complementation studies, mutational analysis and reconstitution of purified protein have now firmly established that the cystic fibrosis gene product, CFTR (cystic fibrosis transmembrane conductance regulator), can function as a chloride channel. The many contributions which helped demonstrate that CFTR can function as a channel have been reviewed in an earlier volume in this series[1] and elsewhere[2–5]. Our laboratory had the privilege of working in collaboration with investigators in Toronto to perform planar lipid bilayer reconstitution studies with CFTR protein purified to homogeneity[6]. The Toronto group has since gone on to compare the channel properties of the wild-type and ΔF508 forms of the purified CFTR proteins after reconstitution into bilayers[7]. The focus of this chapter will be on the preconstitution of CFTR into planar lipid bilayers using native membrane vesicles derived from colonic epithelial cells expressing high levels of CFTR protein. Because native membrane vesicles were used, and not purified CFTR protein, it is perhaps more correct to refer to our studies as preconstitution rather than reconstitution studies[8]. An important caveat when interpreting results obtained with native membrane vesicles is to recognize that other vesicle-associated proteins will coincorporate

*Cystic Fibrosis—Current Topics, Volume 2.* Edited by J. A. Dodge, D. J. H. Brock and J. H. Widdicombe

into the bilayer along with the channel. The possible influence of the coincorporated proteins on the channel can only be determined by performing true reconstitution studies with purified channel protein. A counter-argument to the use of purified channel protein is that the properties of the channel may be altered during purification. Since channels are integral membrane proteins, purification will of necessity involve the use of detergents. This in conjunction with a wide variety of chromatographic separation techniques used for purification may result in altered properties of the channel. These potential changes in channel properties during purification have led Miller[8] to suggest that preconstitution studies should precede reconstitution studies. Below we present the planar lipid bilayer methods used in our laboratory and some results from our reconstitution studies using native membrane vesicles derived from the rat colonic mucosa[9–12] and stripped clathrin-coated vesicles from T84 cells[13], a human colonic chloride secretory cell line[14,15].

## WHY USE PLANAR BILAYERS?

There are two methods available to the electrophysiologist to study ion channels: the bilayer technique and the patch-clamp technique. Each of these techniques has its advantages and limitations. The bilayer technique, as depicted in Figure 1, has several advantages salient to the study of CFTR. These advantages include: (1) the determination of the minimal number of protein molecules comprising a functional channel; (2) the ability to routinely study single channels; (3) access to both the cytoplasmic and extracellular sides of the channel; and (4) channels in subcellular organelles such as endosomes, lysosomes, Golgi and endoplasmic reticulum that are otherwise inaccessible to studies by patch-clamp methods can be studied by bilayer methods. The purification and reconstitution of CFTR into planar lipid bilayers provided strong evidence that CFTR by itself could function as a chloride channel[6]. In addition, estimates of the number of CFTR copies per liposome and the number of liposome fusions necessary to incorporate an active channel suggests CFTR may function as a monomer[6]. However, opponents of the bilayer technique will point out that it is a single molecule assay. Thus, the observed channel activity could result from a minor protein contaminant in the protein fraction and therefore be mistakenly attributed to the abundant protein. One means of overcoming this criticism will be to purify and reconstitute mutant forms of CFTR that display altered channel properties. Patch-clamp studies have indeed shown mutant forms of CFTR to have altered channel properties[16–18]. The success of these studies suggests reconstitution studies with similar mutants will also succeed and thus verify that CFTR protein can by itself function as a chloride channel.

Principal among the difficulties encountered in patch-clamp studies is the inability to routinely obtain patches with a single channel. Because single-channel activity is more readily analysed, electrophysiologists strive to obtain single-channel records. In contrast to patch-clamp studies, the bilayer technique provides several means of obtaining a single channel. Vesicle fusion and channel incorporation into a bilayer generally requires an osmotic gradient and the continuous stirring of the solution[19,20]. Thus, once a channel incorporates the osmotic gradient can be eliminated and stirring discontinued to prevent the incorporation of additional channels. In addition, the bilayer investigator can vary the size (area) of the bilayer, the amount of vesicle protein and the size of the vesicles, hence the number of channels per vesicle, in an effort to obtain a single channel in the bilayer. If multiple channels do appear in the bilayer, lipid may be added or the bilayer deliberately broken and re-formed until a single-channel bilayer is obtained. As shown below, single CFTR channel activity can be readily obtained through the appropriate adjustment of these various parameters.

Most bilayer chambers are designed to allow free access to both sides of the membrane. This arrangement enables the investigator to alter the composition of the solutions bathing the cytoplasmic and extracellular sides of the channel. Thus, in addition to altering the ionic composition on either side the investigator can add reagents that block or activate the channel and with practice remove these reagents by exchanging the solutions in either compartment. For example, as illustrated in Figure 2, by adding protein kinase A (PKA) and ATP to either the *cis* or *trans* compartment the investigator can determine or select the orientation of the CFTR channels in the bilayer. In the upper panel of Figure 2 an outside-out vesicle fuses with the bilayer and a channel is incorporated with its cytoplasmic side facing the *trans* compartment. Only if PKA and ATP are added to the *trans* compartment will the channel be activated. On the other hand, in the lower panel of Figure 2 an inside-out vesicle fuses with the bilayer, incorporates a channel with its cytoplasmic side facing the *cis* compartment and now PKA and ATP are required in the *cis* compartment to activate the channel. Our laboratory has used this advantage of the bilayer technique to document the presence of CFTR in clathrin-coated vesicles—an inside-out vesicle fraction.

The patch-clamp method is largely restricted to the study of ion channels resident in the plasma membrane (but see Hanke et al.[21] and Schmid et al.[22]). In contrast, the bilayer method allows one to study ion channels in any subcellular compartment for which an enriched membrane vesicle fraction can be isolated and fused to the bilayer. We have used this feature of the bilayer method to document the existence of CFTR in plasma membrane-derived clathrin-coated vesicles. We have suggested that acute recruitment of CFTR chloride channels into the plasma membrane via exocytic insertion, and their removal via endocytic retrieval, could provide a mechanism for regulating the

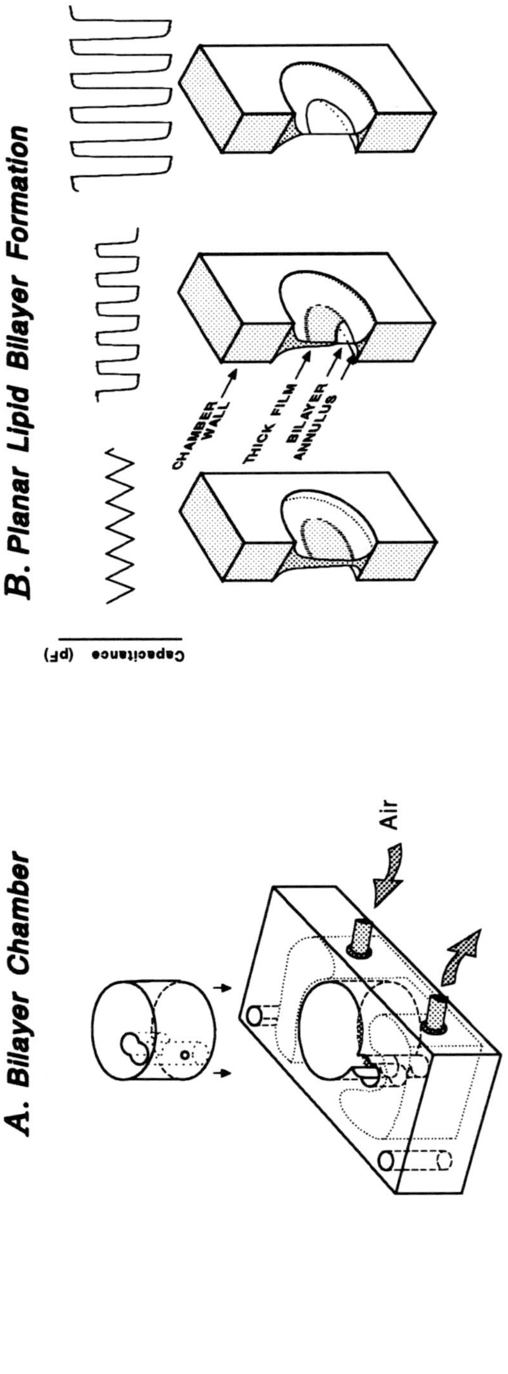
A. Bilayer Chamber
Air
B. Planar Lipid Bilayer Formation
Capacitance (pF)
CHAMBER WALL
THICK FILM
BILAYER ANNULUS

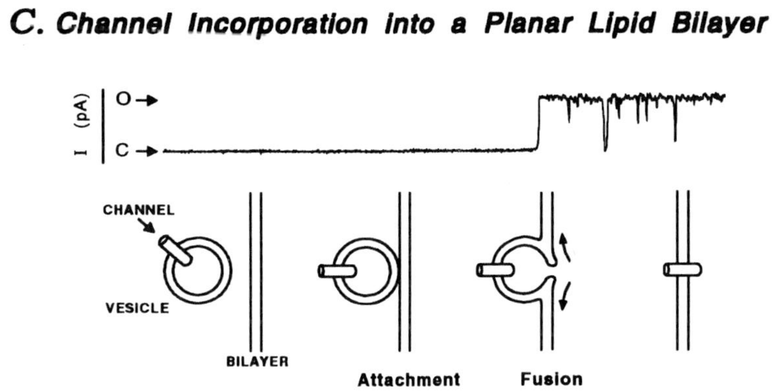


**Figure 1** Illustrations of a bilayer chamber (A), bilayer formation (B) and channel incorporation (C). (A) The unique features of this bilayer chamber are the small volumes (300–400 $\mu$l) required in the *cis* and *trans* compartments and the ability to perfuse the chamber with air to maintain it at 37 °C. (B) Formation of a painted planar lipid bilayer. The thick lipid drop once applied to the septum-hole separating the *cis* and *trans* fluid-filled compartments spontaneously thins to form a bilayer. Bilayer thinning can be monitored as an increase in capacitance (top) as measured by using a triangle wave command potential. (C) Channel incorporation is thought to proceed in two stages: attachment of vesicles to the bilayer and fusion of the two bilayers. Attachment is promoted by the presence of calcium and/or negatively charged lipids (e.g. PS). Once attached to the bilayers, vesicles swell, due to the osmotic gradient, and fuse with the bilayers. Current across the bilayer is monitored and a channel incorporation detected as a sudden jump in current (top). O, open; C, closed

A

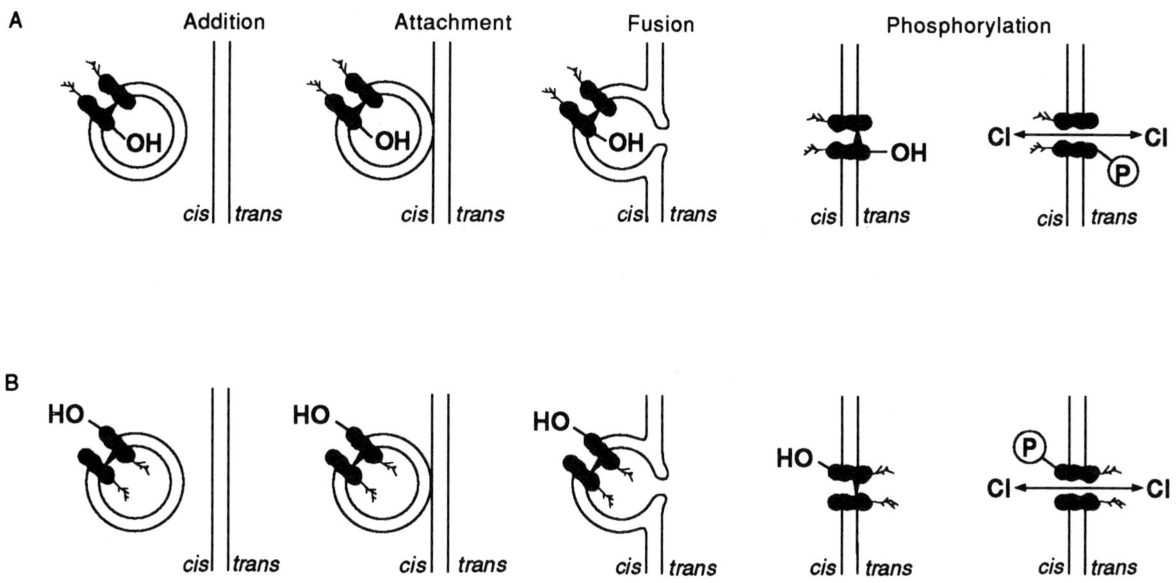


**Figure 2** Two possible orientations of a CFTR channel in the bilayer. The cytoplasmic face of the channel protein is indicated by a phosphorylation site (OH) or phosphate (P) and the glycosylated extracellular face by the tree-like structure. Vesicles, by convention, are added to the *cis* side and often with an imposed *cis* to *trans* osmotic gradient. Part A shows the addition, attachment, fusion and phosphorylation (activation) of a channel from an outside-out vesicle. In this case the cytoplasmic face of the channel is *trans* and intracellular regulators, i.e. PKA and MgATP, must be added to the *trans* bath. Part B shows the addition, attachment, fusion and activation of a channel from an inside-out vesicle. In this case, the cytoplasmic face is *cis* and the regulators must be added to the *cis* bath. Thus, by the selective addition of PKA and ATP it is possible to determine or select the orientation of CFTR in the bilayer

number of plasma membrane resident channels during secretion[13,23,24]. An important tenet of this hypothesis is that CFTR be present within intracellular membrane vesicles of the endocytic/exocytic membrane recycling pathway—a tenet borne out by our bilayer results[13]. Barasch et al.[25] have also suggested that the acidification of intracellular compartments is compromised in CF cells. Because ion channels in subcellular organelles can be studied by bilayer methods the question of whether CFTR contributes to the acidification of these compartments can be addressed in future bilayer studies. Furthermore, there is substantial evidence that several CF mutations prevent the normal processing and delivery of CFTR to the plasma membrane[26]. It is, however, not known whether these same mutations alter the properties of these mutant channel proteins. Bilayer studies using the various subcellular compartments in the biosynthetic pathway will assist in determining the channel competence of these mutant proteins.

One limitation of the planar lipid bilayer method is that due to the larger membrane area the capacitance contribution to the noise level is higher with bilayers compared to patch-clamp membranes. Because CFTR is such a low-conductance channel, this is an important limitation of the bilayer method. While smaller-diameter septum holes can be used to obtain membranes of smaller area, this also reduces the probability of vesicle fusion and channel incorporation. To increase the channel amplitude and thus improve the signal to noise we have modified the bilayer chamber to perform experiments at 37 °C. The bilayer chamber shown in Figure 1 was manufactured so that it could be perfused with air. Laboratory-supplied air is first warmed by circulating through a copper coil set on a hot plate. By adjusting the temperature of the hot plate and the air flow rate the temperature of the bilayer chamber can be maintained at 37 °C. The use of air to warm the chamber greatly reduces the microphonic and electric noise that would otherwise result from the use of alternative perfusion media (e.g. water) or electronic warming devices. As shown below, the conductance of CFTR was increased from 7.8 pS at 20 °C to 11.9 pS at 37 °C with little change in the background noise level, thus providing the hoped for improvement in signal to noise.

An additional important consideration in performing bilayer studies is an appreciation for what one is attempting to reconstitute. In general the bilayer investigator attempts to reconstitute not merely a conductance but rather a set of properties that characterize and preferable uniquely identify the channel of interest. Thus, for example, reconstituted tetrodotoxin (TTX)-sensitive sodium channels should be blocked by TTX and selective for sodium, calcium-activated potassium channels should be activated by calcium and selective for potassium and so on. Since the regulation of several chloride channels with widely different properties had been implicated in CF (for an excellent review of this issue see Hanrahan et al.[27]), it was not certain what properties would (should) be displayed by reconstituted purified CFTR protein. The consensus now is that CFTR is a low-conductance (~ 10 pS) chloride channel with a nearly linear current voltage relation. CFTR channels are activated by PKA and ATP and channel activity in excised patches requires the continued presence of ATP[28,29]. The best blocker of CFTR channel activity is perhaps ADP[28,30,31], although several potassium channel blockers have also been reported to block CFTR in whole cell[32] and excised membrane patches[33,34]. How many other chloride channels share this set of properties is at present not known, but at least one found in the plasma membrane of cardiac muscle[35,36] closely resembles epithelial CFTR.

## BILAYER FORMATION

There are a variety of different methods for forming bilayers and incorporating ion channels, into planar lipid bilayers. The details of these methods have been the subject of several reviews[37–46]. Our laboratory uses the Mueller and Rudin[47,48] painted-bilayer method to form the bilayers and an osmotic gradient to promote vesicle fusion[19,20] as depicted in Figure 1. Lipids of the desired composition (e.g. phosphotidylathanolanine (PE) and phosphatidylserine (PS)) are dissolved in a suitable solvent (e.g. n-decane) and a small droplet is applied with a 'brush', such as a fire-polished glass capillary tube, onto the septum hole separating fluid-filled *cis* and *trans* compartments. The bilayer chamber we have manufactured requires only 300–400 μl of buffer in each compartment and both compartments can be stirred with small magnetic fleas. Once a bilayer of high resistance (200 GΩ) and adequate capacitance (200–300 pF) is obtained, salt from a 3 M stock solution is added to the *cis* compartment to create a *cis* to *trans* osmotic gradient. Membrane vesicles (1–3 μg protein) are then added to the *cis* compartment and the solutions continuously stirred until a channel incorporates. In our experience, a useful set of conditions for the incorporation of CFTR chloride channels is bilayers of PE : PS at a ratio of 7 : 3 (w/w) an osmotic gradient of 300 mM CsCl *cis* to 50 mM CsCl *trans* in a solution of 10 mM bis-tris-propane, 2 mM $MgCl_2$, 1 mM EGTA, 0.6 mM $CaCl_2$, 100 μM ATP, 100 nM PKA at a pH of 7.4 at 37 °C. Typically bilayers are painted in 50 mM CsCl on the *cis* and *trans* sides, and once formed additional CsCl is added to the *cis* side to establish the osmotic gradient. Caesium was selected as the abundant cation since the appearance of conductive cation channels is reduced when compared to the use of potassium or sodium. In addition, caesium, but not n-methyl-D-glucamine (NMDG), allowed for the incorporation of CFTR chloride channels. When PKA and ATP were present, CFTR channels were observed in most experiments within 40 min after vesicle addition and often channels incorporated within 20 min. Incorporation of channels was considerably more frequent at 37 °C compared to room temperature (~ 20 °C). Channel properties including conductance, ion selectivity and kinetics were not altered when using bilayers of pure PE, by the inclusion of cholesterol (e.g. PE : PS : cholesterol, 5 : 1 : 3), when hexane or hexadecane were used as solvents, or by the use of different cations (e.g. Na, K, Cs).

## MEMBRANE VESICLE ISOLATION

One of the first steps in attempting to incorporate an ion channel into a bilayer is to identify a tissue abundant in channel protein and then isolate an enriched membrane vesicle fraction from this tissue. The rat distal colon can generate several hundred microamps per square centimetre of secretory chloride current and sustain these high levels of chloride secretion for many hours[49]. Also, by *in situ* hybridization of $^{35}$S-labelled antisense CFTR mRNA, Trezise and Buchwald[50] have shown high levels of CFTR expression in the bottom two-thirds of rat colonic crypts (Figure 3). Expression of CFTR in the crypts is in good agreement with the notion that these cells are responsible for cAMP-mediated chloride secretion. For these reasons we chose rat colonic crypts as a source of chloride channels for reconstitution studies[9–12]. To perform these studies we first developed methods to isolate the colonic crypts from the mucosa[51]. A scanning electron micrograph of the isolated crypts is shown in Figure 4. Our method enables us to detach the crypts from the mucosa at the basement membrane and thus yields a pure native epithelial preparation free of any subepithelial tissue. To further document the presence of CFTR in the rat colonic crypts we have immunostained, permeabilized crypts with

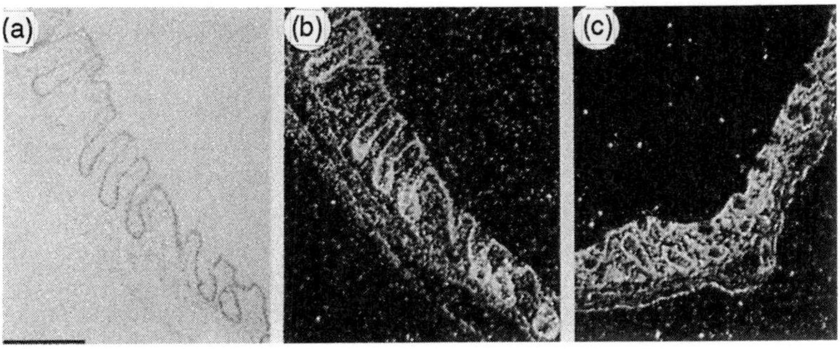


**Figure 3** Photomicrographs of haematoxylin-stained frozen section of rat distal colon (a) and the corresponding bright-field views of sections hybridized to an antisense (b) or sense (c) $^{35}$S-labelled CFTR mRNA in the bottom two-thirds of the crypts. (Reproduced from Trezise and Buchwald[50], with permission)

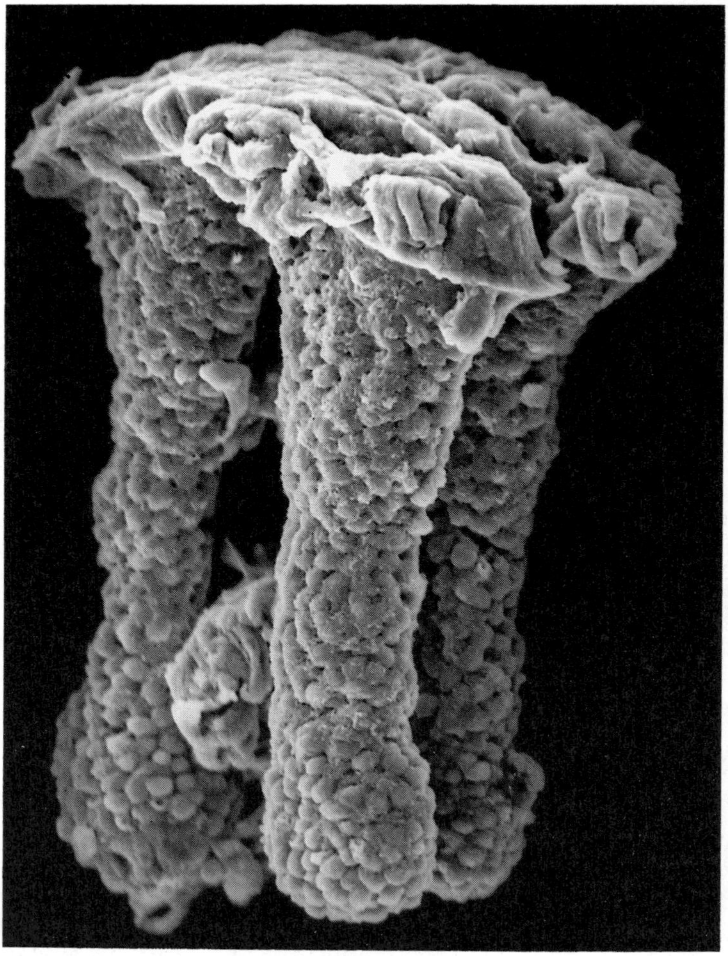

**Figure 4** Scanning electron micrograph of isolated rat colonic crypts. Crypts were isolated from the distal colonic mucosa by calcium chelation and mechanical vibration[9,51]

antibodies to CFTR. Consistent with the expression of CFTR mRNA, immunoreactive staining with anti-CFTR antibodies was localized to the bottom two-thirds of the crypts (Figure 5).

Using the isolated crypts as starting material we have developed a protocol that provides an enriched plasma membrane vesicle fraction[9]. Based on plasma membrane enzyme markers (e.g. $Na^+/K^+$-ATPase, a basal lateral membrane marker) and amiloride-blockable sodium uptake (a marker for apical membrane Na channels), we achieve a 15-fold enrichment in plasma

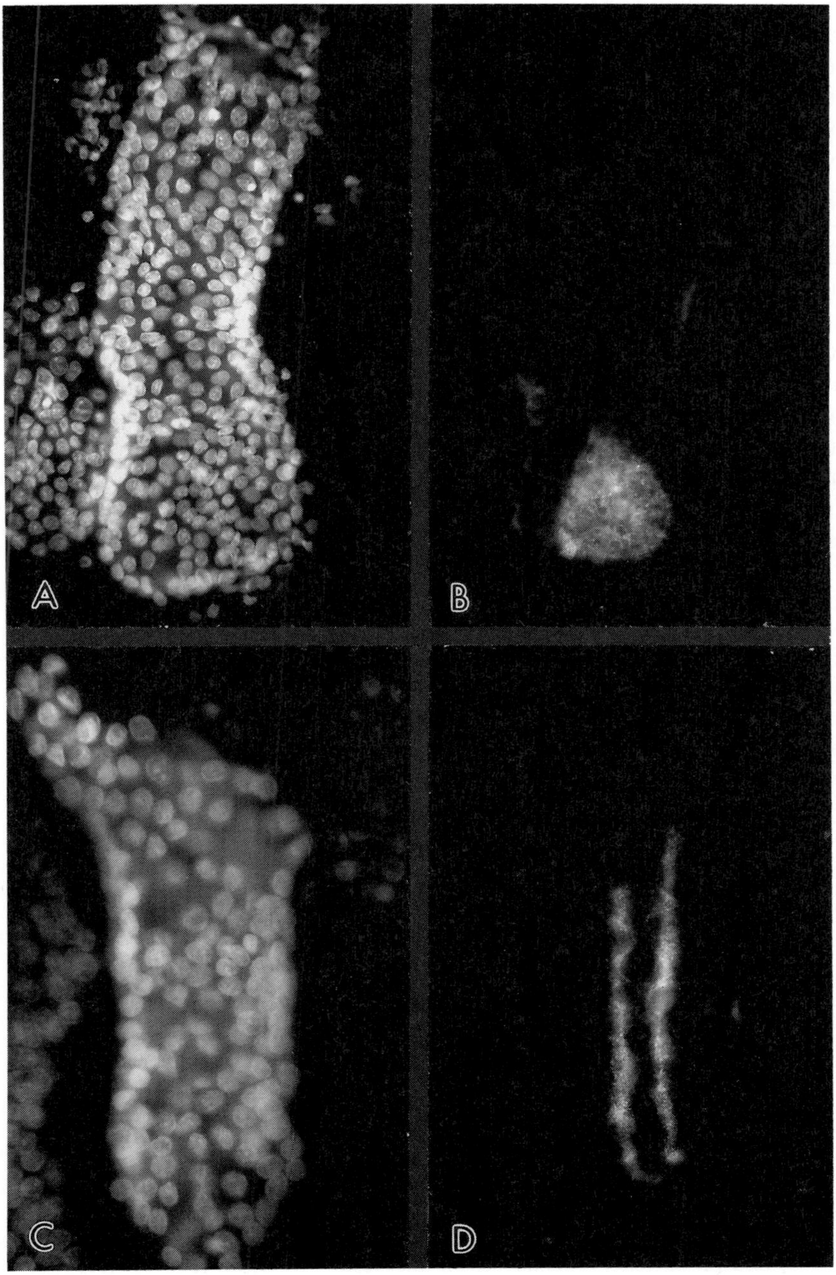


**Figure 5** Immuno-reactive staining of rat colonic crypts with Genzyme monoclonal antibody to CFTR (B and D) and the corresponding micrographs of Hoechst-stained crypts (A and C)

membrane. It is with this fraction that we have performed bilayer studies over the last several years. The only chloride channels we have observed when using this fraction are the outwardly rectifying chloride channel and CFTR. We observe these channels with about equal frequency and often they coincorporate. To further document the presence of CFTR in our plasma membrane vesicle fraction we prepared Western blots and probed with an antibody to a C-terminal peptide of CFTR[52]. As shown in Figure 6, CFTR was significantly enriched in our plasma membrane fraction (lane B3) when compared to crude microsomes (lane B2) derived from rat colonic crypts. Collectively, these results demonstrate the expression of CFTR mRNA in rat colonic crypts, the localization of immunoreactivity to anti-CFTR antibodies in the crypts and the detection of a protein in our plasma membrane-enriched vesicle fraction with a molecular mass that corresponds to CFTR on Western blots. In addition, kinase $^{32}$P-labelling experiments have demonstrated that this band can be phosphorylated (not shown). These results strongly suggest CFTR protein is expressed in rat colonic crypts and that our fractionation protocol provides a plasma membrane preparation enriched in CFTR.

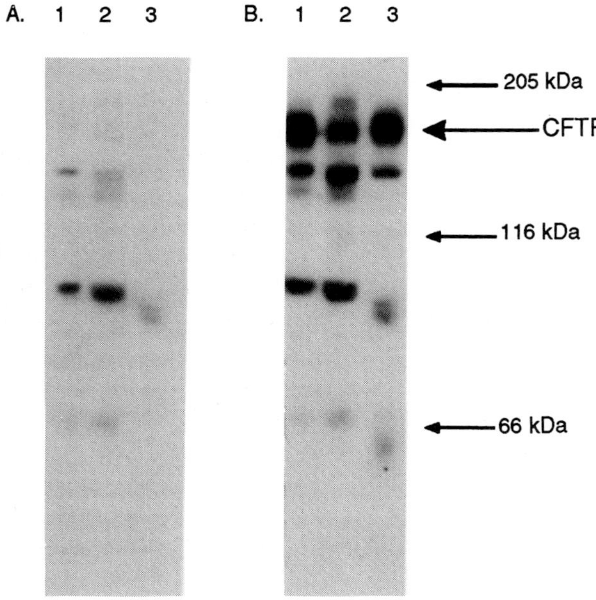


**Figure 6** Western blots of T84 cell lysates (lane 1), crude rat colonic crypt microsomes (lane 2) and an enriched plasma membrane vesicle fraction (lane 3). (A) Immunoreactivity detected without primary antibody and (B) with an antibody to a CFTR C-terminal peptide (residues 1468–1480)[52]. In lanes 1 and 3 25 μg of protein were loaded on the gel and in lane 2 50 μg of protein. Western blots were generously provided by Dr Jonathon Cohn

A second membrane vesicle preparation we have used for our bilayer studies is a highly enriched clathrin-coated vesicle fraction derived from T84 cells[13]. T84 colonic epithelial cells are a well-documented human cell line that has served as an excellent chloride secretory cell model[14,15]. Furthermore T84 cells constitutively express high levels of CFTR[52]. Clathrin-coated vesicles were isolated from confluent monolayers of T84 cells according to the methods of Pearse[53] and Forgac et al.[54]. Several criteria were used to characterize the clathrin-coated vesicle fraction obtained from T84 cells. The clathrin-coated vesicle fraction had a high protein-to-lipid ratio, the basis on which the density gradient isolation was achieved. Secondly, immunoblot analysis of the clathrin-coated vesicles revealed the presence of clathrin heavy chain and the endosome-specific adaptin, $\alpha$-adaptin. Thirdly, electron microscopic examination of the vesicles revealed a homogeneous population of uniformly sized (95 nm) vesicles showing the bristled cage structures characteristic of clathrin-coated vesicles. The presence of CFTR in the clathrin-coated vesicles was documented by immunoblot analysis, PKA $^{32}$P-labelling and tryptic phosphopeptide mapping[13]. Furthermore, as shown below, fusion of uncoated clathrin-coated vesicles with planar lipid bilayers resulted in the incorporation of chloride channel activity characteristic of CFTR.

## CFTR IN BILAYERS

A current record from a bilayer containing three CFTR chloride channels derived from the rat colonic plasma membrane vesicles is shown in Figure 7(A). The amplitude histogram of the record fitted to four Gaussian functions is shown in Figure 7(B). The applied potential was −33 mV (*cis* to *trans*) with a 300 : 50 nm (*cis* to *trans*) Cl gradient (−78 mV total driving force). The amplitudes were 0.22, 0.22 and 0.21 pA. Figure 7(C) shows the linear current voltage relation of the channels under symmetric conditions (300 : 300 mM Cl). The line shows the fit of the data (filled circles) to a straight line. The conductance of the rat colonic channel was 7.6 pS at 20 °C. Plotted on the same axes are data (open triangles) obtained when using purified CFTR protein reconstituted into proteoliposomes and incorporated into a bilayer under the same experimental conditions. The conductance of the purified CFTR protein was 7.2 pS. We have found that the value one assigns to such a low-conductance channel is quite sensitive to the method used to estimate the channel amplitude. Indeed values ranging from 3 to 14 pS have been reported for the CFTR chloride channel[27] and in most cases the method used was not stated. We prefer to use amplitude histograms or data cluster analysis to ensure an unbiased estimate of current amplitude is obtained. Additional points to consider when comparing the conductance reported in different studies are the activity coefficient of the salt solution, the conductance–activity relationship and the temperature. In our experiments the activity coefficient of CsCl at 300 mM is only 0.656, giving a chloride activity of 197 mM. In agreement with Hanrahan et al.[27] we have found that the conductance–activity relationship of CFTR is not linear. In bilayers at room temperature, the channel conductance saturates with a half-maximal conductance reached at an activity of approximately 80 mM. Furthermore, as expected for a diffusion-limited process the conductance of CFTR in bilayers increases to nearly 12 pS when measured at 37 °C (Figure 7D). A final point that may help explain the wide range in conductance values reported for CFTR is illustrated in the

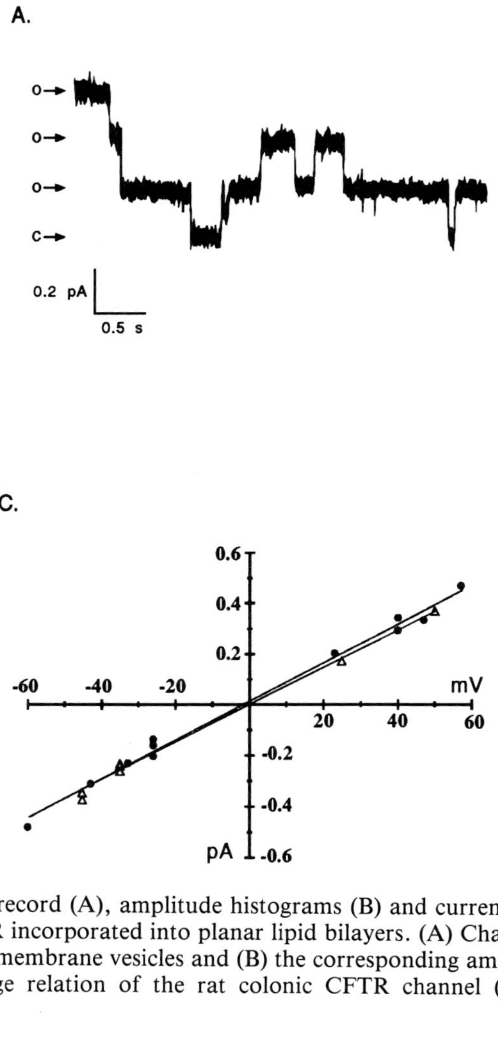


**Figure 7** Current record (A), amplitude histograms (B) and current voltage relations (C and D) of CFTR incorporated into planar lipid bilayers. (A) Channel activity from rat colonic plasma membrane vesicles and (B) the corresponding amplitude histogram. (C) Current–voltage relation of the rat colonic CFTR channel (filled circles) and

current trace shown in Figure 8. In this experiment the channel entered the bilayer in a subconductance state and remained in this state for several minutes before switching to its more fully open state. In other experiments we have observed the channel switch back and forth for several minutes at a time between these two conductances. While many channels display one or more subconductances, the unusual nature of CFTR is that it remains at this subconductance for prolonged periods in planar lipid bilayers. Given these

B.

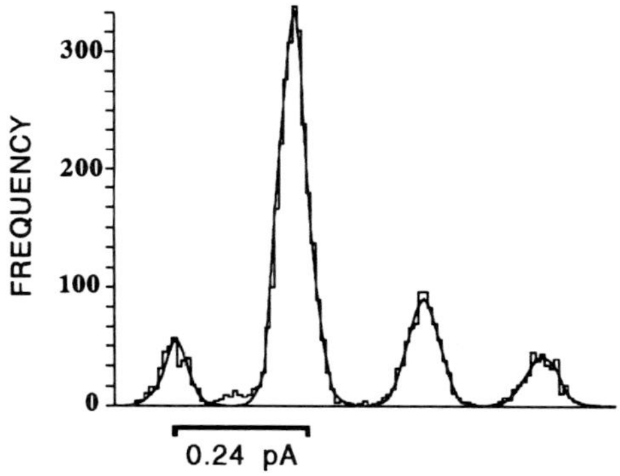


D.

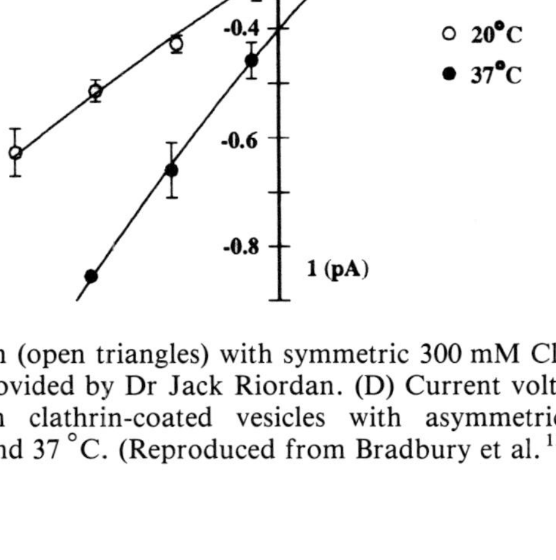


purified CFTR protein (open triangles) with symmetric 300 mM Cl at 20 °C. Purified CFTR protein was provided by Dr Jack Riordan. (D) Current voltage relation of the CFTR channel from clathrin-coated vesicles with asymmetric 300 : 50 mM Cl (*cis* : *trans*) at 20 °C and 37 °C. (Reproduced from Bradbury et al.[13], with permission)

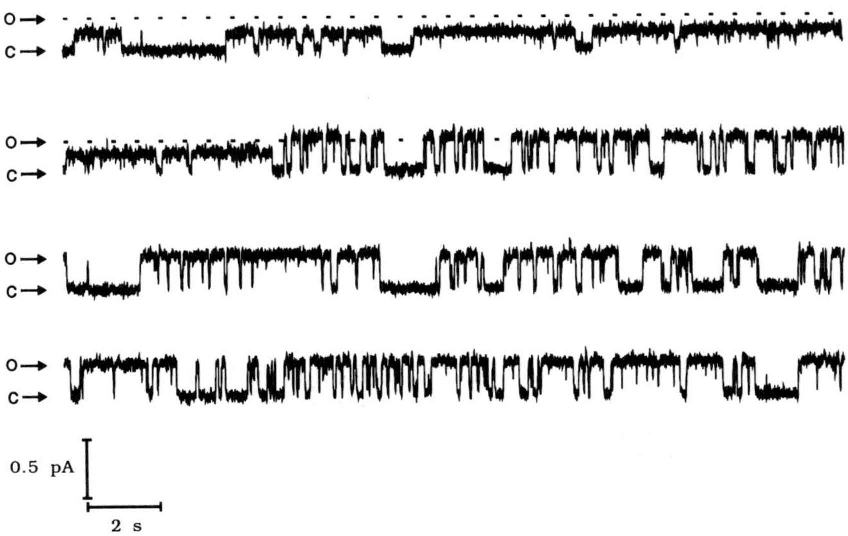


**Figure 8** Prolonged subconductance state of rat colonic CFTR. Only a single channel was observed throughout this experiment lasting more than 20 min. The rapid switch from the subconductance state to the fully open state shown here is a frequent occurrence with CFTR in bilayers. Conditions: 300 : 50 mM Cl (*cis* : *trans*), −30 mV *cis* to *trans*, 37 °C

considerations it is not surprising to find a wide range of conductance values reported from different laboratories for the CFTR chloride channel.

We have also determined that CFTR derived from rat colonic crypts has an anion-to-cation selectivity of at least 10 : 1, a greater permeability to bromide over chloride of 1.4 : 1 and a lower permeability to iodide. It has not been possible to assign a value to the iodide permeability of single channels since iodide appears to cause a fast type block of the channel—results similar to those reported in patch-clamp studies by Tabcharani et al.[55]. We have also found that the frequency of incorporation of CFTR from rat colonic crypts was dramatically increased when PKA and ATP were included in the bathing solutions or by treatment of the vesicles with PKA and ATP prior to their addition to the bilayer chamber. Inclusion of PKA and ATP in either the *cis* or *trans* compartments improved the incorporation of channels, suggesting both outside-out and inside-out vesicles fused with the bilayer when using rat colonic membrane vesicles. In contrast, when stripped clathrin-coated membrane vesicles from T84 cells were used PKA and ATP were required in the *cis* compartment to obtain active channels (Figure 9). Thus, in 18 out of 20 experiments CFTR channels were observed with PKA and ATP on the *cis* side but in only one out of 20 experiments were channels observed when PKA

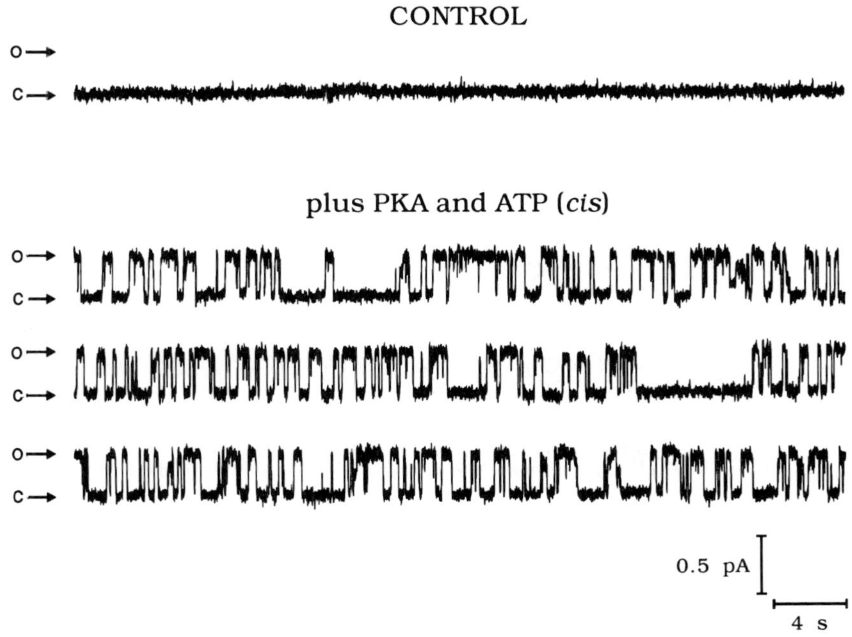


**Figure 9** Activation of clathrin-coated vesicle-derived CFTR by PKA and ATP. Coated vesicles were stripped of clathrin using purified ATP-dependent uncoatase and fused with the bilayer. Upper trace is from the bilayer before the addition of PKA (100 nM) and ATP (1 mM) to the *cis* bath. Conditions as in Figure 8. (Reproduced from Bradbury et al.[13], with permission)

and ATP were added to only the *trans* side. These results are consistent with the fusion of an inside-out vesicle as expected for clathrin-coated vesicle derived CFTR. CFTR chloride channels were also incorporated when using clathrin-coated vesicles from rat colonic crypts. In contrast, CFTR chloride channels were not observed when using clathrin-coated vesicles from brain—a tissue that does not express CFTR. Thus the presence of CFTR in clathrin-coated vesicles is specific to chloride secretory cells.

A current record of a single CFTR chloride channel obtained with stripped clathrin-coated vesicles from T84 cells is shown in Figure 10. Single-channel activity was recorded for over 1 h (only 5 min are shown in Figure 10) in the continued presence of 100 nM PKA and 1 mM ATP in the *cis* bath. Under these conditions the open probability was 0.55. Event duration analysis yielded a single open time constant of 360 ms and one dominant closed time constant of 330 ms (Figure 11A and B). Fluctuation analysis of the same single-channel record yielded a power density spectrum that could be fit to a single Lorentzian function with corner frequency of 0.91 Hz (Figure 11C). This value is in

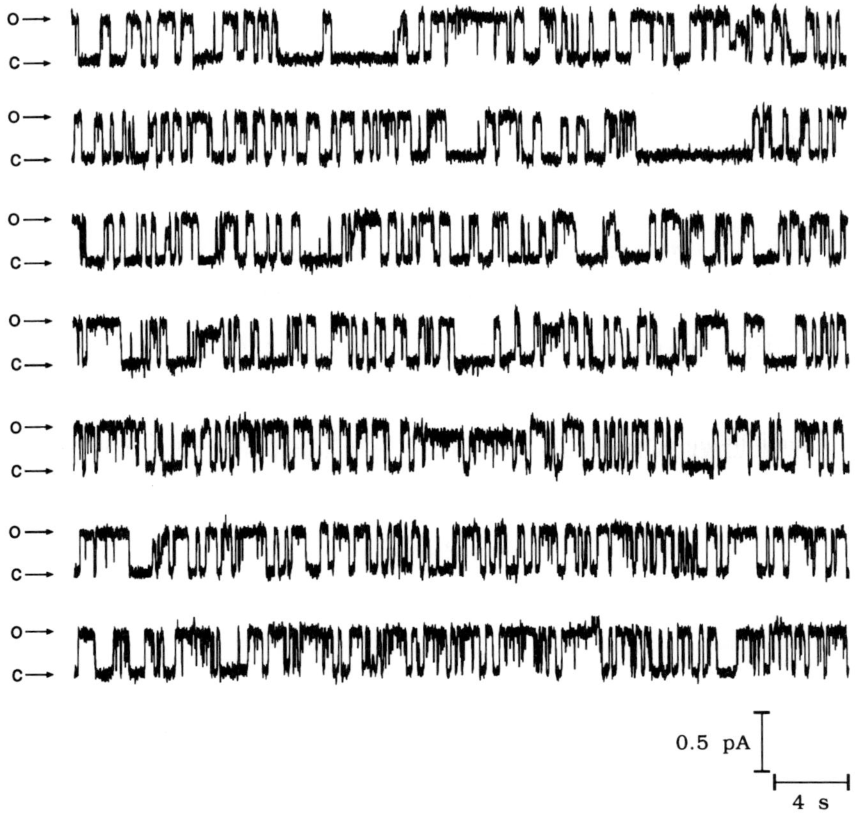


**Figure 10** Current trace of $T_{84}$ clathrin-coated vesicle-derived CFTR. Record is 5 min of data from a single channel that was recorded for more than 1 h. Conditions: 300 : 50 mM Cl (*cis* : *trans*), − 30 mV *cis* to *trans*, 37 °C

excellent agreement with the expected value of 0.92 Hz derived from the open and closed times where $2\pi fc$ equals the sum of $\tau_0^{-1}$ plus $\tau_c^{-1}$. These single-channel kinetics obtained in the bilayer were also in agreement with the range of values obtained in multichannel patches from T84 cells when recorded under similar conditions (Figure 11D). Results from patch-clamp experiments have also shown that the corner frequency changes with the ATP concentration as predicted for a channel activator[29] and that ADP acts as a competitive inhibitor of ATP-dependent channel activation[31]. Preliminary results suggest that ATP and ADP also affect the gating of CFTR in bilayers in a similar manner.

In summary, the above results suggest that CFTR can be reconstituted into planar lipid bilayers. Many of the channel properties of CFTR identified by

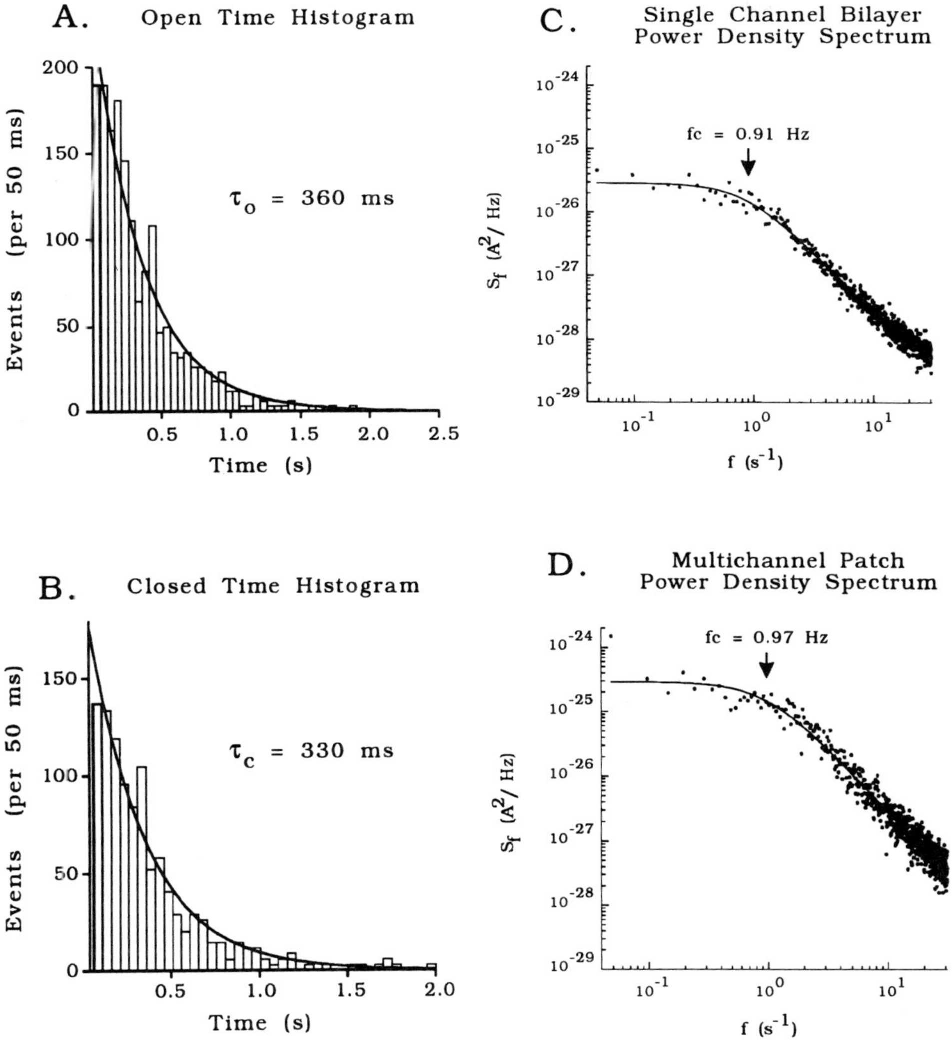


**Figure 11** Open and closed time event duration histograms (A and B) and power density spectra (C and D) of CFTR channel gating. Data for A–C are from the T84 clathrin-coated vesicle-derived CFTR channel shown in Figure 10. Data for D are from a T84 cell-excised membrane patch. Data were filtered at 200 Hz and sampled at 400 Hz. Event duration analysis was performed using a threshold of one-half the channel amplitude and events less than 5 ms were excluded from this analysis. Power density spectra were constructed and fit to Lorenzian functions. All analysis was performed using Biopatch software

patch-clamp studies are retained by the channel after preconstitution from native membrane vesicles. Further reconstitution studies with purified protein will help establish how CFTR is influenced by other membrane proteins and perhaps how CFTR may influence other channels[56]. Bilayer studies reveal that CFTR is in clathrin-coated vesicles and can be functionally activated by PKA and ATP. Additional bilayer studies with other subcellular membrane organelles will help determine the presence and competence of CFTR in these compartments. Thus bilayer studies complement what can be learned by the patch-clamp method and the continued concurrent use of the two methods is certain to further our understanding of CFTR as a chloride channel.

## ACKNOWLEDGEMENTS

We thank Dr John Riordan for the purified CFTR protein used for the studies shown in Figure 7, Dr Jonathan Cohn for performing the Western blots shown in Figure 6 and Albert Tousson and Eugene Arms for their assistance with the immunocytochemistry and scanning electron microscopy. We also acknowledge the excellent technical assistance of Ms Hoa Quang Trummell and Mr Jeff Ervin. Our research was supported by the NIH and CF Foundation.

## REFERENCES

1 Dodge JA, Brock DJH, Widdicombe JH (eds). *Cystic Fibrosis: Current Topics*, Vol 1. Wiley, New York, 1993.
2 Fuller CM, Benos DJ. CFTR! *Am J Physiol* 1992; **263**: C267–86.
3 Marino CR, Gorelick FS. Scientific advances in cystic fibrosis. *Gastroenterology* 1992; **103**: 681–93.
4 Welsh MJ, Anderson MP, Rich DP, et al. Cystic fibrosis transmembrane conductance regulator: a chloride channel with novel regulation. *Neuron* 1992; **8**: 821–9.
5 Riordan JR. The cystic fibrosis transmembrane conductance regulator. *Annu Rev Physiol* 1993; **55**: 609–30.
6 Bear C, Li C, Kartner N, et al. Purification and functional reconstitution of the cystic fibrosis transmembrane conductance regulation (CFTR). *Cell* 1992; **68**: 809–18.
7 Li C, Ramjeesingh M, Reyes E, et al. The cystic fibrosis mutation (ΔF508) does not influence the chloride channel activity of CFTR. *Nature Genet* 1993; **3**: 311–16.
8 Miller C. Ion channel reconstitution. Why bother? In: *Ionic Channels in Cells and Model Systems* (ed R Latorre) Plenum, New York, 1987, pp 257–73.
9 Reinhardt R, Bridges RJ, Rummel W, Lindemann B. Properties of an anion selective channel from rat colonic enterocyte plasma membranes reconstituted into planar phospholipid bilayers. *J Membr Biol* 1987; **95**: 47–54.
10 Bridges RJ, Worrell RT, Frizzell RA, Benos DJ. Stilbene disulfonate blockade of colonic secretory $Cl^-$ channels in planar lipid bilayers *Am J Physiol* 1989; **256**: C902–12.

11 Singh AK, Afink GB, Venglarik CJ, et al. Colonic Cl channel blockade by three classes of compounds. *Am J Physiol* 1991; **261**: C51–63
12 Venglarik CJ, Singh AK, Wang R, Bridges RJ. Trinitrophenyl-ATP blocks colonic chloride channels in planar lipid bilayers: evidence for two nucleotide binding sites. *J Gen Physiol* 1993; **101**: 545–69.
13 Bradbury NA, Cohn JA, Venglarik CJ, Bridges RJ. Biochemical and biophysical identification of the cystic fibrosis transmembrane conductance regulator chloride channel as components of clathrin coated vesicles. *J Biol Chem* 1994 **269**: 8296–302.
14 Dharmsathaphorn K, Mandel KG, McRoberts JA, et al. A human colonic tumor cell line that maintains vectorial electrolyte transport. *Am J Physiol* 1984; **246**: G204–8.
15 Barrett KE. Positive and negative regulation of chloride secretion in T84 cells. *Am J Physiol* 1993; **265**: C859–68.
16 Dalemans W, Barbry P, Champigny G, et al. Altered chloride ion channel kinetics associated with delta F508 cystic fibrosis mutation. *Nature* 1991; **354**: 526–8.
17 Sheppard DN, Rich DP, Ostedgaard LS, et al. Mutations in CFTR associated with mild disease form $Cl^-$ channels with altered pore properties. *Nature* 1993; **363**: 160–4.
18 Tabcharani JA, Rommens JM, Hou YX, et al. Multi-ion pore behavior in the CFTR chloride channel. *Nature* 1993; **366**: 79–82.
19 Miller C, Arvan P, Telford JN, Racker E. $Ca^{2+}$-induced fusion of proteoliposomes: dependence on transmembrane osmotic gradient. *J Membr Biol* 1976; **30**: 271–82.
20 Miller C, Racker E. Calcium-induced fusion of fragmented sarcoplasmic reticulum with artificial planar bilayers. *J Membr Biol* 1976; **30**: 283–300.
21 Hanke W, Methfessel C, Wilmsen HO, Boheim G. Ion channel reconstitution into planar lipid bilayers on glass pipettes. *Biochem Bioeng J* 1984; **12**: 329–39.
22 Schmid A, Gogelein H, Kemmer TP, Schultz I. Anion channels in giant liposomes made of endoplasmic reticulum vesicles from rat exocrine pancreas. *J Membr Biol* 1988; **104**: 275–82.
23 Bradbury NA, Jilling T, Kirk KL, Bridges RJ. Regulated endocytosis in chloride secretory epithelial cell line. *Am J Physiol* 1992; **262**: C752–9.
24 Bradbury NA, Jilling T, Berta G, et al. Regulation of plasma membrane recycling by CFTR. *Science* 1992; **256**: 530–2.
25 Barasch J, Kiss B, Prince A, et al. Defective acidification of intracellular organelles in cystic fibrosis. *Nature* 1991; **352**: 70–3.
26 Welsh MJ, Smith AE. Molecular mechanisms of CFTR chloride channel dysfunction in cystic fibrosis. *Cell* 1993; **73**: 1251–4.
27 Hanrahan JW, Tabcharani JA, Gryorczyk R. Patch clamp studies of apical membrane chloride channels. In: *Cystic Fibrosis: Current Topics*, Vol 1 (eds JA Dodge, DJH Brock, JH Widdicombe) Wiley, New York, 1993, pp 93–137.
28 Anderson MP, Berger HA, Rich DP, et al. Nucleoside triphosphates are required to open the CFTR chloride channel. *Cell* 1991; **67**: 775–84.
29 Venglarik CJ, Schultz BD, Frizzell RA, Bridges RJ. ATP alters current fluctuations of cystic fibrosis transmembrane conductance regulator: evidence for a three state activation mechanism. *J Gen Physiol* 1994; **104**: 123–46.
30 Anderson MP, Welsh MJ. Regulation by ATP and ADP of CFTR chloride channels that contain mutant nucleotide-binding domains. *Science* 1992; **257**: 1701–4.
31 Schultz BD, Venglarik CJ, Bridges RJ, Frizzell RA. Regulation of CFTR by adenine nucleotide phosphates. *FASEB J* 1993; **7**: A426.

32 Sheppard DN, Welsh MJ. Effect of ATP-sensitive K channel regulators on cystic fibrosis transmembrane conductance regulator chloride currents. *J Gen Physiol* 1992; **100**: 573–91.
33 DeRoos ADG, Schultz BD, Venglarik CJ, et al. Glybenclamide blockade of CFTR. *Pediatr Pulmonol* 1993 (Suppl 9): 213.
34 Venglarik CJ, DeRoos ADG, Singh AK, Bridges RJ. Tolbutamide causes a fast-flickery block of CFTR. *Pediatr Pulmonol* 1993 (Suppl 9): 216.
35 Nagel G, Hwang TZ, Nastiuk KL, et al. The protein kinase A-regulated cardiac $Cl^-$ channel resembles the cystic fibrosis transmembrane conductance regulator. *Nature* 1992; **360**: 81–4.
36 Levesque PC, Hart PJ, Hume JR, et al. Expression of cystic fibrosis transmembrane regulator $Cl^-$ channels in heart. *Circ Res* 1992; **71**: 1002–7.
37 Alvarez O, Benos DJ, Latorre R. The study of ion channels in planar lipid bilayer membranes. *J Electrophysiol Tech* 1985; **12**: 159–77.
38 Bridges RJ, Benos DJ. Epithelial ion channel reconstitution. In: *Current Topics in Membrane Transport, Vol. 37: Channels and Noise in Epithelial Tissues* (eds SI Helman, W van Driessche) Academic Press, New York, 1990. pp 285–312.
39 Bridges RJ, Benos DJ. Reconstitution of epithelial ion channels. In: *Textbook of Secretory Diarrhea* (eds E Lebenthal, M Duffy) Raven Press, New York, 1990, pp 67–79.
40 Coronado R. Recent advances in planar phospholipid bilayer techniques for monitoring ion channels. *Annu Rev Biophys Chem* 1986; **15**: 259–77.
41 Darszon A. Planar bilayers: a powerful tool to study membrane proteins involved in ion transport. In: *Methods of Enzymology*, Vol. 127 (ed L Packer) Academic Press, Orlando, FL, 1986, pp 486–502.
42 Ehrlich BE. Planar lipid bilayers on patch pipettes; bilayer formation and ion channel incorporation. In: *Methods of Enzymology* (eds B Rudy, LE Iverson) Academic Press, San Diego, 1992, pp 463–70.
43 Hanke W, Eibl H, Boheim G. A new method for membrane reconstitution: fusion of protein-containing vesicles with planar bilayer membranes below the phase transition temperature. *Biophys Struct Mech* 1981; **7**: 131–7.
44 Labarca P, Latorre R. Insertion of ion channels into planar lipid bilayers by vesicle fusion. In: *Methods of Enzymology*, Vol 207 (eds B. Rudy, LE Iverson) Academic Press, San Diego, 1992, pp 447–63.
45 Miller C (ed). *Ion Channel Reconstitution*. Plenum, New York, 1986.
46 Wonderlin WF, Finkel A, French RJ. Optimizing planar lipid bilayer single channel recordings for high resolution with rapid voltage steps. *Biophys J* 1990; **58**: 289–97.
47 Mueller P, Rudin DO. Bimolecular lipid membranes: techniques of formation, study of electrical properties, and induction of ionic gating phenomena. In: *Laboratory Techniques in Membrane Biophysics* (eds H Passow, R Stamplfi) Springer-Verlag, Berlin, 1968, 141–56.
48 Mueller P, Rudin DO, Tren HT, Westcott WC. Reconstitution of cell membrane structure in vitro and its transformation into an excitable system. *Nature* 1962; **194**: 979–80.
49 Bridges RJ, Rummel W, Simon B. Forskolin induced chloride secretion across isolated mucosa of rat colon descendens. *Naunym-Schmiedebergs Arch Pharmacol* 1983; **328**: 355–60.
50 Trezise AEO, Buchwald M. In vivo cell-specific expression of the cystic fibrosis transmembrane conductance regulator. *Nature* 1991; **353**: 434–7.
51 Bridges RJ, Rack M, Schreiner J, Rummel W. Mucosal plexus and electrolyte transport across the rat colonic mucosa. *J Physiol* 1985; **364**: 301–12.

52 Cohn JA, Nairn AC, Marino CR, et al. Characterization of the cystic fibrosis transmembrane conductance regulator in a colonocyte cell line. *Proc Natl Acad Sci USA* 1992; **89**: 2340–4.
53 Pearse BMF. Coated vesicles from pig brain: purification and characterization. *J Mol Biol* **97**: 93–8.
54 Forgac M, Cantley L, Wiedenmann B, et al. Clathrin-coated vesicles contain a ATP-dependent proton pump. *Proc Natl Acad Sci USA* 1983; **80**: 1300–3.
55 Tabcharani JA, Chang XB, Riordan JR, Hanrahan JW. The cystic fibrosis transmembrane conductance regulator chloride channel: iodide block and permeation. *Biophys J* 1992; **62**: 1–4.
56 Egan M, Flotte T, Afiones, et al. Defective regulation of outwardly rectifying $Cl^-$ channels by protein kinase A corrected by insertion of CFTR. *Nature* 1992; **358**: 581–4.

Chapter Eight

# Functions of CFTR other than as a Plasma Membrane Chloride Channel

Joachim Biwersi and A. S. Verkman
*Departments of Medicine and Physiology, Cardiovascular Research Institute, University of California, San Francisco, California, USA*

## INTRODUCTION

Although an extensive body of information has been acquired over the last five years on the genetic defect in cystic fibrosis (CF) and the function and tissue distribution of CFTR (cystic fibrosis transmembrane conductance regulator), the cellular abnormalities that link CFTR genotype to clinical disease are not understood. There is definitive evidence from studies of CFTR expression in mammalian cells[1,2] and *Xenopus* oocytes[3,4], and direct reconstitution experiments[5], that CFTR functions as a cAMP-regulated non-rectifying chloride channel. The tissue distribution of CFTR is consistent with its role in transepithelial salt and fluid transport, although the level of CFTR expression in various tissues does not correlate well with the severity of organ disease in CF.

*Cystic Fibrosis—Current Topics, Volume 2.* Edited by J. A. Dodge, D. J. H. Brock and J. H. Widdicombe

A fundamental question in CF research remains how the CF genotype leads to clinical disease. A number of cellular abnormalities have been associated with CF including defective chloride conductance[6,8], abnormal post-translational reactions in the secretory pathway[9,11], abnormal bacterial adhesion[12] and others. While it is possible that defective plasma membrane chloride conductance can account for all of the cellular abnormalities in CF it seems difficult to reconcile these pleiotropic abnormalities with a single plasma membrane ion transport defect.

A number of other cellular sites of CFTR function, and other (non-chloride-transporting) roles for CFTR have been proposed as summarized in Figure 1. In addition to its role as a plasma membrane chloride channel, CFTR may function as a chloride channel in subcellular vesicles in the endosomal and secretory pathways. Functional intracellular CFTR may modulate vesicular acidification[13,14] and trafficking[15] mechanisms. CFTR may itself have other distinct functions, such as the transport of nucleotides[16], water[17], and other ions, or it may regulate the functioning of other cellular components, such as the outwardly rectifying chloride channel[18] or a sulphate transporter[19]. Although there is little experimental evidence, roles for CFTR in the transport of intracellular toxins[20] and second messengers have been proposed. The purpose of this chapter is to review the evidence for the existence of functions of CFTR that are distinct from its well-established role as an apical membrane chloride channel in epithelial cells.

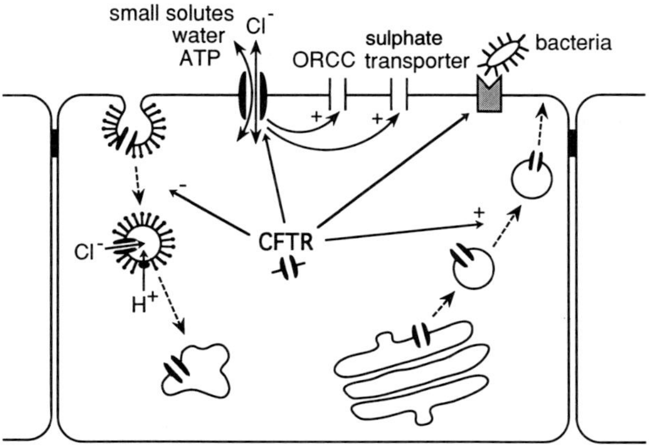


**Figure 1** Possible cellular functions of CFTR. In addition to its well-established role as a cAMP-regulated plasma membrane chloride channel, CFTR may function as an intracellular chloride channel that regulates endosomal acidification, a regulator of the outwardly rectifying chloride channel and sulphate transporter, a transporter for small polar solutes and ATP, and a regulator of vesicular trafficking

# ROLE OF CFTR AS AN INTRACELLULAR CHLORIDE CHANNEL

## CHLORIDE CHANNELS IN SUBCELLULAR VESICLES

It has been proposed that chloride channels play a role in acidification of intracellular organelles. Chloride channels could facilitate and possibly regulate the action of the electrogenic proton pump (vacuolar $H^+$ ATPase) by providing an electrical shunt to dissipate the interior positive diffusion potential produced by inward proton pumping (Figure 2). Functional studies suggest that chloride channels are present in a variety of organelles, including Golgi[21], lysosomes[22], clathrin-coated vesicles[23], zymogen granules[24] and endosomes[25].

There is functional evidence that chloride conductance in some organelles may be regulated. Bae and Verkman[26] found that endosomes from renal cortex contained a chloride conductance that was activated by protein kinase A-dependent phosphorylation and inhibited by phosphatase action. Chloride conductance was measured by a stopped-flow fluorescence technique in which endosomes labelled *in vivo* by SPQ[27] were subjected to defined electrochemical chloride gradients. Reenstra et al.[28] demonstrated that phosphorylation of an ~65 kDa protein in purified endosomes correlated well with chloride conductance. Mulberg et al.[29] reported similar studies for a chloride channel in clathrin-coated vesicles from brain whose activity was modulated by the state of phosphorylation. In these studies, SPQ was used to measure chloride transport in proteoliposomes reconstituted with partially purified coated vesicle proteins. There were several earlier indirect studies that suggested a regulated intracellular chloride conductance. Barasch et al.[30] found evidence for chloride-dependent ATP-induced acidification in granules isolated from thyroid parafollicular cells. Acidification was strongest when the thyroid cells

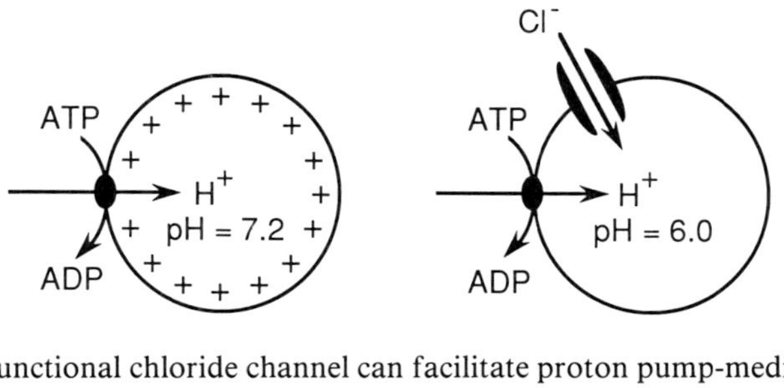


**Figure 2** A functional chloride channel can facilitate proton pump-mediated vesicular acidification. In the absence of a chloride conductance, an interior positive potential develops and inhibits inward proton pumping (left). The potential is dissipated by inward chloride movement (right)

were treated with secretagogues prior to granule isolation. Similar experiments suggested a role for regulated chloride channels in zymogen granules from pancreatic cells[24]. Granules isolated from rats pretreated with secretory antagonists had very low ion permeability, whereas pretreatment with secretagogues resulted in an activation or induction of a high chloride permeability.

The molecular identity of intracellular chloride channels is not known with certainty. Chloride channels cloned to date can be divided into five distinct gene families (for review, see Jentsch[31]). Their functions involve regulation of cell volume and intracellular pH (in combination with $Cl/HCO_3$ exchangers), and more specialized functions including transepithelial chloride transport and regulation of muscle and nerve excitability. The superfamily of ligand-gated chloride channels includes the $\gamma$-aminobutyric acid (GABA) and glycine receptors[32,33]. The first member of the family of voltage-gated chloride channels to be cloned was ClC-0 from *Torpedo* electric organ[34]. The ClC-0 gene was used to clone the major chloride channel of the mammalian skeletal muscles, ClC-1[35]. Mutations in ClC-1 lead to myotonia. The homologous chloride channel ClC-2 is expressed in all tissues and cell lines examined. The $I_{Cln}$ protein is a voltage- and nucleotide-dependent chloride channel that was obtained by expression cloning from a dog kidney epithelial cell line[36]. Phospholemman is a small polypeptide of 72 amino acids with a single predicted transmembrane region that may form an oligomeric chloride channel in membranes[37]. The final class contains CFTR and possibly MDR-1, both of which are members of the ABC (ATP-binding cassette) transporter superfamily. There is evidence that MDR-1 functions as a hypotonicity-activated chloride channel[38,39] in addition to its well-established role as a drug transporter.

Landry et al.[40] used antiserum against a putative 64 kDa kidney chloride channel[41] to clone the cDNA encoding protein p64. The antiserum was shown to deplete chloride transport activity from solubilized kidney membranes[42]. The p64 message was expressed in all cells tested. When injected into *Xenopus* oocytes, cRNA encoding p64 produced protein expression in microsomes but not in the plasma membrane. It was proposed that p64 encodes an intracellular chloride channel. Direct expression and localization studies will be required to establish the function and cellular distribution of p64.

## EVIDENCE FOR CFTR IN THE ENDOSOMAL COMPARTMENT

CFTR may play a role in endosomal acidification and trafficking if it is present and functional in the endosomal compartment or, less likely, if it exerts a secondary effect from a distant location. It should first be pointed out that even a single CFTR molecule that is partially functional might have a major effect on the membrane potential, pH and function of an intracellular organelle. For example, if CFTR-mediated chloride transport is rate limiting across a 200 nm diameter vesicle containing a single 10 pS CFTR chloride channel, the equilibration time for dissipation of an electrochemical chloride gradient would be $<50$ ms. Therefore, it might be difficult to identify single CFTR molecules on endosomes by conventional morphological or biochemical techniques. Nevertheless, several recent morphological, biochemical and functional studies suggest that CFTR is present in endosomes in at least some CFTR-expressing cells.

Initial antibody-staining studies showed localization of CFTR primarily in the apical membrane of epithelial cells[43,44]. Several recent reports suggest that some CFTR is present in intracellular membranes. Dalemans et al.[45] found CFTR in the perinuclear area of CFTR-transfected L cells by immunofluorescence; Puchelle et al.[46] located CFTR in vesicles beneath the apical membrane in airway epithelia from polyps by immunogold electron microscopy. CFTR was also identified in secretory granules of glandular serous cells of human and bovine tracheal tissues. In CFTR-transfected CFPAC cells, CFTR was localized by immunoperoxidase staining to multivesicular bodies, with occasional staining in endoplasmic reticulum cisternae, nuclear envelope and Golgi complex[48]. In preliminary studies, CFTR has been detected by immunoblotting in endosomes from rabbit kidney cortex[49] and by immunogold in endosomes of rat salivary duct epithelia cells[50].

Biochemical studies suggest the presence of intracellular CFTR. Prince et al.[51] found that a significant quantity of mature, fully glycosylated CFTR was present in an intracellular compartment. They labelled surface CFTR by biotin, and quantified biotinylated and non-biotinylated CFTR by immunoprecipitation, *in vitro* phosphorylation and autoradiography. Approximately half of the immunoreactive CFTR was biotinylated in both control and forskolin-stimulated cells. Assuming a 100% biotinylation efficiency, it was concluded that approximately 50% of mature CFTR molecules in T84 cells were not exposed at the cell surface. These results are consistent with the presence of CFTR on specific intracellular membranes; however, the data might also be interpreted in terms of non-selective constitutive processing of plasma membrane transport proteins, or incomplete biotinylation of surface CFTR. In preliminary studies, Bradbury et al.[52] reported immunoreactive CFTR in purified clathrin-coated vesicles. However, these studies must be viewed cautiously because of the non-quantitative nature of CFTR immunoblotting and the possible contamination of coated vesicle preparations with CFTR-containing membranes.

Two studies have reported functional evidence for CFTR in endosomes. Lukacs et al.[53] labelled the endosomal compartment of CFTR- and mock-transfected CHO cells with FITC–dextran. The endosomal chloride conductance was measured from the rate of dissipation of the endosomal pH gradient after addition of the protonophore CCCP. In intact labelled CHO cells studied in suspension, cAMP stimulation by CPT–cAMP or forskolin resulted in an approximately two-fold increase in the rate of alkalinization after CCCP addition in CFTR- but not mock-transfected cells. Cell-free measurements were carried out using a microsomal preparation derived from the CFTR-transfected cells. In fluorescently labelled endosomes present in the microsomal preparation, the endosomal pH gradient produced by ATP was dissipated by CCCP at a significantly faster rate when microsomes were pretreated with protein kinase A. These results suggested that endosomes from CFTR-transfected cells contained a functional cAMP-dependent conductance, presumably CFTR. However, the difficulty in extrapolating these results to native CFTR-expressing epithelial cells is that foreign proteins expressed in transfected cells are often misdirected to compartments in which they are normally excluded, particularly when the protein is expressed at high levels.

Biwersi and Verkman[54] recently used a similar approach to determine whether functional CFTR was present in the endosomal compartment in transfected Swiss 3T3 fibroblasts and T84 cells. Adherent fibroblasts on glass coverslips were labelled with FITC–dextran, and rate of endosomal alkalinization after CCCP addition was measured by quantitative microfluorimetry. Prestimulation by forskolin increased the rate of alkalinization by 1.5–2-fold in T84 cells and CFTR-expressing fibroblasts, but had no significant effect in mock-transfected and ΔF508 CFTR-expressing fibroblasts. Figure 3(A) shows representative data for the kinetics of the endosomal alkalinization and the effect of CCCP. Fluorescence data for the CFTR-expressing fibroblasts are shown on an expanded time scale in Figure 3(B), and the rates of alkalinization after CCCP addition are summarized in Figure 3(C). There was no effect of forskolin on alkalinization in any of the cell types in the absence of chloride, indicating that endosomes from CFTR-expressing fibroblasts and T84 cells contained a functional cAMP-dependent CFTR chloride conductance. Analysis of the alkalinization curve shapes suggested that the majority of endosomes contained at least one functional CFTR molecule.

## THE 'DEFECTIVE ACIDIFICATION' HYPOTHESIS

Barasch et al.[13] advanced an interesting hypothesis in which acidification in the endosomal and secretory compartments is defective in CF because of lack of activation of a Cl channel. The hypothesis is potentially attractive because it provides a unifying theme to account for the multiplicity of cellular defects in CF[55]. For example, the decreased sialylation of secreted proteins may result from decreased activity of pH-dependent sialyltransferases in Golgi; sialyltransferase enzymes generally have pH optima near 6[56]. Although the pH optima of sulphotransferases and fucosyltransferases are higher, it is conceivable that sulphation and fucosylation reactions can be affected by Golgi pH if terminal glycosylation reactions are competitive[57]. Another class

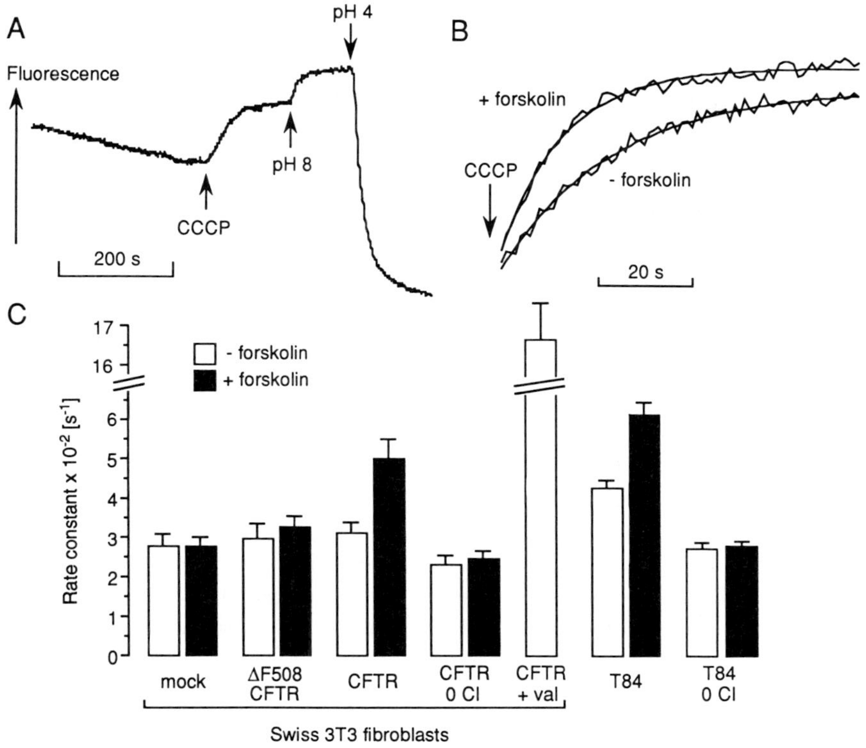


**Figure 3** Functional CFTR chloride channels in endosomes from CFTR-expressing Swiss 3T3 fibroblasts and T84 cells. Endosomes were labelled with FITC–dextran and fluorescence was measured in response to CCCP addition[54]. (A) Time course of fluorescence, showing rapid alkalinization after CCCP addition. The rate of alkalinization in the presence of CCCP provided a measure of chloride conductance (see text). (B) Expanded view of time course of change in fluorescence on addition of CCCP in CFTR-expressing fibroblasts with and without forskolin stimulation. (C) Summary of the initial rates of alkalinization after CCCP addition. Where indicated, chloride was replaced by isethionate (0 Cl), or valinomycin was added (+val). The fast rate of alkalinization after addition of valinomycin shows that the perfusion system and the CCCP-induced proton conductance were not rate limiting

of defects in CF involves abnormal bacterial adhesion leading to chronic *Pseudomonas* colonization. It was proposed that alkalinization of Golgi in CF might lead to undersialylation of a cell surface *Pseudomononas* receptor which might be involved in bacterial adhesion[58]. The 'defective acidification' hypothesis provides a provocative explanation for multiple cellular defects in CF. However, it is difficult to understand how very small pH differences (see below) could cause profound effects on cell function, particularly when there is considerable heterogeneity in vesicular pH in different cell types from normal tissues. A defect in organelle acidification which is significant enough to cause the above defects would likely affect multiple other cellular processes related to receptor trafficking, protein processing and degradation, and others. Finally, some of the proposed mechanisms linking Golgi pH to abnormalities in post-translational protein reactions and changes in bacterial adhesion should be considered speculative at this time.

The principle evidence cited by Barasch et al.[13] for defective organelle acidification was: (a) the pH in early endosomes and secretory vesicles in CF cells, measured by DAMP immunoelectron microscopy, was 0.2–0.3 units alkaline relative to that in normal cells; and (b) ATP-dependent acidification in cell-free endosomal preparations suggested a functional Cl channel in endosomes from normal but not from CF cells. Possible caveats in the interpretation of these results are the difficulties in quantifying small pH differences by the DAMP method and in comparing organelle pH values in unmatched normal and CF cell lines.

In the study of Lukacs et al.[53] discussed above, endosomal pH in control and CFTR-expressing CHO cells in suspension was estimated by fluorescence. There was no difference in average endosomal pH in the control and CFTR-expressing cells, nor was there an effect of forskolin. They concluded that factors other than endosomal CFTR chloride conductance were dominant in regulation of endosomal pH. However, because average pH measurements were made in suspended cells labelled with FITC–dextran, pH differences may have been missed because: (a) much of the fluorescence may have originated from late endosomes; (b) a subpopulation of endosomes with altered pH was not detected; and (c) there may have been an undetermined amount of extra-endosomal fluorescent marker. In a study of ATP-dependent acidification in lysosomes isolated from CFTR-transfected cells, Van Dyke et al.[59] concluded that CFTR did not play a role in lysosomal acidification.

Zen et al.[60] developed a quantitative imaging method to measure pH in individual fluorescently labelled endocytic vesicles in intact adherent cells. Cells were labelled with dual-wavelength fluorescent markers, such as carboxyfluorescein–tetramethylrhodamine (Cf–TMR) transferrin to visualize early endosomes, and Cf–TMR dextran and Cf–TMR macroglobulin to visualize both early and late endosomes. Cells were imaged at high magnification using an epifluorescence microscope equipped with a cooled charge-coupled device camera. Software was developed to identify endosomes and to quantify background-subtracted fluorescence for pH determination by ratio imaging. The distribution of endosomal pH values was determined as a function of time after pulse labelling with the fluorescent indicator and in response to addition of various agonists or changes in solution composition. The pH in transferrin-labelled endosomes in Swiss 3T3 fibroblasts was 6.2, with a tight distribution in the range 6.0–6.4; the pH distribution in dextran-labelled endosomes was very broad, with some pH values below 5.0. It was found that cAMP agonists caused mild alkalinization of early endosomes, $Na^+/K^+$-ATPase inhibition by ouabain and protein kinase C activation by phorbol esters caused acidification of early endosomes, and calcium elevation had no effect. It was concluded that multiple second messengers were involved in the regulation of endosomal pH.

Biwersi and Verkman[54] applied the imaging methods developed by Zen et al.[60] to measure the pH distribution of transferrin-labelled early endosomes in control, and CFTR and ΔF508 CFTR-expressing Swiss 3T3 fibroblasts. There was little difference in endosomal pH distributions in each of the cell types before or after forskolin stimulation. In addition, no subpopulation of endosomes was identified in which acidification was different in the various cell types before or after forskolin stimulation. These results supported the conclusion that factors other than the endosomal CFTR chloride conductance were responsible for regulation of pH in early endosomes. Measurements of pH in the endosomal and secretory compartments in native normal and CF cells will be required to definitively prove or disprove the defective acidification hypothesis.

## OTHER TRANSPORTING FUNCTIONS OF CFTR

### CFTR AS A MULTIFUNCTIONAL AQUEOUS PORE

Hasegawa et al.[17] reported evidence that CFTR can transport not only anions but also water and urea. CFTR was expressed in *Xenopus* oocytes and water permeability was measured by a swelling assay. Expression of CFTR was maximized by placing the *Xenopus* globin 5′ untranslated region just upstream from the CFTR translation initiation codon. In CFTR-expressing oocytes, cAMP agonists induced a chloride conductance of 94 μS and an increase in osmotic water permeability of $4 \times 10^{-4}$ cm/s. There was no effect of cAMP agonists in water-injected control oocytes. The increase in water permeability in the CFTR-expressing oocytes was inhibited by a chloride channel blocker and was dependent upon anion composition. Transport of urea but not the larger solute sucrose was increased in oocytes expressing CFTR, suggesting that CFTR forms an aqueous channel that is able to pass urea-sized molecules. Although the aqueous pore properties of CFTR are interesting in terms of CFTR structure, the low density of CFTR molecules in cell membranes makes CFTR ineffective as a water transporter. Instead, there are selective water transporters including CHIP28 (for review, see reference 61) and a recently identified lung water transporter (MIWC[62]) that is probably responsible for water movement in secretory and absorptive epithelia[63]. Because water movement is driven by osmotic forces produced by active and secondary active ion and solute transport, it is unlikely that defective water transport plays a role in the pathophysiology of CF.

### CFTR AS AN ATP CHANNEL

CFTR belongs to the ABC superfamily of membrane transporters that are responsible for the active transport of various substrates including amino acids, peptides and proteins[64]. The most closely related ABC family member to CFTR is the MDR-1 multidrug transporter. Because of this relationship, it has been proposed that CFTR transports substrates other than chloride. MDR-1 has multiple transporting functions, including transport of hydrophobic drugs, ATP[65], and possibly chloride (under hypotonic conditions)[38,39]. Reisin et al.[16] have shown in preliminary studies that expression of CFTR in mouse mammary carcinoma cells was associated with a three-fold increase of cAMP-inducible release of ATP and an increase in whole-cell chloride currents compared to mock-transfected cells. Patch-clamp experiments suggested a single anionic conductive pathway for both ATP and Cl. Cantiello et al.[66] reported CFTR-mediated ATP currents in patch clamp studies of CFTR-expressing mouse mammary carcinoma cells. If CFTR is able to transport ATP, then multiple ATP-dependent intracellular processes might be altered in CF.

## CFTR AS A REGULATOR OF CELLULAR FUNCTIONS

### THE 'DEFECTIVE TRAFFICKING' HYPOTHESIS

Bradbury et al.[15] proposed that CFTR is a general regulator of vesicular trafficking and that the pleiotropic nature of the defect in CF might be due to abnormal vesicular trafficking in CF cells. The principal evidence that CFTR is important for cAMP-regulated endocytosis and exocytosis was that forskolin altered trafficking in CFTR-transfected CFPAC cells, but had little effect in the non-transfected cells. Endocytosis, as assayed by horseradish peroxidase uptake[67], was decreased by approximately three-fold in the forskolin-treated CFTR-expressing cells. Exocytosis, as assayed by recycling of a biotinylated wheat-germ agglutinin marker, was increased two- to three-fold in CFTR-transfected cells after cAMP stimulation. Although the defective trafficking hypothesis may provide a link between CFTR genotype and cellular dysfunction, there are several issues that should be considered. Are the effects of CFTR transfection in the CFPAC cells specific for CFTR and does CFTR regulate vesicular trafficking in native epithelial cells? What is the mechanism by which CFTR affects vesicular trafficking? What is the link between defective vesicular trafficking and altered post-translational protein processing in CF cells? Why is the CF genotype not lethal if a process so general as vesicular trafficking is defective? Additional studies in native CFTR-expresing normal and CF cells are warranted to evaluate the significance of the defective trafficking hypothesis in CF pathophysiology.

## REGULATION OF THE OUTWARDLY RECTIFYING CHLORIDE CHANNEL (ORCC)

The ORCC is a high-conductance chloride channel (25–50 pS) that is distributed widely in epithelia and non-epithelial tissues, including fibroblasts and lymphocytes[68,69]. Prior to identification of the CF gene, the ORCC was believed to be the principal defective chloride channel in CF[7,8,70]. Based on single-channel characteristics and tissue distribution, it is clear that the ORCC and CFTR are distinct proteins[71]. Gabriel et al.[72] reported that the ORCC is present in CFTR (−/−) knock-out mice. Egan et al.[18] reported that CFTR can regulate the ORCC. Upon expression of CFTR in CF bronchial epithelia, they found that protein kinase A activation resulted in the appearance of both small linear conductance chloride channels (presumably CFTR) and the ORCC channel. In cells lacking CFTR (uncorrected cells and cells transfected with a plasmid having a frameshift mutation), the ORCC was not activated by PKA. These studies provided evidence that CFTR can influence the activity of another protein. It was proposed that CFTR may regulate the ORCC by either affecting the post-translational processing of the ORCC or interacting with another substance that regulates the ORCC. Based on these observations, it is conceivable that CFTR may regulate other cellular functions indirectly. It will be important to define the precise mechanism by which the ORCC and CFTR interact.

## REGULATION OF A SULPHATE ANION EXCHANGER BY CFTR

It was suggested that there is increased sulphation of bronchial mucous secretions in CF compared to normal controls[9,73]. Because inorganic sulphate is the major substrate for sulphation, changes in intracellular sulphate concentration might be important for altered mucous secretions in CF bronchial and pancreatic epithelia. Elgavish and Meezan[19] found that sulphate transport in CFPAC cells—a pancreatic cell line homozygous for ΔF508 CFTR—and PANC-1 cells—an epithelioid cell line from a pancreatic carcinoma—occurs by an anion-exchange mechanism. The rate of sulphate transport was markedly reduced in CFPAC cells compared to PANC-1. To test the hypothesis that the absence of functional CFTR in CFPAC cells was responsible for the altered sulphate transport, sulphate transport in mock- and CFTR-transfected CFPAC cells was compared. There was a 10-fold increase in sulphate transport in CFTR-expressing CFPAC cells compared to the control cells; however, cAMP stimulation did not affect the rate of sulphate transport. These results suggested that expression of CFTR was necessary for sulphate transport in pancreatic epithelial cells. It was proposed that altered sulphate transport may be related to the over-sulphation of glycoproteins in CF. A sulphate transporter has also been reported in human bronchial epithelial cells[74]; however sulphate transport rates in native normal and CF cells have not been compared.

## SUMMARY AND PERSPECTIVE

Although many of the observations described above are provocative and many provide causal relationships between CF genotype and cellular dysfunction, the data remain inconclusive. It is important to understand how mutant CFTRs affect cell function for the further development of non-gene replacement modes of therapy and to define the appropriate cells for gene targeting. Further analysis of CFTR function in intracellular organelles is warranted. These studies would be facilitated by the development of methods to measure chloride activity and membrane potential *in situ* in organelles, and to label vesicular compartments in the secretory pathway with pH and ion indicators. Further analysis of non-chloride-transporting roles of CFTR is warranted, particularly transport studies in well-defined systems containing only CFTR or CFTR plus a putative target protein that may be regulated by CFTR. Finally, the possibility remains that the cellular defects in CF may arise as a direct or indirect consequence of defective plasma membrane chloride conductance without ascribing novel function(s) to CFTR.

## NOTE ADDED IN PROOF

Several relevant studies have been reported since submission of this review. Bradbury et al.[75] detected functional CFTR in clathrin coated vesicles from T84 cells by immunoblotting, tryptic phosphopeptide mapping and bilayer fusion. Using a two-step biotinylation procedure to label cell surface glycoconjugates, Prince et al.[76] found CFTR in a rapidly recycling endocytic compartment in T84 cells. CFTR internalization and fluid-phase endocytosis were inhibited by cAMP stimulation. The inhibition was not observed in Cl-depleted cells and in cells expressing G551D CFTR, a mutant in which CFTR is targeted to the plasma membrane but lacks Cl-channel activity. Dunn et al.[77] reported that CFTR expression did not affect endosomal acidification and cAMP-mediated endocytosis in CFPAC-1 cells expressing CFTR and ΔF508 CFTR. Similarly, Dho et al.[78] found no influence of CFTR expression on endocytosis and exocytosis in transfected CHO cells. Dosanjh et al.[79] showed that expression of ΔF508 CFTR but not wt-CFTR resulted in decreased sialylation of membrane glycoconjugates in mouse mammary epithelia cells. In a preliminary study, Seksek et al.[80] developed a novel approach to label selectively the aqueous compartment of trans-Golgi in living cells and found no difference between trans-Golgi pH of mock transfected, CFTR and ΔF508 CFTR expressing 3T3 fibroblasts.

## ACKNOWLEDGEMENTS

This work was supported by grant HL42368 from the National Institutes of Health and a grant from the National Cystic Fibrosis Foundation.

## REFERENCES

1 Anderson MP, Rich DP, Gregory RJ, et al. Generation of cAMP-activated chloride currents by expression of CFTR. *Science* 1991; **251**: 205–7.
2 Rommens JM, Dho S, Bear CE, et al. cAMP-inducible chloride conductance in mouse fibroblast lines stably expressing the human cystic fibrosis transmembrane conductance regulator. *Proc Natl Acad Sci USA* 1991; **88**: 7500–4.
3 Drumm ML, Wilkinson DJ, Smit LS, et al. Chloride conductance expressed by the ΔF508 and other mutant CFTRs in *Xenopus* oocytes. *Science* 1991; **254**: 1797–9.
4 Bear CE, Duguay F, Naismith AL, et al. $Cl^-$ channel activity in *Xenopus* oocytes expressing the cystic fibrosis gene. *J Biol Chem* 1991; **266**: 19142–5.
5 Bear CE, Li C, Kartner N, et al. Purification and functional reconstitution of the cystic fibrosis transmembrane conductance regulator (CFTR). *Cell* 1992; **68**: 809–18.
6 Quinton PM. Chloride impermeability in cystic fibrosis. *Nature* 1983; **301**: 421–2.
7 Li M, McCann JD, Liedtke CM, et al. Cyclic AMP opens chloride channels in normal but not cystic fibrosis airway epithelium. *Nature* 1988; **331**: 358–60.
8 Schoumacher RA, Shoemaker RL, Halm DR, et al. Phosphorylation fails to activate chloride channels from cystic fibrosis airway cells. *Nature* 1987; **330**: 752–4.
9 Cheng PW, Boucher RC, Yankaskas JM, Boat TF. Glycoconjugates secreted by cultured human nasal epithelial cells. In: *Cellular and Molecular Basis of Cystic Fibrosis* (eds G Mastella, PM Quinton). San Francisco Press, San Francisco, 1988. pp 233–8.
10 Rose MC. Epithelial mucous glycoproteins and cystic fibrosis. *Horm Metab Res* 1988; **20**: 601–8.
11 Boat TF, Kleinerman JL, Carlson DM, et al. Human respiratory tract secretions. 1. Mucous glycoproteins secreted by cultured nasal polyp epithelium from subjects with allergic rhinitis and with cystic fibrosis. *Am Rev Respir Dis* 1974; **110**: 428–41.
12 Woods DE, Bass JA, Johanson WG Jr, Straus DC. Role of adherence in the pathogenesis of *Pseudomonas aeruginosa* lung infection in cystic fibrosis patients. *Infect Immun* 1980; **30**: 694–9.

13 Barasch J, Kiss B, Prince A, et al. Defective acidification of intracellular organelles in cystic fibrosis. *Nature* 1991; **352**: 70–3.
14 Al-Awqati Q, Barasch J, Landry D. Chloride channels of intracellular organelles and their potential role in cystic fibrosis. *J Exp Biol* 1992; **172**: 245–66.
15 Bradbury NA, Jilling T, Berta G, et al. Regulation of plasma membrane recycling by CFTR. *Science* 1992; **256**: 530–2.
16 Reisin IL, Prat AG, Abraham EH, et al. Expression of CFTR results in the appearance of an ATP-conductive channel. *Pediatr Pulmonol* 1992; **14**: 262.
17 Hasegawa H, Skach W, Baker O, et al. A multifunctional aqueous channel formed by CFTR. *Science* 1992; **258**: 1477–9.
18 Egan M, Flotte T, Afione S, et al. Defective regulation of outwardly rectifying Cl channels by protein kinase A corrected by insertion of CFTR. *Nature* 1992; **358**: 581–4.
19 Elgavish A, Meezan E. Altered sulfate transport via anion exchange in CFPAC is corrected by retrovirus-mediated CFTR gene transfer. *Am J Physiol* 1992; **263**: C176–86.
20 Kunzelmann K, Tilmann M, Hansen CP, Greger R. Inhibition of epithelial chloride channels by cytosol. *Pflugers Arch* 1991; **418**: 479–90.
21 Glickman J, Croen K, Kelly S, Al-Awqati Q. Golgi membranes contain an electrogenic $H^+$ pump in parallel to a chloride conductance. *J Cell Biol* 1983; **97**: 1303–8.
22 Harikumar P, Reeves JP. The lysosomal proton pump is electrogenic. *J Biol Chem* 1983; **258**: 10403–10.
23 Stone DK, Xie X-S, Racker E. An ATP-driven proton pump in clathrin-coated vesicles. *J Biol Chem* 1983; **258**: 4059–62.
24 Gasser KW, DiDomenico J, Hopfer U. Secretagogues activate chloride transport pathways in pancreatic zymogen granules. *Am J Physiol* 1988; **254**: G93–9.
25 Schmid A, Burckhardt G, Gogelein H. Single chloride channels in endosomal vesicle preparations from rat kidney cortex. *J Membr Biol* 1989; **111**: 265–75.
26 Bae H-R, Verkman AS. Protein kinase A regulates chloride conductance in endocytic vesicles from the proximal tubule. *Nature* 1990; **348**: 637–9.
27 Verkman AS, Biwersi J. Chloride-sensitive fluorescent indicators. In: *Methods in Neuroscience* (eds J Kraicer, DJ Dixon) Academic Press, New York, 1994 (in press).
28 Reenstra WW, Sabolic I, Bae H-R, Verkman AS. Phosphorylation of endosome membrane proteins by protein kinase A. *Biochemistry* 1992; **31**: 175–81.
29 Mulberg AE, Tulk BM, Forgac M. Modulation of coated vesicle chloride channel activity and acidification by reversible protein kinase A-dependent phosphorylation. *J Biol Chem* 1991; **266**: 20590–3.
30 Barasch J, Gershon MD, Nunez EA, et al. Thyrotropin induces the acidification of the secretory granules of parafollicular cells by increasing the chloride conductance of the granular membrane. *J Cell Biol* 1988; **107**: 2137–47.
31 Jentsch TJ. Chloride channels. *Curr Opin Neurobiol* 1993; **3**: 316–21.
32 Schofield PR, Darlison MG, Fujita N, et al. Sequence and functional expression of the $GABA_A$ receptor shows a ligand gated receptor superfamily. *Nature* 1987; **328**: 221–7.
33 Grenningloh G, Rienitz A, Schmitt B, et al. The strychnine-binding subunit of the glycine receptor shows homology with nicotinic acetylcholine receptor. *Nature* 1990; **328**: 215–20.
34 Jentsch TJ, Steinmeyer K, Schwarz G. Primary structure of *Torpedo marmorata* chloride channel isolated by expression cloning in *Xenopus* oocytes. *Nature* 1990; **348**: 510–14.

35 Steinmeyer K, Ortland C, Jentsch TJ. Primary structure and functional expression of a developmentally regulated skeletal muscle chloride channel. *Nature* 1991; **354**: 301–4.
36 Paulmichl M, Li Y, Wickman K, et al. New mammalian chloride channel identified by expression cloning. *Nature* 1992; **356**: 238–41.
37 Moorman JR, Palmer CJ, John JE, et al. Phospholemman expression induces a hyperpolarization-activated chloride current in *Xenopus* oocytes. *J Biol Chem* 1992; **267**: 14551–4.
38 Valverde MA, Diaz M, Sepulveda FV, et al. Volume-regulated chloride channels associated with the human multidrug resistance P-glycoprotein. *Nature* 1992; **355**: 830–3.
39 Gill DR, Hyde SC, Higgins CF, et al. Separation of drug transport and chloride channel functions of the human multidrug resistance P-glycoprotein. *Cell* 1992; **71**; 23–32.
40 Landry D, Sullivan S, Nicolaides M, et al. Molecular cloning and characterization of p64: a chloride channel protein from kidney microsomes. *J Biol Chem* 1993; **268**: 14948–55.
41 Landry DW, Akabas MH, Redhead C, et al. Purification and reconstitution of chloride channels from kidney and trachea. *Science* 1989; **244**: 1469–72.
42 Redhead CR, Edelman AE, Brown D, et al. A ubiquitous 64-kDa protein is a component of a chloride channel of plasma and intracellular membranes. *Proc Natl Acad Sci USA* 1992; **89**: 3716–20.
43 Crawford I, Maloney PC, Zeitlin PL, et al. Immunocytochemical localization of the cystic fibrosis gene product CFTR. *Proc Natl Acad Sci USA* 1991; **88**: 9262–6.
44 Denning GM, Ostedgaard LS, Cheng SH, et al. Localization of cystic fibrosis transmembrane conductance regulator in chloride secretory epithelia. *J Clin Invest* 1992; **89**: 339–49.
45 Dalemans W, Hinnrasky J, Slos P, et al. Immunocytochemical analysis reveals differences between the subcellular localization of normal and ΔPhe508 recombinant cystic fibrosis transmembrane conductance regulator. *Exp Cell Res* 1992; **201**: 235–40.
46 Puchelle E, Gaillard D, Ploton D, et al. Differential localization of the cystic fibrosis transmembrane conductance regulator in normal and cystic fibrosis airway epithelium. *Am J Respir Cell Mol Biol* 1992; **7**: 485–91.
47 Jacquot J, Puchelle E, Hinnrasky J, et al. Localization of the cystic fibrosis transmembrane conductance regulator in airway secretory glands. *Eur Respir J* 1993; **6**: 169–76.
48 Yang Y, Janich S, Cohn JA, Wilson JM. The common variant of cystic fibrosis transmembrane conductance regulator is recognized by hsp70 and degraded in a pre-golgi nonlysosomal compartment. *Proc Natl Acad Sci USA* 1993; **90**: 9480–4.
49 Crawford IT, Beardmore C, Beck JC, et al. Identification of CFTR-immunoreactive material in renal endosomes. *Pediatr Pulmonol* 1992; **14**: 261.
50 Marino CR, Webster P. Ultrastructural localization of CFTR to endosomes in a ductal epithelium. *Pediatr Pulmonol* 1994 (in press).
51 Prince LS, Tousson, A, Marchase RB. Cell surface labeling of CFTR in T-84 cells. *Am J Physiol* 1993; **264**: C491–8.
52 Bradbury NA, Cohn JA, Venglarik CJ, Bridges RJ. CFTR is in clathrin coated vesicles. *Pediatr Pulmonol* 1992; **14**: 261.

53 Lukacs GL, Chang XB, Kartner N, et al. The cystic fibrosis transmembrane conductance regulator is present and functional in endosomes: role as a determinant of endosomal pH. *J Biol Chem* 1992; **267**: 14568–72.
54 Biwersi J, Verkman AS. Functional CFTR in the endosomal compartment of CFTR-expressing fibroblasts and T84 cells. *Am J Physiol* 1994; **266**: C149–56.
55 Barasch J, Landry D, Al-Awqati Q. The chloride channel of intracellular organelles and potential role in cystic fibrosis. In: *Cystic Fibrosis: Current Topics* Vol 1 (eds JA Dodge, DJH Brock, JH Widdicombe) Wiley, Chichester, 1993, pp 191–213.
56 Roseman S, Carlson DM, Jourdian GW, et al. Animal sialic acid transferases (sialyltransferases). In: *Methods in Enzymology* (eds EF Neufeld, V Ginsburg) Academic Press, New York, 1966, pp. 354–72.
57 Paulson JC, Prieels JP, Glasgow LR, Hill RL. Sialyl and fucosyltransferases in the biosynthesis of asparaginyl-linked oligosaccharides in glycoproteins: mutually exclusive glycosylation by $\beta$-galactoside $\alpha$-2,6-sialyltransferase and *N*-acetyl glucosaminide $\beta$-1,6,3-fucosyltransferase. *J Biol Chem* 1978; **253**: 5617–24.
58 Krivan HC, Ginsburg V, Roberts DD. *Pseudomonas aeruginosa* and *Pseudomonas cepacia* isolated from cystic fibrosis patients bind specifically to gangliotetraosylceramide (Asialo GM1) and gangliotriaosylceramide (Asialo GM2). *Arch Biochem Biophys* 1988; **260**: 493–6.
59 Van Dyke RW, Root KV, Schreiber JH, Wilson JM. Role of CFTR in lysosome acidification. *Biochem Biophys Res Commun* 1992; **184**: 300–5.
60 Zen K, Biwersi J, Periasamy N, Verkman AS. Second messengers regulate endosomal acidification in Swiss 3T3 fibroblasts. *J Cell Biol* 1992; **119**: 99–110.
61 Verkman AS. *Water Channels*, RG Landes Company, Austin, TX, 1993.
62 Hasegawa H, Ma T, Skach W, et al. Molecular cloning of a mercurial-insensitive water channel (MIWC30) expressed in selective water transporting epithelia. *J Biol Chem* 1994; **269**: 5497–5500.
63 Folkesson HG, Matthay MA, Hasegawa H, et al. Transcellular water transport in lung alveolar epithelium through mercurial sensitive water channels. *Proc Natl Acad Sci USA* 1994; **91**: 4970–4.
64 Hyde SC, Emsley P, Hartshorn MJ, et al. Structural model of ATP-binding proteins associated with cystic fibrosis, multidrug resistance and bacterial transport. *Nature* 1990; **346**: 362–5.
65 Abraham EH, Prat AG, Gerweck L, et al; The multidrug resistance (MDR1) gene product functions as an ATP channel. *Proc Natl Acad Sci USA* 1993; **90**: 312–16.
66 Cantiello HF, Prat AG, Reisih IL, et al. External ATP and its analogs activate the cystic fibrosis transmembrane conductance regulator by a cyclic AMP-independent mechanism. *J Biol Chem* 1994; **269**: 11224–32.
67 Bradbury NA, Jilling T, Kirk KL, Bridges RJ. Regulated endocytosis in a chloride secretory epithelial cell line. *Am J Physiol* 1992; **262**: C752–9.
68 Bear CE. Phosphorylation-activated chloride channels in human skin fibroblasts. *FEBS Lett* 1988; **237**: 145–9.
69 Chen JH, Schulman H, Gardner P. A cAMP regulated chloride channel in lymphocytes that is affected in cystic fibrosis. *Science* 1989; **243**: 657–60.
70 Hwang TC, Lu L, Zeitlin PL, et al. Cl-channels in CF: lack of activation by protein kinase C and cAMP dependent protein kinase. *Science* 1989; **244**: 1351–3.
71 Ward CL, Krouse ME, Gruenert DC, et al. Cystic fibrosis gene expression is not correlated with rectifying Cl-channels. *Proc Natl Acad Sci USA* 1991; **88**: 5277–81.

72 Gabriel SE, Clarke LL, Boucher RC, Stutts MJ. CFTR and outward rectifying chloride channels are distinct proteins with a regulatory relationship. *Nature* 1993; **363**: 263–6.
73 Cheng PW, Boat TF, Cranfill K, et al. Increased sulfation of glycoconjugates by cultured nasal epithelial cells from patients with cystic fibrosis. *J Clin Invest* 1989; **84**: 68–72.
74 Mohapatra NK, Cheng PW, Parker JC, et al. Sulfate concentrations and transport in human bronchial epithelial cells. *Am J Physiol* 1993; **264**: C1231–7.
75 Bradbury NA, Cohn JA, Venglarik CJ, Bridges RJ. Biochemical and biophysical identification of cystic fibrosis transmembrane conductance regulator chloride channels as components of endocytic clathrin-coated vesicles. *J Biol Chem* 1994; **269**: 8296–302.
76 Prince LS, Workman RB, Marchase RB. Rapid endocytosis of the cystic fibrosis transmembrane conductance regulator chloride channel. *Proc Natl Acad Sci USA* 1994; **91**: 5192–6.
77 Dunn KW, Park J, Semrad CE, et al. Regulation of endocytic trafficking and acidification are independent of the cystic fibrosis transmembrane regulator. *J Biol Chem* 1994; **269**: 5336–45.
78 Dho S, Grinstein S, Foskett JK. Plasma membrane recycling in CFTR-expressing CHO cells. *Biochim Biophys Acta* 1993; **1225**: 78–82.
79 Dosanjh A, Lencer W, Brown D, et al. Heterologous expression of ΔF508 CFTR results in decreased sialylation of membrane glycoconjugates. *Am J Physiol* 1994; **266**: C360–6.
80 Seksek O, Biwersi J, Verkman AS. A novel method to label the aqueous compartment of trans-Golgi in living cells: influence of CFTR expression on Golgi pH. *Pediatr Pulmonol* 1994: in press.

Chapter Nine

# CFTR Localization: Implications for Cell and Tissue Pathophysiology

Jonathan A. Cohn

*Departments of Medicine and Cell Biology, Duke University and Veterans Administration Medical Centers, Durham, North Carolina, USA*

## INTRODUCTION

Cystic fibrosis (CF) is an inherited disease in which many epithelial tissues show defective secretory responses to cAMP-mediated stimuli[1–6]. By 1989, experimental data generated using two general approaches suggested that the primary defect in CF involves a protein that normally controls $Cl^-$ channel activation by undergoing cAMP-dependent phosphorylation. First, cAMP responses and cAMP-dependent protein kinase (PKA) isozymes were normal in CF epithelial cells, suggesting that the early steps in cAMP-mediated intracellular signalling are unaffected by CF[7,8]. Second, electrophysiological studies found that a 40 pS outwardly rectifying $Cl^-$ channel could be activated by PKA in normal, but not in CF, epithelial cells[9,10]. Accordingly, when the CF gene was identified in 1989, it was designated *CFTR* (for CF transmembrane conductance regulator) to reflect the prediction that the protein product of this gene (CFTR) functions either as a component or as a regulator of the $Cl^-$ channel that is defective in CF[1,2].

The initial characterization of the *CFTR* gene provided much information about the properties of CFTR. Based on cDNA sequence data, CFTR was

*Cystic Fibrosis—Current Topics, Volume 2.* Edited by J. A. Dodge, D. J. H. Brock and J. H. Widdicombe

predicted to be a glycoprotein of 168 kDa containing 12 membrane-spanning domains, two ATP-binding domains (NBF 1 and NBF 2), and a putative regulatory (R) domain including a cluster of PKA consensus sequences[2]. Initial genetic studies showed that CF most commonly results from the ΔF508 mutation in which the phenylalanine normally in position 508 in NBF 1 is deleted[11], and an initial Northern blot tissue survey identified pancreas as the human tissue showing highest levels of *CFTR* expression[2]. Methods were rapidly developed to express CFTR in a variety of heterologous expression systems and this generated the models and reagents used for the initial characterization of CFTR as a protein[12–14].

## STUDIES OF CFTR EXPRESSED IN TRANSFECTED CELLS

One major conclusion from studies of recombinant CFTR is that CFTR is, itself, a non-rectifying $Cl^-$ channel with a unitary conductance of approximately 8 pS. Three findings support this conclusion: CFTR expression (based on mRNA analyses) correlates closely with the occurrence of the 8 pS $Cl^-$ channel and does not correlate with the previously described rectifying 40 pS $Cl^-$ channel[15–18]; mutagenesis of CFTR membrane-spanning domains affects the ion selectivity of the 8 pS channel[19]; and insertion of purified CFTR into bilayers reconstitutes the 8 pS channel[20]. Related studies have shown that CFTR can also function as a regulator of the 40 pS $Cl^-$ channel[21,22], that ATP hydrolysis occurs at NBF 1[23], that the CFTR $Cl^-$ channel is regulated both by PKA and by high concentrations of ATP[24], and that either deletion of the R domain or mutations at specific PKA phosphorylation sites affect the ability of the CFTR $Cl^-$ channel to be regulated by PKA[25,26].

A second conclusion from studies of transfected cells is that expression of wild-type CFTR can correct the defect in ion transport exhibited by CF cell lines[13,14]. One implication of this finding is that somatic gene transfer may provide a strategy to correct the defects in ion transport that occur in CF patients and to thereby delay the onset of the clinical manifestations of this disease. A further implication of the phenotypic correction of CF cell lines is that transfected cells can be used to study the mechanism by which CFTR mutations lead to defective ion transport.

## MATURATION AND TRAFFICKING OF RECOMBINANT CFTR

The mechanism by which CFTR mutations lead to defective ion transport was first addressed in a seminal series of experiments by Cheng and colleagues[27,28].

In this work, COS-7 cells were transfected to express high levels of wild-type versus ΔF508 CFTR. Immunoprecipitation and metabolic labelling studies showed that there was a difference in intracellular processing when the two forms of CFTR were compared. The wild-type protein occurred predominantly as a mature glycoprotein, while ΔF508 CFTR was detected only as an immature, incompletely glycosylated protein. This unexpected finding suggested that newly synthesized ΔF508 CFTR might be trapped in the endoplasmic reticulum and led to the hypothesis 'that the molecular basis of most CF is the absence of mature CFTR at the correct cellular location'. In this context, preliminary immunostaining data were presented suggesting that the distribution of CFTR is different in COS-7 cells expressing wild-type versus ΔF508 CFTR. Even though the sites of CFTR within these cells could not be identified, these data provided an impetus for more definitive efforts to compare the localization of wild-type and ΔF508 CFTR.

Additional studies have confirmed and extended these data using two general approaches. First, CF-causing mutations other than ΔF508 were tested to determine whether they also affected the intracellular processing of CFTR[27,28]. Most CFTR variants resulting from CF-causing mutations showed the same defect in glycosylation seen with ΔF508. However, one exception was noted: the G551D mutation results in a CFTR variant showing normal maturation. Second, different forms of CFTR have been studied in other heterologous expression systems to test whether the processing of CFTR variants by COS-7 cells is representative of what occurs in other cell types and to test the prediction that the ΔF508 mutation prevents the delivery of CFTR to the cell membrane. Using confocal microscopy and immunoelectron microscopy to localize different forms of CFTR, the wild-type protein has been detected as a component of the plasma membrane in transfected mouse fibroblasts (L cells), CF pancreatic adenocarcinoma (CFPAC) cells and Sf9 cells[15,29–31]. The ΔF508 variant differs from wild-type CFTR in that it has been detected only in an intracellular compartment corresponding to the endoplasmic reticulum[29–31]. Thus, each of these findings supports the concept that the ΔF508 mutation affects the intracellular trafficking of CFTR in transfected cells.

## MOLECULAR BASIS FOR DEFECTIVE PROCESSING OF ΔF508 CFTR

Transected cells have proved to be particularly useful for studying how the ΔF508 mutation may affect the intracellular processing of CFTR. As noted by Denning and colleagues[32], functional studies of CFTR showed that when ΔF508 CFTR was expressed in cells grown at reduced temperatures (*Xenopus* oocytes, Sf9 cells and Vero cells), CFTR $Cl^-$ channel activity occurred at the plasma membrane, while CFTR $Cl^-$ channels were not detected at this site in other types of transfected cells grown at 37 °C. This discrepancy led to two studies in which the glycosylation and function of ΔF508 CFTR was systematically compared in cells grown at temperatures ranging from 26 °C to 37 °C. These studies demonstrated that ΔF508 functions as a temperature-sensitive mutation in that ΔF508 CFTR showed normal maturation and function in cells grown at reduced temperature[29,32]. The mislocalization of ΔF508 CFTR was corrected in cells grown at reduced temperature[29], further supporting the correlation of the CF phenotype in cells expressing only ΔF508 CFTR (defective cAMP-regulated $Cl^-$ transport) with the failure of ΔF508 CFTR to be delivered to the plasma membrane when these cells are grown under routine conditions (at 37 °C).

The temperature dependence of the localization of ΔF508 CFTR provides an important clue about the mechanism by which ΔF508 affects CFTR. It suggests that the ΔF508 mutation may cause CFTR to misfold such that the mutant protein is targeted for accelerated degradation by a quality-control mechanism in the endoplasmic reticulum. To test this hypothesis, Yang and colleagues have examined the biosynthesis and degradation of wild-type versus ΔF508 CFTR[30]. Both forms of newly synthesized CFTR initially occur as complexes with the chaperone protein, hsp70. For wild-type CFTR, these complexes rapidly dissociate, enabling CFTR to transfer to the Golgi and then to the plasma membrane. Wild-type CFTR functions as a $Cl^-$ channel at the plasma membrane and is subsequently transferred to lysosomes, where it is degraded. By contrast, ΔF508 CFTR forms a more stable complex which prevents the misfolded protein from being transferred to the Golgi. Instead, ΔF508 CFTR is transferred to a non-lysosomal compartment, where it is rapidly degraded. Thus, these findings implicate hsp70 as a component of the quality-control mechanism responsible for recognizing misfolded variants of CFTR and targeting them for accelerated degradation.

These studies of recombinant CFTR suggest an explanation for the difference between ion transport responses of transfected cells expressing ΔF508 versus wild-type CFTR: ΔF508 CFTR is trapped in the endoplasmic reticulum and therefore cannot be delivered to the plasma membrane where the wild-type protein is required for cAMP-regulated $Cl^-$ transport. More importantly, these studies suggest that the ΔF508 mutation may cause similar defects in the maturation and intracellular trafficking of CFTR when the variant protein is expressed at endogenous levels in human tissues from patients with CF. Even though this working hypothesis is a direct extension from the properties of ΔF508 versus wild-type CFTR in transfected cells, this type of extrapolation must be viewed with caution due to uncertainties about the fidelity of CFTR quality control in cells driven to over-express the protein. This is an inherent limitation of studies of CFTR processing in transfected cells. To definitively test how CF-causing mutations affect the maturation and trafficking of CFTR in tissues of CF patients, it was necessary to develop methods to detect endogenous CFTR in these tissues.

## LOCALIZATION OF ENDOGENOUS CFTR: GENERAL CONSIDERATIONS

The localization of CFTR in tissues has been studied at both the cellular and the subcellular levels. Cellular localization studies aim to identify populations of cells within a tissue in which CFTR is most abundant, while subcellular localization studies aim to identify the predominant sites of the protein within CFTR-expressing cells. Corroboration for cellular localization data can be provided by *in situ* hybridization studies which identify cells containing high levels of CFTR mRNA. To corroborate subcellular localization data, alternative approaches are used, including cell fractionation, cell surface labelling and the detection of functional CFTR as a cAMP-regulated $Cl^-$ channel.

Most CFTR localization studies rely primarily on the immunodetection of CFTR by cell or tissue staining. For this purpose, several laboratories have developed antibodies capable of recognizing CFTR with varying degrees of sensitivity and specificity. When highly specific antibodies are used to stain tissues, localization data can be extremely informative. Unfortunately, it can be difficult to determine whether individual CFTR antibodies provide sufficient specificity to generate reliable immunostaining data in any particular tissue. Since there is no single criterion or control experiment which can conclusively validate a CFTR antibody for use in immunostaining, data for each tissue or cell line must be evaluated using a combination of indirect approaches. This caveat is particularly important in reviewing cell staining data for tissues containing low levels of CFTR because of the possibility that staining patterns may reflect contributions from cross-reacting proteins other than CFTR.

## ANTIBODY VALIDATION USING RECOMBINANT CFTR

Several groups have developed antibodies capable of recognizing CFTR in specimens containing high levels of the protein. Most of these antibodies were initially validated in two stages using CFTR-expressing transfected cells. The first stage has been to use Western blotting or immunoprecipitation to show that the antibodies detect a signal of the appropriate electrophoretic mobility as the predominant immunoreactive protein. When individual antibodies detect no other immunoreactive proteins using these biochemical methods, this suggests that staining with these antibodies should reflect the distribution of CFTR in this cell preparation. The second stage of validating CFTR antibodies has been to use them to compare staining of CFTR-expressing cells versus cells lacking the protein. Even antibodies showing limited specificity and sensitivity often can be used to reliably detect recombinant CFTR by immunostaining because of the high levels of CFTR expression in transfected cells. An additional advantage of transfected cells for optimizing CFTR staining methods is that mock-transfected cells can be used to control for non-specific staining and for cross-reacting proteins. Nonetheless, it is important to perform a variety of technical controls when trying to detect either recombinant or endogenous CFTR by immunostaining. These controls include sections (or cytospins) stained with serial dilutions of the primary antibody, sections stained using the antibody in the presence of an excess of the immunogen (often a synthetic or recombinant peptide) to competitively block binding of the antibody, sections stained using different methods to detect binding of the primary antibody, and sections prepared using different fixation and embedding procedures.

## CFTR ANTIBODY VALIDATION IN HUMAN TISSUES

Only a limited number of antibodies have been validated for use in staining endogenous CFTR. To date, only one antibody has been shown to detect CFTR as the predominant immunoblot or immunoprecipitation signal in human tissues[33]. This antibody, $\alpha$-1468, was raised as a rabbit polyclonal antibody against a synthetic peptide containing the C-terminal amino acid sequence of CFTR and was affinity purified using this same peptide; $\alpha$-1468 binds the immunizing peptide with high affinity and recognizes a single heterodisperse protein of 155–170 kDa in immunoblots of T84 cells (a human colonocyte cell line) and of human pancreas and intestine[33–35]. A similar protein was detected in immunoprecipitation PKA-labelling experiments using $\alpha$-1468, and the $^{32}$P-labelled protein was shown to be identical to the immunoblot signal based on mobility shifts following deglycosylation. Finally, the $^{32}$P-labelled protein immunoprecipitated by $\alpha$-1468 was unequivocally identified as human CFTR by two-dimensional tryptic phosphopeptide mapping using synthetic phosphopeptides containing authentic CFTR sequences as internal standards for mixing-comigration studies[36].

To date, similar biochemical validation studies have not been performed for other CFTR antibodies in human tissues. The potential importance of this is illustrated by immunoblot data for one of the CFTR antibodies in wide use at this time. As shown in Figure 2 of reference 37, this CFTR antibody was able to recognize a protein resembling CFTR as the predominant immunoblot signal in CFTR-expressing COS-1 cells and this signal was absent in cells transfected with the vector alone. Thus, this antibody should be a reliable reagent for staining CFTR in these transfected COS-1 cells (see Figure 3C of reference 37) and in other cells containing similarly high levels of CFTR. However, when this antibody was used for immunoblots of untransfected epithelial cells (T84 cells and fetal tracheal airway cells), the signal at the correct molecular weight for CFTR was less intense than signals generated by other proteins in the same samples. Since proteins other than endogenous CFTR apparently account for the predominant immunoblot signals in these cells, it seems unlikely that CFTR will be the only protein in these cells contributing to the immunostaining pattern when this antibody is used to stain tissues containing low levels of CFTR. Some component of the detected staining pattern would probably result from binding of the antibody to cross-reacting proteins, and such cross-reacting proteins may account for the predominant immunostaining signals in some cases. Similar uncertainties about specificity exist concerning the reagents used for many published CFTR localization studies because antibodies have been used for tissue staining without showing that they detect CFTR as the predominant immunoreactive protein in the tissues of interest.

A general challenge in this field is the low abundance of CFTR in many tissues. This factor has precluded the use of biochemical criteria to validate CFTR antibodies in some of the tissues that are of greatest interest regarding the pathophysiology of CF (e.g. lung). Beyond this, it is likely that no CFTR antibody will ultimately prove to be completely dependable with respect to specificity. It therefore seems prudent to examine individual CFTR localization experiments in the context of other corroborating data for the same tissue including localization studies using other CFTR antibodies and *in situ* hybridization studies. When individual immunostaining studies are not supported by such corroborating data, these studies should probably be considered preliminary.

## CFTR IN HUMAN PANCREAS

The first localization of CFTR as an endogenously expressed protein was performed in human pancreas[35]. High levels of CFTR were anticipated in this tissue based on the Northern blot survey of human tissues that accompanied the original description of the CFTR gene[2]. By now, studies using a total of 10 unrelated CFTR antibodies have been reported, indicating that the predominant site of CFTR in human pancreas is the apical domain of the intralobular duct cell[34,35,37,38]. Intense staining occurs at this site, with much lower levels of CFTR being detected in the cells lining larger ducts, and with no immunoreactivity occurring in pancreatic acinar cells, islets or nerves. The localization of CFTR in pancreas is supported by biochemical evidence that one of the antibodies used to stain human pancreas detects CFTR as the predominant immunoreactive protein in human pancreas[28,30]. The cellular localization of CFTR is further corroborated by *in situ* hybridization data in rodent and human pancreas[39,40] and by double-immunofluorescence studies confirming the identity of the stained cells as duct cells[35]. The subcellular localization of CFTR to the apical plasma membrane is further supported by double-immunofluorescence staining showing colocalization of different CFTR antibodies to the same subcellular sites[35] and by electrophysiological studies of cAMP-regulated $Cl^-$ channels in isolated pancreatic duct cells[41,42].

The pathophysiological implications of the occurrence of CFTR in the proximal pancreatic ductular system have been separately reviewed[35]. Briefly, the subcellular localization of CFTR in pancreatic duct cells supports the concept that the CFTR $Cl^-$ channel is required at the duct cell apical membrane to permit cAMP-regulated $HCO_3^-$ secretion via apical $Cl^-/HCO_3^-$ exchangers. This model explains how the absence of functional CFTR in CF could lead to decreased $HCO_3^-$ and fluid secretion into the proximal pancreatic duct lumen, and is consistent with independent evidence that CF results in impaired alkalinization and dilution of pancreatic juice[43,44]. The cellular localization of CFTR in pancreas suggests that the proximal ducts are the site of the primary defect leading to pancreatic insufficiency in CF. This conclusion agrees well with prior studies of the natural history of CF which showed that the earliest pathological finding in CF pancreatic disease is obstruction of the proximal ducts with protein plugs[45].

## CFTR IN HUMAN SWEAT GLANDS

The occurrence of CFTR in sweat glands was suggested by Northern blots[2] and by the characteristic ion transport abnormalities shown by sweat glands isolated from patients with CF[3,46]. The predominant site of CFTR in eccrine sweat glands is the luminal reabsorptive duct cell[34,37,38]. Within these luminal duct cells, CFTR occurs primarily at the apical domain. This localization of CFTR has been detected using antibodies to a variety of CFTR domains, including monoclonal and monospecific antibodies which are likely to show minimal binding to other components of the luminal cells of the sweat gland reabsorptive duct (e.g. cytokeratins). To date, the cellular localization of CFTR in sweat glands has not been confirmed by *in situ* hybridization, and the specificity of CFTR antibodies in sweat glands has not been evaluated by Western blot or by double-immunofluorescence colocalization. Nonetheless, the reproducibility of the staining pattern detected using multiple CFTR antibodies suggests that this staining accurately represents the distribution of CFTR in sweat glands. As discussed below, the validity of CFTR localization data in human sweat gland is further supported by evidence that the CFTR staining pattern is altered in sweat glands from patients homozygous for the ΔF508 mutation[38].

## CFTR IN HUMAN INTESTINE AND ENTEROCYTES

Several aspects of the localization of CFTR in intestine agree well with the concept that CFTR functions to regulate apical $Cl^-$ conductance and to thereby permit cAMP-regulated secretion of either $Cl^-$ or $HCO_3^-$ by the enterocyte. *In situ* hybridization studies in human and rat intestine indicate that CFTR expression gradually decreases along both the proximal-to-distal and crypt-to-villus axes, with highest levels of mRNA generally occurring in the crypts and submucosal (Brunner's) glands of the proximal small intestine[39,40]. Immunostaining data from several laboratories tend to support these predictions concerning the cellular localization of CFTR[37,38,47]. Within the enterocyte, CFTR staining is primarily apical, and this finding agrees well with cell fractionation studies showing that CFTR occurs in apical plasma membranes prepared from isolated enterocytes[48,49]. Immunostaining, cell fractionation, cell surface labelling and electrophysiological studies in polarized enterocyte cell lines further support the conclusion that CFTR occurs, at least in part, as a component of the apical plasma membrane[33,48,50–53].

In $Cl^-$-secreting enterocytes, such as colonic crypt cells, the apical localization of CFTR suggests that this protein functions either as a cAMP-regulated $Cl^-$ channel or as a regulator of other apical $Cl^-$ channels to control electrogenic $Cl^-$ secretion. Activation of apical $Cl^-$ channels in these cells is likely to be important in secretory diarrhoeal diseases such as cholera which are associated with increased cAMP levels in enterocytes[54]. This role for CFTR is consistent with evidence that cAMP-mediated enterocyte $Cl^-$ secretion is defective in patients with CF[8,55–59] and with the concept that the high prevalence of CF may result from a heterozygote advantage with respect to resistance to certain diarrhoeal diseases[60,61]. At other sites in the intestine, including the proximal crypts and Brunner's glands, CFTR is also apical. Some of these sites are known to secrete $HCO_3^-$ in response to stimuli acting via cAMP[62]. It therefore seems likely that in these enterocytes CFTR contributes to cAMP-regulated $HCO_3^-$ secretion in a manner resembling that discussed for the pancreatic duct cell.

However, other aspects of the localization of CFTR in intestine suggest that CFTR may have additional roles in this tissue. First, relatively high levels of CFTR mRNA and of immunoreactive CFTR have been detected in a subpopulation of enterocytes scattered throughout the villi of human and rodent proximal intestine[39,40,47]. These cells occur infrequently ($<5\%$ of the cell population) and cannot be distinguished from other enterocytes based on either routine morphological criteria or special stains for enteroendocrine cells. Within these cells, several CFTR antibodies generate an equivalent punctate staining pattern in the cytoplasm with subapical accentuation, suggesting that CFTR occurs as a component of subapical vesicles[47]. The role of CFTR in these infrequent cells is unknown. Finally, several studies in colonocyte cell lines indicate that a significant proportion of total cellular CFTR occurs in an intracellular compartment[50,63]. Clathrin-coated vesicles have been identified as one intracellular site of CFTR[63] and this finding supports the concept that CFTR may participate in endocytic recycling[64].

## CFTR IN HUMAN LUNG AND AIRWAY CELLS

Because CFTR protein and mRNA are less abundant in lung than in many other tissues, initial efforts to localize CFTR in lung were unsuccessful[37,38]. More recently, three studies have described different aspects of the distribution of CFTR in pulmonary tissues. The first study used *in situ* hybridization and immunostaining to show that submucosal glands are the predominant site of CFTR expression in human large airways, with only low levels of the protein being detected in the bronchial surface epithelium[65]. Within the submucosal glands, CFTR is uniformly expressed by the epithelial cells comprising the serous tubules. By contrast, CFTR expression in the collecting and ciliated ducts of the glands is not uniform and CFTR is only detected in a distinct subpopulation representing 1–3% of the cells. Within the CFTR-containing epithelial cells at all sites in the submucosal gland, CFTR occurs at or near the apical plasma membrane. The validity of CFTR staining in airway submucosal glands is supported by studies of lung specimens from ΔF508 homozygous patients with CF (see below)[65] and by an additional study performed using other CFTR antibodies[66].

The abundance of CFTR in airway submucosal glands is important because it suggests that submucosal glands play a major role in the pathogenesis of CF lung disease[65]. This concept is supported by prior studies showing that obstruction of the airway submucosal glands occurs as an early manifestation of CF lung disease[45] and that airway submucosal glands isolated from CF patients show defective ion transport[67]. Nonetheless, the abundance of CFTR in airway submucosal glands was initially unanticipated because most studies of airway ion transport in CF have focused on the surface epithelium. In any event, one consequence of the observed distribution of CFTR in airways has been a concentrated effort to clarify the normal role of CFTR during mucous secretion in airway submucosal glands[68,69].

Additional CFTR localization studies have been performed at two other sites in the human respiratory tract. In distal airways[70], both CFTR mRNA and protein occur primarily in a subpopulation of non-ciliated cells representing about 5% of the cells lining the proximal and terminal bronchioles. In these larger bronchioles, the distribution of CFTR resembles that of CC10, a Clara cell marker. In smaller (respiratory) bronchioles and alveoli, CFTR gene expression also occurs in a distinct subpopulation of cells; immunolocalization studies have not been possible at these sites due to technical factors. Within CFTR-expressing cells of the proximal and terminal bronchioles, the protein occurs at or near the apical plasma membrane, suggesting that CFTR may function to regulate ion and fluid movement across the bronchiolar epithelium. A role for CFTR at this site seems to be generally consistent with the occurrence of obstructive disease in the distal airways in patients with CF, although further study will be required to clarify this role.

An additional site where CFTR immunoreactivity has been detected in the human respiratory tract is the nasal epithelium. Northern blots indicate that CFTR mRNA occurs in nasal polyps[2] and one group has reported immunostaining data for CFTR within these polyps[71]. This study concludes that CFTR is uniformly expressed by the ciliated surface epithelial cells of human nasal and tracheal epithelia based on staining with two CFTR antibodies. When these antibodies were used for confocal and electron microscopy, a subapical vesicular compartment was identified as the predominant site of immunostaining in these cells. Two caveats seem pertinent concerning this study. First, *in situ* hybridization studies of CFTR expression have not been reported for nasal polyps. Second, the antibodies used to detect CFTR were validated using recombinant CFTR only[31,66,71]. (When a related CFTR antibody was used for Western blotting of human tissues, proteins other than CFTR accounted for most of the detected immunoreactivity[66].)

## CFTR IN HUMAN LIVER

In both humans and rats, the predominant site of hepatobiliary CFTR expression is the intrahepatic bile duct cell based on *in situ* hybridization and immunostaining studies[72–74]. Within bile duct cells, CFTR occurs as an apical protein. The validity of these CFTR immunostaining data is supported by biochemical evidence that one of the antibodies used for tissue staining detects CFTR as the predominant immunoreactive protein in liver[72]. The localization of CFTR in liver can be interpreted in the context of emerging information about the electrophysiological properties of isolated bile duct cells[72,75–78] to develop a model explaining the normal role of CFTR during biliary secretion[73]. Briefly, this model suggests that the intrahepatic bile duct cell resembles the intralobular pancreatic duct cell in that CFTR plays a similar role during cAMP-mediated $HCO_3^-$ secretion at both sites. One implication of this model is that the regulation of biliary $HCO_3^-$ secretion may be affected in patients with CF and this prediction should be testable. A second implication of these findings is that bile duct epithelial cells appear to be the site of the primary defect leading to hepatobiliary disease in CF. This concept is consistent with pathological data indicating that obstruction of the intrahepatic ducts is the earliest pathological feature of CF in the liver[79].

## CFTR LOCALIZATION DATA IN OTHER HUMAN TISSUES

A limited amount of immunostaining data exists concerning the distribution of CFTR as an endogenous protein in other tissues and cell types, including intestinal goblet cells[80], kidney[37] and choroid plexus[81]. At this time, it seems unlikely that intestinal goblet cells are the predominant site of CFTR in intestine since this conclusion is inconsistent with *in situ* hybridization data[39,40] and with subsequent immunolocalization data[37,38,47]. By contrast, *in situ* hybridization data have not been reported for CFTR expression in kidney or choroid plexus. However, the absence of prominent renal or neurological manifestations in patients with CF seems to argue against a major role for CFTR in these sites.

## CFTR LOCALIZATION IN TISSUES FROM PATIENTS WITH CF

One goal of several studies has been to compare the subcellular localization of CFTR in tissues from patients expressing wild-type versus ΔF508 CFTR. Even though the ΔF508 mutation clearly affects the processing of ΔF508 CFTR when it is over-expressed in transfected cells (see above), conflicting evidence exists concerning whether ΔF508 has a similar effect on endogenous ΔF508 CFTR. In CF airway cells, an indirect assay of CFTR localization suggests that ΔF508 does affect protein delivery to the cell membrane[82]; this is supported by one observation related to CFTR maturation in airway cells[66], while two other studies suggest that CFTR maturation is unaffected by ΔF508[48,83].

Three CFTR localization studies have been performed in tissues from genotyped patients with CF. Taken together, these studies indicate that the ΔF508 mutation results in the absence of CFTR at the subcellular site, where it is normally most abundant in eccrine sweat gland[38], bronchial submucosal gland[65] and nasal polyp[71]. An informative control experiment in two of these studies[38,65] was the use of tissues from compound heterozygotes in which endogenously expressed G551D CFTR shows normal intracellular trafficking. This finding confirms predictions based on the maturation and localization of G551D CFTR in transfected cells[27,29] and suggests that secondary changes related to long-standing CF (e.g. due to tissue injury in lung) are not responsible for the abnormality in CFTR localization seen in ΔF508 homozygous patients. A second prediction based on data in transfected cells[28,30] is that ΔF508 CFTR may undergo accelerated degradation in tissues from patients with CF. The markedly reduced immunostaining signals observed in eccrine sweat glands and bronchial submucosal glands from ΔF508 homozygous CF patients[38,65] are consistent with this prediction. A third prediction based on studies of recombinant CFTR[27,30] is that ΔF508 CFTR may accumulate at an intracellular site in cells from patients with CF. This concept of mislocalization is supported by a limited amount of immunostaining data in eccrine sweat gland[38] and in nasal polyps[71] However, these data seem somewhat preliminary because different patterns of intracellular staining occurred when different antibodies were used to detect CFTR immunoreactivity.

## DIRECTIONS FOR FURTHER STUDY

One gap in existing studies of CFTR localization concerns detection of the endogenous protein by immunoelectron microscopy. To date, several groups have described the localization of recombinant CFTR at the ultrastructural level[15,30,31]. By contrast, only limited data exist concerning the immunoelectron microscopic localization of endogenous CFTR in human or animal tissues[66,71,80,84,85]. As this methodology is optimized and more rigorously validated, it should generate more definitive information about the subcellular distribution of endogenous CFTR in different tissues.

A second aspect of CFTR localization where rapid advances are anticipated concerns gene therapy for CF. One strategy for preventing the clinical manifestations of CF is to try to correct the ion transport defect in tissues of CF patients by reconstituting functional CFTR at the sites where the protein is normally most abundant by somatic gene transfer. For this approach to be feasible, it is essential that recombinant wild-type CFTR be expressed at the correct subcellular sites and in the correct populations of cells when vectors are delivered to tissues. CFTR localization studies are playing a central role in efforts to develop this type of therapy by identifying target cell populations for gene transfer, by identifying the subcellular sites at which CFTR reconstitution will be important, and by providing methods to monitor the targeting selectivity and efficacy of individual vectors in experimental models and in patients with CF[74,86–90].

## SUMMARY

Much has been learned about the pathophysiology of CFTR from studies of CFTR localization. In several tissues, including pancreas, liver and intestine,

CFTR has been mainly localized to sites where cAMP-regulated $Cl^-$ channels are known to participate directly in the control of transepithelial ion and fluid transport. In these tissues, CFTR localization data can be integrated with physiological and pathological data to develop models explaining the normal roles of CFTR and the mechanisms by which tissue injury results from the absence of functional CFTR in CF patients. By contrast, the predominant site of CFTR expression in the proximal airway is the submucosal gland—a structure in which cAMP-regulated $Cl^-$ channels have not been recognized as important effectors. The unanticipated abundance of CFTR at this site suggests that these glands may contribute to the pathogenesis of CF lung disease and has led to efforts by several groups to define the role of CFTR during submucosal gland secretion.

A second theme emerging from CFTR localization studies is that the most common CF-causing *CFTR* mutation ($\Delta$F508) apparently brings about defective ion transport in CF epithelial cells by blocking the maturation and intracellular trafficking of newly synthesized CFTR. This mechanism was proposed based on comprehensive studies of the glycosylation and localization of recombinant CFTR and is supported by all available data concerning the localization of endogenous $\Delta$F508 CFTR in tissues from patients with CF. Thus, the subcellular localization of CFTR variants can provide information about the mechanism by which *CFTR* mutations affect CFTR function both in transfected cells and in human tissues. These studies imply that it may be feasible to correct the ion transport defect in tissues of CF patients by reconstituting functional CFTR at the sites where the protein is normally most abundant by somatic gene transfer. CFTR localization studies are contributing to the effort to develop this type of therapy by identifying the sites at which CFTR reconstitution will be important and by providing methods to monitor the targeting selectivity and efficacy of individual vectors in experimental models and in patients with CF.

## ACKNOWLEDGEMENTS

This work was supported in part by grants from the Cystic Fibrosis Foundation, the National Institutes of Health, and the Department of Veterans Affairs.

## REFERENCES

1 Rommens JM, Iannuzzi MC, Kerem B, et al. Identification of the cystic fibrosis gene: chromosome walking and jumping. *Science* 1989; **245**: 1059–65.
2 Riordan JR, Rommens JM, Kerem B, et al. Identification of the cystic fibrosis gene: cloning and characterization of complementary DNA. *Science* 1989; **245**: 1066–73.

3 Quinton PM. Cystic fibrosis: a disease in electrolyte transport. *FASEB J* 1990; **4**: 2709–17.

4 Welsh MJ. Abnormal regulation of ion channels in cystic fibrosis epithelia. *FASEB J* 1990; **4**: 2718–25.

5 Collins FS. Cystic fibrosis: molecular biology and therapeutic implications. *Science* 1992; **256**: 774–9.

6 Marino CR, Gorelick FS. Scientific advances in cystic fibrosis. *Gastroenterology* 1992; **103**: 681–93.

7 Barthelson RA, Widdicombe J. Cyclic adenosine monophosphate-dependent kinase in cystic fibrosis tracheal epithelium. *J Clin Invest* 1987; **80**: 1799–802.

8 Goldstein JL, Nash NT, Al-Bazzaz F, et al. Rectum has abnormal ion transport but normal cAMP-binding proteins in cystic fibrosis. *Am J Physiol* 1988; **254**: C719–24.

9 Schoumacher RA, Shoemaker RL, Halm DR, et al. Phosphorylation fails to activate chloride channels from cystic fibrosis airway cells. *Nature* 1987; **330**: 752–4.

10 Li M, McCann JD, Liedtke CM, et al. Cyclic AMP-dependent protein kinase opens chloride channels in normal but not cystic fibrosis airway epithelium. *Nature* 1988; **331**: 358–60

11 Kerem B, Rommens JM, Buchanan JA, et al. Identification of the cystic fibrosis gene: genetic analysis. *Science* 1989; **245**: 1073–80.

12 Gregory RJ, Cheng SH, Rich DP, et al. Expression and characterization of the cystic fibrosis transmembrane conductance regulator. *Nature* 1990; **347**: 382–6.

13 Drumm ML, Pope HA, Cliff WH, et al. Correction of the cystic fibrosis defect in vitro by retrovirus-mediated gene transfer. *Cell* 1990; **62**: 1227–33.

14 Rich DP, Anderson MP, Gregory RJ, et al. Expression of cystic fibrosis transmembrane conductance regulator corrects defective chloride channel regulation in cystic fibrosis airway epithelial cells. *Nature* 1990; **347**: 358–63.

15 Kartner N, Hanrahan JW, Jensen TJ, et al. Expression of the cystic fibrosis gene in non-epithelial invertebrate cells produces a regulated anion conductance. *Cell* 1991; **64**: 681–91

16 Ward CL, Krouse ME, Gruenert DC, et al. Cystic fibrosis gene expression is not correlated with rectifying $Cl^-$ channels. *Proc Natl Acad Sci USA* 1991; **88**: 5277–81.

17 Berger HA, Anderson MP, Gregory RJ, et al. Identification and regulation of the cystic fibrosis transmembrane conductance regulator-generated chloride channel. *J Clin Invest* 1991; **88**: 1422–31.

18 Anderson MP, Rich DP, Gregory RJ, et al. Generation of cAMP-activated chloride currents by expression of CFTR. *Science* 1991; **251**: 679–82.

19 Anderson MP, Gregory RJ, Thompson S, et al. Demonstration that the CFTR is a chloride channel by alteration of its anion selectivity. *Science* 1991; **253**: 202–5.

20 Bear CE, Li C, Kartner N, et al. Purification and functional reconstitution of the cystic fibrosis transmembrane conductance regulator (CFTR). *Cell* 1992; **66**: 809–18.

21 Egan M, Flotte T, Afione S, et al. Defective regulation of outwardly rectifying $Cl^-$ channels by protein kinase A corrected by insertion of CFTR. *Nature* 1992; **358**: 581–4.

22 Gabriel SE, Clarke LL, Boucher RC, Stutts MJ. CFTR and outward rectifying chloride channels are distinct proteins with a regulatory relationship. *Nature* 1993; **363**: 263–6.

23 Anderson MP, Berger HA, Rich DP, et al. Nucleoside triphosphates are required to open the CFTR chloride channel. *Cell* 1991; **67**: 775–84.
24 Quinton PM, Reddy MM. Control of CFTR chloride conductance by ATP levels through non-hydrolytic binding. *Nature* 1992; **360**: 79–81.
25 Rich DP, Gregory RJ, Anderson MP, et al. Effect of deleting the R domain on CFTR-generated chloride channels. *Science* 1991; **253**: 205–7.
26 Cheng SH, Rich DP, Marshall J, et al. Phosphorylation of the R domain by cAMP-dependent protein kinase regulates the CFTR chloride channel. *Cell* 1991; **66**: 1027–36.
27 Cheng SH, Gregory RJ, Marshall J, et al. Defective intracellular transport and processing of CFTR is the molecular basis of most cystic fibrosis. *Cell* 1990; **63**: 827–34.
28 Gregory RJ, Rich DP, Cheng SH, et al. Maturation and function of cystic fibrosis transmembrane conductance regulator variants bearing mutations in putative nucleotide-binding domains 1 and 2. *Mol Cell Biol* 1991; **11**: 3886–93.
29 Yang Y, Devor DC, Engelhardt JF, et al. Molecular basis of defective anion transport in L cells expressing recombinant forms of CFTR. *Hum Mol Genet* 1993; **2**: 1253–61.
30 Yang Y, Janich S, Cohn JA, Wilson JM. The common variant of cystic fibrosis transmembrane conductance regulator is recognized by hsp70 and degraded in a pre-Golgi nonlysosomal compartment. *Proc Natl Acad Sci USA* 1993; **90**: 9480–4.
31 Dalemans W, Hinnrasky J, Slos P, et al. Immunocytochemical analysis reveals differences between the subcellular localization of normal and ΔF508 recombinant cystic fibrosis transmembrane conductance regulator. *Exp Cell Res* 1992; **201**: 235–40.
32 Denning GM, Anderson MP, Amara JF, et al. Processing of mutant cystic fibrosis transmembrane conductance regulator is temperature-sensitive. *Nature* 1992; **358**: 761–4
33 Cohn JA, Nairn AC, Marino CR, et al. Characterization of the cystic fibrosis transmembrane conductance regulator in a colonocyte cell line. *Proc Natl Acad Sci USA* 1992; **89**: 2340–4.
34 Cohn JA, Melhus O, Page LJ, et al. CFTR development of high-affinity antibodies and localization in sweat gland. *Biochem Biophys Res Commun* 1991; **181**: 36–43.
35 Marino CR, Matovcik LM, Gorelick FS, Cohn JA. Localization of the cystic fibrosis transmembrane conductance regulator in pancreas. *J Clin Invest* 1991; **88**: 712–16.
36 Picciotto M, Cohn JA, Bertuzzi G, et al. Phosphorylation of the cystic fibrosis transmembrane conductance regulator. *J Biol Chem* 1992; **267**: 12742–52.
37 Crawford I, Maloney PC, Zeitlin PL, et al. Immunocytochemical localization of the cystic fibrosis gene product CFTR. *Proc Natl Acad Sci USA* 1991; **88**: 9262–6.
38 Kartner N, Augustinas O, Jensen TJ, et al. Mislocalization of ΔF508 CFTR in cystic fibrosis sweat gland. *Nature Genet* 1992; **1**: 321–7.
39 Trezise AE, Buchwald M, *In vivo* cell-specific expression of the CFTR. *Nature* 1991; **353**: 434–7.
40 Strong TV, Boehm K, Collins FS. Localization of cystic fibrosis transmembrane conductance regulator mRNA in the human gastrointestinal tract by *in situ* hybridization. *J Clin Invest* 1994; **93**: 347–54.
41 Gray MA, Greenwell JR, Argent BE. Secretin-regulated chloride channel on the apical plasma membrane of pancreatic duct cells. *J Membr Biol* 1988; **105**: 131–42.

42 Gray MA, Harris A, Coleman L, et al. Two types of chloride channels on duct cells cultured from human fetal pancreas. *Am J Physiol* 1989; **257**: C240–C51.
43 Gaskin KJ, Durie PR, Corey M, et al. Evidence for a primary defect in bicarbonate secretion in cystic fibrosis. *Pediatr Res* 1982; **16**: 554–7.
44 Kopelman H, Forstner G, Durie P, Corey M. Origins of chloride and bicarbonate secretory defects in the cystic fibrosis pancreas as suggested by pancreatic function studies on control and CF subjects with preserved pancreatic function. *Clin Invest Med* 1989; **12**: 207–11.
45 Oppenheimer EH, Esterly JR. Pathology of cystic fibrosis: review of the literature and comparison with 146 autopsied cases. *Perspect Pediatr Pathol* 1975; **2**: 241–78.
46 Quinton PM. Missing Cl conductance in cystic fibrosis. *Am J Physiol* 1986; **251**: C649–52.
47 Ameen NA, West AB, Marino CR. The localization of CFTR to a distinct subpopulation of intestinal epithelial cells. *Gastroenterology* 1993; **104**: A233.
48 Zeitlin PL, Crawford I, Lu L, et al. CFTR protein expression in primary and cultured epithelia. *Proc Natl Acad Sci USA* 1992; **89**: 344–7.
49 Cohn JA, Nguyen TD, Kaz AM, Kole J. The cystic fibrosis transmembrane conductance regulator in rat enterocytes. *Gastroenterology* 1994; **106**: A229.
50 Prince LS, Tousson A, Marchase RB. Cell surface labeling of CFTR in T84 cells. *Am J Physiol* 1993; **264**: C491–8.
51 Denning GM, Ostedgaard L, Cheng SH, et al. Localization of cystic fibrosis transmembrane conductance regulator in chloride secretory epithelia. *J Clin Invest* 1992; **89**: 339–49.
52 Tabcharani JA, Low W, Elie D, Hanrahan JW. Low-conductance chloride channel activated by cAMP in the epithelial cell line T84. *FEBS Lett* 1990; **270**: 157–64.
53 Bear CE, Reyes EF. cAMP-activated chloride conductance in the colonic cell line, Caco-2. *Am J Physiol* 1992; **262**: C251–6.
54 Field M, Rao MC, Chang EB. Intestinal electrolyte transport and diarrheal disease. *N Engl J Med* 1989; **321**: 800–6.
55 Goldstein JL, Shapiro AB, Rao MC, Layden TJ. In vivo evidence of altered chloride but not potassium secretion in cystic fibrosis rectal mucosa. *Gastroenterology* 1991; **101**: 1012–19.
56 Orlando RC, Powell DW, Croom RD, et al. Colonic and esophageal transepithelial potential difference in cystic fibrosis. *Gastroenterology* 1989; **96**: 1041–8.
57 Berschneider HM, Knowles MR, Azizkhan RG, et al. Altered intestinal chloride transport in cystic fibrosis. *FASEB J* 1988: **2**: 2625–9.
58 Taylor CJ, Baxter PS, Hardcastle J, Hardcastle PT. Absence of secretory response in jejunal biopsy samples from children with cystic fibrosis. *Lancet* 1987; **ii**: 107–8.
59 O'Loughlin EV, Hunt DM, Gaskin KJ, et al. Abnormal epithelial transport in cystic fibrosis jejunum. *Am J Physiol* 1991; **260**: G758–63.
60 Wine JJ. Basic aspects of cystic fibrosis. *Clin Rev Allergy* 1991; **9**: 1–28.
61 Baxter PS, Goldhill J, Hardcastle J, et al. Accounting for cystic fibrosis. *Nature* 1988; **335**: 311.
62 Odes HS, Hogan DL, Ballesteros MA, et al. Human duodenal mucosal bicarbonate secretion. *Gastroenterology* 1990; **98**: 867–72.
63 Bradbury NA, Cohn JA, Venglarik CJ, Bridges RJ. Biochemical and biophysical identification of the cystic fibrosis transmembrane conductance regulator chloride channel clathrin coated vesicles. *J Biol Chem* 1994; **269**: 8296–302.
64 Bradbury NA, Jilling T, Berta G, et al. Regulation of plasma membrane recycling by CFTR. *Science* 1992; **256**: 530–2.

65 Engelhardt JF, Yankaskas JR, Ernst SA, et al. Submucosal glands are the predominant site of CFTR expression in the human bronchus. *Nature Genet* 1992; **2**: 240–8.
66 Jacquot J, Puchelle E, Hinnrasky J, et al. Localization of the cystic fibrosis transmembrane conductance regulator in airway secretory glands. *Eur Respir J* 1993; **6**: 169–76.
67 Yamaya M, Finkbeiner WE, Widdicombe JH. Altered ion transport by tracheal glands in cystic fibrosis. *Am J Physiol* 1991; **261**: L491–4.
68 Widdicombe JH, Yamaya M, Finkbeiner WE. Ion transport by cultures of human submucosal glands. *Pediatr Pulmonol Suppl* 1993; **9**: 143–4.
69 Engelhardt JF, Wilson JM. CFTR expression in submucosal glands: model systems. *Pediatr Pulmonol Suppl* 1993; **9**: 145–7.
70 Engelhardt JF, Zepeda M, Cohn JA, et al. Expression of the cystic fibrosis gene in adult human lung. *J Clin Invest* 1994; **93**: 737–49.
71 Puchelle E, Gaillard D, Ploton D, et al. Differential localization of the cystic fibrosis transmembrane conductance regulator in normal and cystic fibrosis airway epithelium. *Am J Respir Cell Mol Biol* 1992; **7**: 485–91.
72 Fitz JG, Basavappa S, McGill JM, et al. Regulation of membrane chloride currents in rat bile duct epithelial cells. *J Clin Invest* 1993; **914**: 319–28.
73 Cohn JA, Strong TV, Picciotto M, et al. Localization of the cystic fibrosis transmembrane conductance regulator in human bile duct epithelial cells. *Gastroenterology* 1993; **105**: 1857–64.
74 Yang Y, Raper SE, Cohn JA, et al. An approach to treating the hepatobiliary disease of cystic fibrosis by somatic gene transfer. *Proc Natl Acad Sci USA* 1993; **90**: 4601–5.
75 Nathanson MH, Boyer JL. Mechanisms and regulation of bile secretion. *Hepatology* 1991; **14**: 551–66.
76 Lenzen R, Alpini G, Tavoloni N. Secretin stimulates bile ductular secretory activity through cAMP system. *Am J Physiol* 1992; **263**: G527–32.
77 Basavappa S, Middleton JP, Mangel AW, et al. Chloride and potassium transport in human biliary cell lines. *Gastroenterology* 1993; **104**: 1796–805.
78 McGill JM, Basavappa S, Gettys TW, Fitz JG. Secretin activates chloride channels in bile duct epithelial cells through a cAMP-dependent mechanism. *Am J Physiol* 1994; **266**: G731–6.
79 Oppenheimer EH, Esterly JR. Hepatic changes in young infants with cystic fibrosis: possible relation to focal biliary cirrhosis. *J Pediatr* 1975; **86**: 683–9.
80 Hoogeveen AT, Keulemans J, Willemsen R, et al. Immunological localization of cystic fibrosis candidate gene products. *Exp Cell Res* 1991; **193**: 435–7.
81 Hincke MT, Nairn AC, Staines WA. Cystic fibrosis transmembrane conductance regulator is found within brain ventricular epithelium and choroid plexus. *Pediatr Pulmonol Suppl* 1993; **9**: 207.
82 Denning GM, Ostedgaard LS, Welsh MJ. Abnormal localization of cystic fibrosis transmembrane conductance regulator in primary cultures of cystic fibrosis airway epithelia. *J Cell Biol* 1992; **118**: 551–9.
83 Sarkadi B, Bauzon D, Huckle WR, et al. Biochemical characterization of the cystic fibrosis transmembrane conductance regulator in normal and cystic fibrosis epithelial cells. *J Biol Chem* 1991; **267**: 2087–95.
84 Marino CR, Webster P. A subapical vesicular compartment of the cystic fibrosis transmembrane conductance regulator is present in a duct epithelial cell population. *Clin Res* 1993; **41**: 219a.

85 Ernst SA, Post MA, Crawford KM, Cohn JA. Osmotic stress increases the abundance and glycosylation of a CFTR homologue at the apical membrane of avian salt gland secretory cells. *Am J Physiol* (in press).
86 Rosenfeld MA, Yoshimura K, Trapnell BC, et al. In vivo transfer of the human CFTR gene to the airway epithelium. *Cell* 1992; **68**: 143–55.
87 Engelhardt JF, Yankaskas JR, Wilson JM. In vivo retroviral gene transfer into human bronchial epithelia of xenografts. *J Clin Invest* 1992; **90**: 2598–607.
88 Engelhardt JF, Yang Y, Stratford-Perricaudet LD, et al. Direct gene transfer of human CFTR into human bronchial epithelia of xenografts with E1 deleted adenoviruses. *Nature Genet* 1993; **4**: 127–34.
89 Engelhardt JF, Simon RH, Yang Y, et al. Adenovirus-mediated transfer of the CFTR gene to lung of non-human primates: biological efficacy study. *Hum Gene Ther* 1994; **4**: 759–69.
90 Flotte TR, Afione SA, Solow R, et al. In vivo delivery of adeno-associated virus vectors expressing the cystic fibrosis transmembrane conductance regulator to the airway epithelium. *Nature Genet* 1994 (in press).

Chapter Ten

# Regulation of the CFTR $Cl^-$ Channel by cAMP-dependent Phosphorylation

Michael J. Welsh, Herbert A. Berger, Sue M. Travis, Seng Cheng[a] and Alan E. Smith[a]

*Howard Hughes Medical Institute, Department of Internal Medicine and Physiology and Biophysics, University of Iowa College of Medicine, Iowa City, Iowa, and [a]Genzyme Corporation, Framingham, Massachusetts, USA*

## INTRODUCTION

A characteristic abnormality in cystic fibrosis (CF) epithelia is a loss of cAMP-stimulated transepithelial $Cl^-$ secretion[1,2]. With the identification of the gene encoding the cystic fibrosis transmembrane conductance regulator (CFTR)[3] as that which is mutated in CF, and with the discovery that CFTR is a regulated $Cl^-$ channel (for reviews see references 4–6), several studies have attempted to understand how an increase in the cellular levels of cAMP causes the CFTR $Cl^-$ channel to open. In this chapter, we briefly review some of our current understanding of this problem. We focus on regulation of CFTR $Cl^-$ channels by phosphorylation by cAMP-dependent kinases (PKA). The reader may consult several studies[7–12] for information on regulation by other protein kinases.

---

*Cystic Fibrosis—Current Topics, Volume 2.* Edited by J. A. Dodge, D. J. H. Brock and J. H. Widdicombe

# A MODEL OF CFTR

With the elucidation of the primary amino acid sequence of CFTR, a model for the domains of the protein was developed. The model was based on predictions made from the amino acid sequence and a comparison of the sequence of CFTR with that of a family of proteins called the ATP-Binding Cassette (ABC) transporters[13], or traffic ATPases[14]. CFTR is predicted to consist of two motifs, each containing a membrane-spanning domain and a nucleotide-binding domain. These two motifs are separated by a unique segment called the R domain.

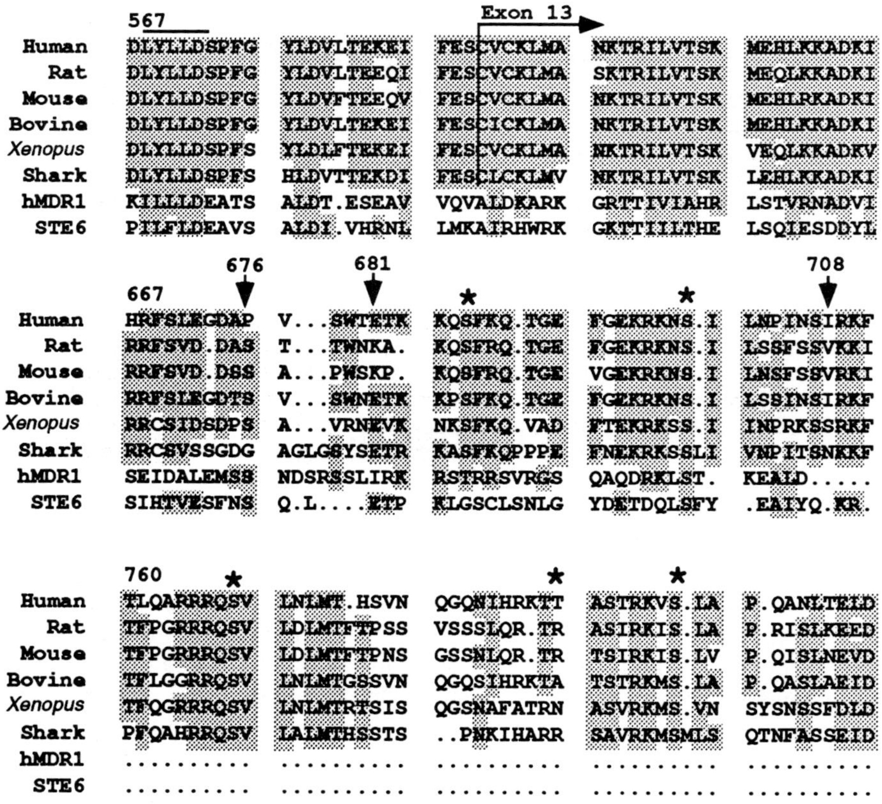


**Figure 1** Amino acid alignment of exon 13 and surrounding sequences of human CFTR with five different species of CFTR, human MDR1 and yeast STE6. Amino acid sequences are shown in single-letter code. Identical and conservatively substituted residues are shaded. Dots represent shifts in the amino acid sequence necessary for

Figure 1 shows the amino acid sequence of the R domain, which was originally defined as the sequence encoded by exon 13[3]. The R domain contains a number of consensus PKA phosphorylation sites. PKA favours the consensus phosphorylation sequence R-R/K-X-S*/T* > R-X-X-S*/T* = R-X-S*/T*, where amino acids are designated using the single-letter amino acid code, with X being any amino acid and the phosphoacceptor site indicated by an asterisk[15]. There are 10 'classic' R-R/K-X-S*/T* PKA consensus sequences within CFTR: eight serines plus one threonine within the R domain (these are indicated by asterisks in Figure 1) and one serine just prior to NBD 1.

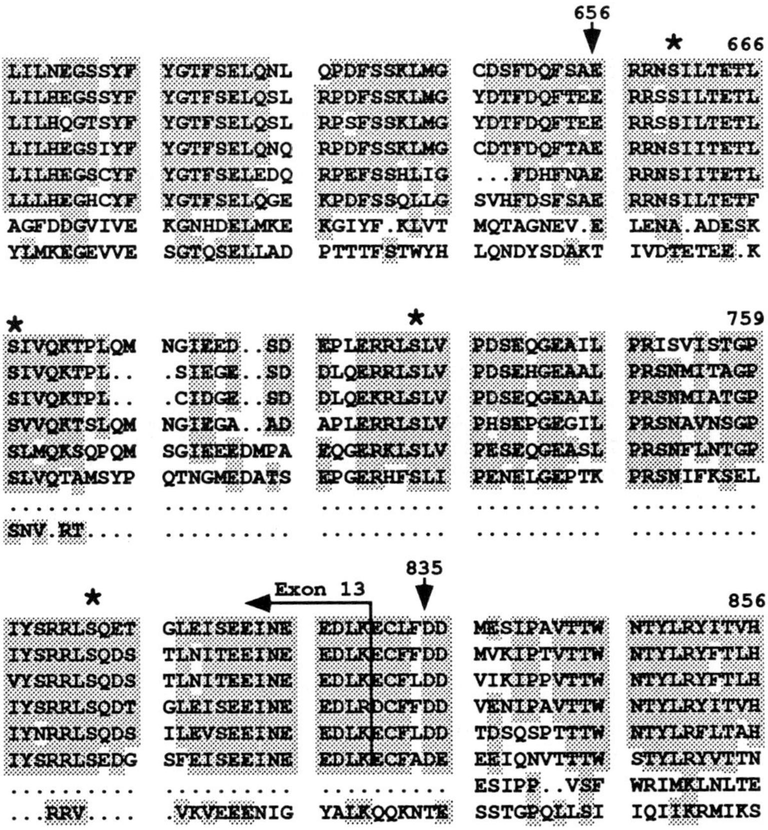


'best' alignment. The Walker B motif in nucleotide-binding domain −1 is indicated by an overline and the nine potential consensus *in vivo* PKA phosphorylation sites are labelled with asterisks. The small arrows indicate residues significant for the R domain deletion mutants. (Reproduced from Rich et al.[30], with permission)

These observations about the sequence of the R domain, as well as the observation that cAMP-stimulated $Cl^-$ secretion is lost in CF epithelia, suggested that the CFTR $Cl^-$ channel may be regulated by PKA-dependent phosphorylation.

## PKA PHOSPHORYLATES CFTR AND ACTIVATES CFTR $Cl^-$ CHANNELS

Some of the first evidence that CFTR might be regulated by phosphorylation was the observation that CFTR can be phosphorylated *in vitro* by PKA[16]. Additional studies using the whole-cell patch-clamp technique showed that expression of recombinant CFTR generated $Cl^-$ channels that could be activated by an increase in intracellular levels of cAMP[17–19]. Addition of cAMP increased current and then, when cAMP agonists were withdrawn, current returned to basal values. These results suggested that the effect of phosphorylation was reversible and that protein phosphatases also controlled activity.

More direct evidence that the CFTR $Cl^-$ channel was regulated by phosphorylation came from studies of single CFTR $Cl^-$ channels. In cell-attached patches, an increase in cellular levels of cAMP reversibly activated CFTR $Cl^-$ channels[20,21]. Additional evidence that phosphorylation was responsible came from studies in cell-free, inside-out patches of membrane. Addition of the catalytic subunit of PKA (in the presence of ATP) activated single channels. An example is shown in Figure 2. When CFTR $Cl^-$ channels were excised from cells expressing endogenous or recombinant CFTR[20–22] there was little reversal of the effect of the kinase, suggesting that the phosphatases that regulate CFTR did not remain in the membrane patch after excision from the cell.

## REVERSAL OF THE EFFECT OF PKA BY SPECIFIC PROTEIN PHOSPHATASES

Stimulation of $Cl^-$ secretion in airway or intestinal epithelia is reversible; once the agonist is removed, the rate of secretion returns to basal values, and subsequent readdition of agonist can once again stimulate $Cl^-$ secretion. This observation implies that phosphorylation is reversible and suggests that specific phosphatases dephosphorylate CFTR.

The role of several specific protein phosphatases in regulating CFTR has now been investigated. Protein phosphatase 2A (PP2A) has been found in the cytoplasm of many types of cells[23]. Addition of PP2A to CFTR that had been phosphorylated *in vitro* by PKA caused a dephosphorylation that was blocked

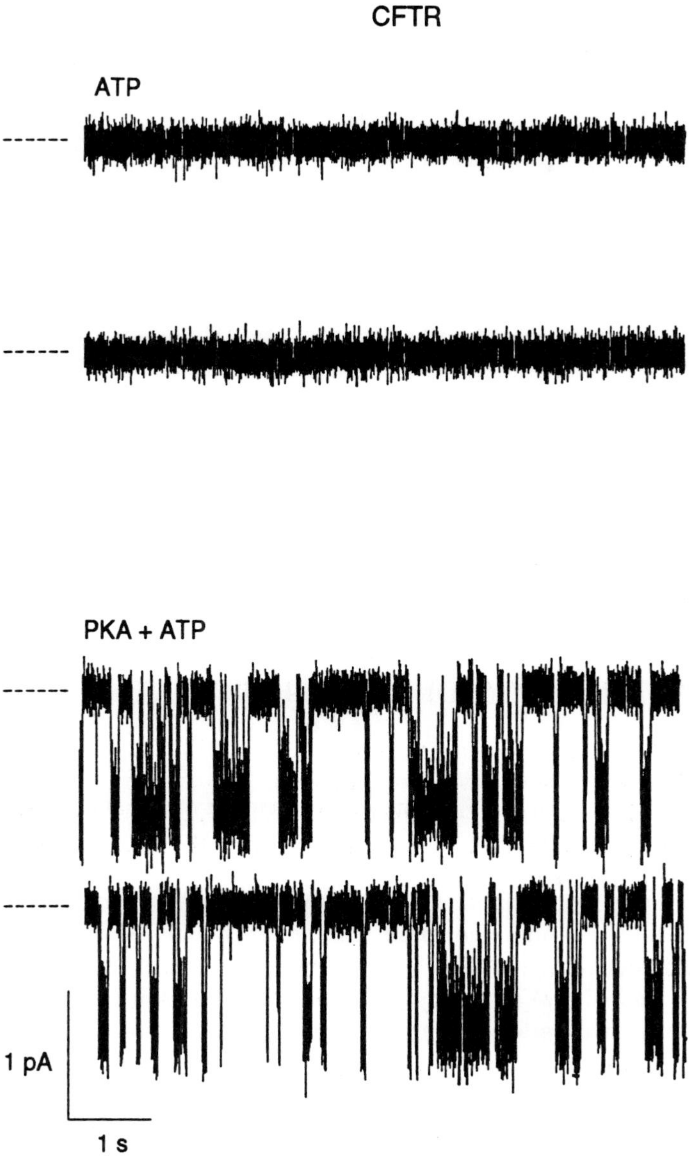


**Figure 2** Single-channel recording of a CFTR $Cl^-$ channel. Tracing was from an excised, inside-out membrane patch. MgATP (0.88 mM) and the catalytic subunit of PKA (75 nM) were present in the intracellular solution, as indicated. (Courtesy of Dr David N. Sheppard)

by the phosphatase inhibitors okadaic acid (1 μM) and by calyculin-A (0.1 μM)[11]. When PP2A was added to the cytosolic surface of excised membrane patches containing CFTR $Cl^-$ channels, it also inhibited current to near-basal levels. After PP2A was removed and PKA was readded, the channels reopened. Calyculin-A blocked the effect of PP2A on $Cl^-$ currents.

In contrast to the effect of PP2A, neither PP1 nor PP2B dephosphorylated CFTR nor closed CFTR $Cl^-$ channels that had been activated by PKA and ATP[11]. These results suggest that the effect of PP2A is specific.

Alkaline phosphatase may also dephosphorylate and inactivate CFTR, although reports have been conflicting. In one report, alkaline phosphatase was shown to inactivate $Cl^-$ channels from shark rectal gland and recombinant CFTR expressed in CHO cells[21]. However, another study found no direct effect of alkaline phosphatase[11]. Although alkaline phosphatase decreased CFTR $Cl^-$ current, it appeared that the effect was at least in some cases due to alkaline phosphatase-dependent hydrolysis of ATP in the bathing solution. As a result the ATP concentration decreased and, because ATP is required for activity of CFTR $Cl^-$ channels, the channels closed. However, they could be reactivated by addition of fresh ATP, even in the absence of PKA. Additional studies will be required to investigate the effect and specificity of alkaline phosphatases.

## IDENTIFICATION OF PHOSPHORYLATED SITES IN CFTR

Specific sequences of CFTR that are phosphorylated have begun to be identified in studies in which CFTR is phosphorylated by an increase in cAMP *in vivo* or by addition of PKA *in vitro*. In order to identify each phosphorylation site in CFTR, variants were produced in which each of the 10 potential phosphoserines was mutated to an alanine[24]. The CFTR variants were then expressed in heterologous cells. The protein was immunoprecipitated, labelled with PKA and [$^{32}$P]ATP, the protein was digested with trypsin, and then a two-dimensional cryptic phosphopeptide map of wild-type CFTR and each of the variants was assessed.

Although CFTR contains 10 'classic' PKA consensus sequences, PKA does not phosphorylate all 10 of the sites. Immunoprecipitation of CFTR, followed by phosphorylation *in vitro* shows that seven sites (S660, S700, S712, S737, S768, S795 and S813) are phosphorylated. Of the three that were not phosphorylated, S422 lies outside the R domain before the first nucleotide-binding domain. Serine 686 does not contain a consensus phosphorylation sequence that is conserved in CFTR from other species (Figure 1). Finally, T788 is not conserved across species and phosphoamino acid analysis indicates that only serines are phosphorylated; there is no evidence of phosphotyrosine or phosphothreonine[24].

When similar studies were done under *in vivo* conditions in which labelling was stimulated by addition of cAMP agonists, four major phosphopeptides were identified, corresponding to residues S660, S737, S795 and S813[24]. Additional studies using CFTR from T84 intestinal epithelial cell line, or using a peptide containing part of the R domain, reported that an additional serine within the R domain (S700) was phosphorylated *in vivo* after stimulation with cAMP agonists.

## FUNCTIONAL CONSEQUENCES OF MUTATING PHOSPHORYLATION SITES IN CFTR

As a way to address the functional consequences of PKA-dependent phosphorylation, CFTR variants containing various serines mutated to alanine were studied using isotope efflux assays and the patch-clamp technique[12,24,25]. Initial studies from our laboratory showed that mutation of any one serine to alanine did not prevent activation of $Cl^-$ channels following addition of cAMP agonists. Further, we initially reported that mutation of four serines that were identified as *in vivo* phosphorylation sites (S660/737/795/813A, named S-Quad-A) caused the loss of response to cAMP[24]. However, in subsequent studies, when the expression level of CFTR-S-Quad-A was increased, it became apparent that stimulation by cAMP agonists opened the channels[12,25]. These results suggested that the activity of the S-Quad-A mutant was decreased relative to that of wild-type CFTR but not abolished.

To test this hypothesis more directly, the patch-clamp technique was used to examine single $Cl^-$ channels[12,25]. Figure 3 shows the open-state probability ($P_o$) of wild-type CFTR and CFTR containing mutations of several of the serines. In the S-Quad-A variant, the $P_o$ was decreased compared to that of wild-type CFTR. By contrast, the response to changes in cytosolic ATP, which interacts with the nucleotide-binding domains, was unaltered, and the conductive properties of the variant, which are predominantly determined by the membrane-spanning domains, were unchanged. These data suggested a specific effect of the mutations in S-Quad-A on regulation by the R domain.

The fact that the S-Quad-A mutant remained responsive to cAMP seemed surprising because the mutation removed the four major *in vivo* phosphorylation sites. Therefore, we asked whether mutation of the four major serine phosphorylation sites allowed PKA-dependent phosphorylation at new sites within the R domain or elsewhere within CFTR. To test this possibility we mapped sites phosphorylated *in vivo* in CFTR S-Quad-A after stimulation by cAMP agonists[25]. As expected, the data showed that the mutant indeed lacked all of the mutated phosphopeptides, but, more importantly, no new

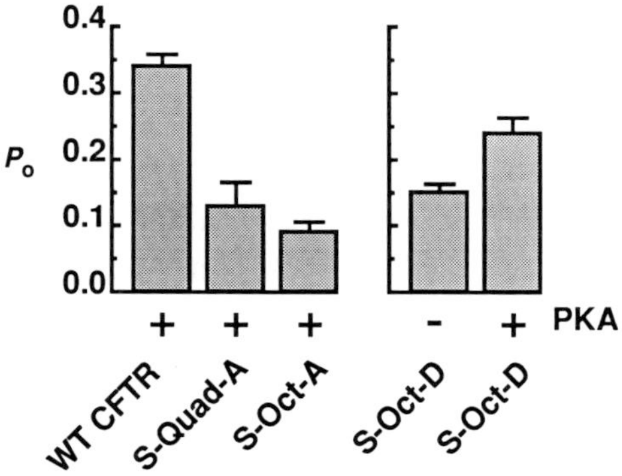


**Figure 3** Single-channel open-state probability of wild-type and mutant CFTR $Cl^-$ channels. The single-channel open-state probability for wild-type CFTR ($n = 14$), CFTR S-Quad-A (S660/737/795/813A) ($n = 5$), CFTR S-Oct-A (S660/686/700/712/737/768/795/813A) ($n = 7$), or CFTR S-Oct-D (S660/686/700/712/737/768/795/813D) ($n = 7$ in ATP alone (– PKA); $n = 10$ in PKA and ATP (+ PKA)) $Cl^-$ channels is shown. Data are mean ± s.e.m. of $n$ experiments measured before (–) or after (+) phosphorylation by PKA. (Reproduced from Rich et al.[25], with permission)

phosphopeptides were identified. Although the S-Quad-A mutant was still phosphorylated *in vivo*[12,25], no new specific phosphopeptides could be identified.

In a further attempt to identify sites that might be involved in the regulation, we constructed an S-Oct-A mutant (S660, S700, S712, S737, S768, S795 and S813) in which all seven of the sites that are phosphorylated *in vitro* plus the potential phosphorylation site, S686, were mutated to alanine[25]. Chang et al.[12] mutated those eight sites plus S422 and T788 to alanine. Data from both laboratories indicated that the variant CFTR was phosphorylated *in vivo* and that the channels retained residual, albeit reduced activity (Figure 3). Thus, it appears that there may be residual phosphorylation that can regulate the channel, but that the level of phosphorylation at any one site is too low to allow detection and identification of the corresponding phosphopeptide.

We considered the possibility that activation of CFTR containing multiple serine to alanine mutations might not be the result of phosphorylation; perhaps cAMP had some other effect. However, this possibility seems unlikely because the S-Quad-A and S-Oct-A mutants were still phosphorylated *in vivo* and because the channels were activated only by addition of PKA and ATP to excised membrane patches.

## ACTIVATION OF CFTR BY SUBSTITUTION OF ASPARTATE FOR PHOSPHOSERINE

One mechanism by which phosphorylation may open the CFTR $Cl^-$ channel is by the addition of negative charge to the R domain. To assess this, the hypothesis that phosphoserines could be replaced by negatively charged residues was tested[25]. Serine-to-aspartate mutations have been used in a variety of other proteins to mimic the functional effects of phosphorylation of serine residues[26–28]. When four or five of the serines were mutated to aspartate, channel activity was only observed after addition of cAMP agonists. However, when six, seven or eight serines were mutated to aspartate, channels were found to be open, even without the addition of cAMP. Figure 3 shows the effects on $P_o$ when channels were studied with the patch-clamp technique: CFTR S-Oct-D $Cl^-$ channels opened immediately upon addition of ATP, although subsequent addition of PKA produced a further increase in $Cl^-$ current.

## EFFECT OF DELETING PORTIONS OF THE R DOMAIN

The data presented above suggest that phosphorylation of the R domain opens the CFTR $Cl^-$ channel. To test the hypothesis that the R domain has a negative effect that keeps the channel closed, the effect of deleting the R domain was tested[29]. As shown in Figure 1 the R domain was originally defined as 241 amino acids (residues 590–830) encoded by exon 13. We tested the effect of deleting parts or all of exon 13. Comparison of the amino acid sequence of human CFTR with that of several different species and with that of two other members of the traffic ATPase/ABC transporter family, MDR and STE6, is shown in Figure 1. It is apparent that CFTR contains a segment of over 120 amino acids that is not found in any of those other family members. Therefore, we created an R domain deletion mutant (CFTRΔR) which deleted only the unique segment (residues 708–835). Deletion of this part of the R domain produced channels that were active even in the absence of cAMP-dependent stimulation or stimulation by PKA. However, subsequent addition of cAMP *in vivo* or application of PKA in excised membrane patches produced a further increase in activity measured as open-state probability.

To further define this unique segment and the 'functional' R domain, additional deletion mutants were constructed[30]. Figure 1 shows the extent of these deletions. When we deleted 154 amino acids (residues 681–835), 159 amino acids (residues 676–835), 179 amino acids (residues 656–835), or all 241 amino acids encoded by exon 13 (residues 590–830), we found that none generated cAMP-stimulated opening of CFTR $Cl^-$ channels. These deletions did not appear to cause a loss of $Cl^-$ channel activity by producing a grossly misfolded protein that could not be delivered to the plasma membrane, because protein was detected at the membrane in unpermeabilized cells. Thus, we concluded that trafficking of CFTR to the plasma membrane requires neither the R domain nor active CFTR $Cl^-$ channel activity. We cannot exclude the possibility, however, that the deletion of extensive portions of the R domain alters the juxtaposition of the transmembrane domains and this alters $Cl^-$ channel activity of the deletion mutants.

The increase in channel $P_o$ observed on addition of PKA to the CFTRΔR mutant resulted from phosphorylation of at least one additional site within the protein. Of the reported major phosphorylation sites, the CFTRΔR variant retains S660 and S700. When the S660A mutation was made in CFTRΔR, the PKA-dependent increase in $P_o$ was abolished although activity in the absence of phosphorylation persisted. That data suggest that S660 is involved in regulation of R domain function, whereas perhaps S700 is not involved in all cell types.

## FUNCTION OF THE R DOMAIN IN REGULATION OF CFTR

The data presented above show that regulation of CFTR by the R domain is complex. In the following, we speculate about several aspects of this complexity.

### HOW DOES THE R DOMAIN REGULATE CFTR?

One simple (certainly overly simplistic) interpretation of the data is that the R domain has a negative influence, keeping the channel closed. In such a case the role of the R domain might be analogous to that of the N-terminal 'ball' of the Shaker $K^+$ channel, which inactivates or closes that channel[31,32]. It should be noted, however, that the N-terminal ball of the $K^+$ shaker channel and the R domain of CFTR differ greatly in size. In Shaker $K^+$ channels, inhibition can be relieved by deleting or altering the charge of the amino terminal sequences in the 'ball' region. In CFTR, inhibition of the R domain can be relieved in three different ways as shown in Figure 4: by phosphorylation, by addition of negatively charged amino acids, or by deleting a large part of the domain.

The observation that substitution of negatively charged aspartate for serine in the R domain generated $Cl^-$ channels that were open, even without phosphorylation by PKA, suggests that electrostatic interactions within the protein may be important for channel activation. We speculate that addition of negative charges might generate charge–charge interactions between the R domain and another part of the protein to either push or pull the R domain away from the pore and open the channel. However, we cannot rule out the alternative explanation that charge-induced conformational charges in the

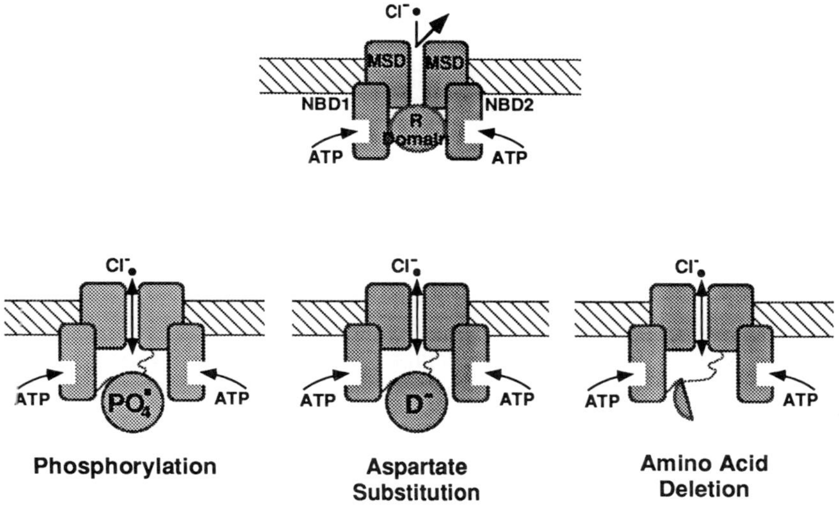


**Figure 4** Model of regulation of CFTR by the R domain. Top panel shows model of CFTR and bottom panels show mechanisms by which the R domain can open CFTR $Cl^-$channels. Hatched area represents cell membrane, MSD refers to membrane-spanning domains, and NBD refers to nucleotide-binding domains

R domain open the channel. In either case, it is unclear whether the important factor for channel activation is the number of charges introduced by addition of aspartate or by PKA phosphorylation, or charge density within the R domain.

However, the model shown in Figure 4 is probably overly simplistic based on the observation that deletion of the R domain and mutation of S660A to alanine (CFTRΔR-S660A) produces $Cl^-$ channels that tend to have a lower open-state probability than do wild-type channels after phosphorylation. If the R domain only had a negative effect, then one would expect that its removal might produce a channel that had a $P_o$ similar to or even greater than that of phosphorylated wild-type CFTR. Thus, in addition to negative effects, the presence of the R domain most likely has positive effects on the function of the channel. An alternative interpretation inherent in any study using site-directed mutations is that the mutation caused some unanticipated alteration in the structure of the protein that in some way reduced activity.

## WHICH PHOSPHORYLATION SITES ARE IMPORTANT IN REGULATING THE CHANNEL?

We propose that four or perhaps five serines are the major regulatory sites for PKA-dependent phosphorylation *in vivo* for two reasons. First, S660, S737,

S795, S813[24] and S700[10] were phosphorylated *in vivo* following stimulation by cAMP agonists. Even when phosphorylation of those residues is prevented by mutation to alanine, we did not detect any additional phosphorylation sites by tryptic phosphopeptide mapping. Second, most of the decrease in $P_o$ occurred with simultaneous mutation of those serines to alanine. Concomitant mutation of those serines plus an additional four serines produced only a small additional decrement in $P_o$.

Yet, PKA phosphorylated and regulated CFTR both *in vivo* and *in vitro* in the absence of eight or 10 consensus PKA sites. One interpretation of these results is that PKA phosphorylated several sites within the R domain (or elsewhere within CFTR), but that no one site predominated and, hence, was not detected in our phosphopeptide maps. For example, within the population of CFTR proteins, one serine might be phosphorylated in some channels, a different one in other channels, yet another one in still other channels, and so on. If true, this interpretation predicts that *in vivo* the four or five previously identified serines normally regulate CFTR $Cl^-$ channel activity. But, in their absence, phosphorylation of any one of the additional unidentified sites can open the channel.

## WHERE MIGHT UNIDENTIFIED PHOSPHORYLATION SITES BE?

It is likely that the unidentified sites are located within the R domain because we found that CFTRΔR-S660A $Cl^-$ channels were regulated by ATP, but not by PKA. Thus, any residual PKA regulatory phosphorylation sites were either removed by deletion of part of the R domain or their influence on channel activation was eliminated by the deletion. Alternatively, it is possible that PKA phosphorylates 'non-classic' sites within other parts of CFTR which interact with the R domain; thus deletion of part of the R domain would disrupt those interactions whether or not additional sites were phosphorylated. Another possibility is that the many non-classic sites scattered throughout CFTR might be phosphorylated. Finally, we cannot rule out the possibility that PKA cannot interact with CFTRΔR-S660A even though it does interact with CFTR.

## WHAT RESIDUES COMPRISE THE FUNCTIONAL R DOMAIN?

The R domain was originally defined as those amino acids encoded by exon 13 in the CFTR gene. Such exon/intron boundaries provide a convenient way to define the R domain, but that does not necessarily reflect the corresponding functional domain within CFTR. As shown in Figure 1, exon 13 is the site of the greatest amino acid sequence divergence between CFTR from different species. However, Figure 1 also shows that most of the sequence variation occurs in the second half of exon 13. Indeed, there is sequence similarity between CFTR and MDR and STE6 within the initial portion of the R domain.

One interpretation of the amino acid sequence comparison shown in Figure 1 and the data on the effect of deletions is that the unique segment of 127 amino acids from the second half of exon 13 defines, at least in part, a 'functional' domain within CFTR. Deletion of this unique segment to produce CFTRΔR does not alter the biophysical properties of the CFTR $Cl^-$ channel but does produce a channel that is open even in the absence of phosphorylation. However, other parts of exon 13 appear to be required for CFTR $Cl^-$ channel function. As indicated above, PKA may phosphorylate five serines in exon 13 *in vivo* to cause the channel to open. However, two of those sites (S660 and S700) lie outside the unique sequence that can be deleted (residues 708–835). Thus, the actual *functional* R domain may consist of amino acids 708–835 plus additional parts of the protein defined by its overall three-dimensional structure. This observation is further supported by the fact that more extensive deletions of exon 13 abolish CFTR $Cl^-$ channel function. It is also consistent with the identification of a mutation in exon 13 that is reported to cause CF: this mutation deletes 28 amino acids corresponding to residues 607–635[33].

## WHY ARE THERE RELATIVELY FEW CF MUTATIONS IN THE R DOMAIN?

Relatively few nonsense mutations associated with CF map to the R domain, whereas other parts of the molecule with important functional roles appear to have many more CF-associated mutations. Perhaps the observation that mutation of any one or indeed all of the major *in vivo* phosphorylation sites is without major effect on $Cl^-$ channel activity, even though phosphorylation is clearly important, means that the R domain of CFTR is somewhat plastic within the structure of CFTR and can accommodate structural alteration without measurable effect on function. This would support a model arguing that regulation by the R domain is brought about by charge–charge interactions and that these are degenerate. In other words, charge may be important in regulation but its precise location, at least in the primary sequence, is less critical.

## WHY IS REGULATION OF CFTR BY THE R DOMAIN SO COMPLEX?

There are several possibilities. It might be that multiple phosphorylation sites provide a mechanism by which graded phosphorylation of CFTR could provide graded activation of CFTR $Cl^-$ channels and, hence, graded regulation of transepithelial $Cl^-$ secretion. It is possible to test this hypothesis using single-channel patch-clamp techniques and the study of CFTR variants containing various numbers of serines available for phosphorylation.

It is also possible that different sites within CFTR provide substrates for different protein kinases and phosphatases. For example, the presence of multiple phosphoserines within CFTR might tend to slow the effect of a phosphatase. Alternatively, different kinases and phosphatases might regulate different phosphorylation sites within the protein. Finally, there may be interactions between the phosphorylation sites and a pattern of hierarchical phosphorylation that is important in control of the channel.

In the end, there are many questions that remain to be answered about how phosphorylation regulates CFTR. One frustrating problem is that we do not yet understand how the R domain interacts with the rest of the protein. As with so many other channels and transporters a notion of the three-dimensional structure of the channel would be particularly valuable.

## ACKNOWLEDGEMENTS

We thank our laboratory colleagues for helpful discussions. Michael J. Welsh is an investigator of the Howard Hughes Medical Institute. Herbert A. Berger is a Fellow of the Parker B. Francis Foundation. Work from the authors' laboratories was supported by grants from the Howard Hughes Medical Institute, the National Heart, Lung and Blood Institute and the Cystic Fibrosis Foundation.

## REFERENCES

1 Boat TF, Welsh MJ, Beaudet AL. Cystic fibrosis. In: *The Metabolic Basis of Inherited Disease*, 6th (eds CR Scriver, AL Beaudet, WS Sly, D Valle). McGraw-Hill, New York, 1989, pp 2649–80.
2 Quinton PM. Cystic fibrosis: a disease in electrolyte transport. *FASEB J* 1990; **4**: 2709–17.
3 Riordan JR, Rommens JM, Kerem B-S, et al. Identification of the cystic fibrosis gene: cloning and characterization of complementary DNA. *Science* 1989; **245**: 1066–73.
4 Welsh MJ, Anderson MP, Rich DP, et al. Cystic fibrosis transmembrane conductance regulator: a chloride channel with novel regulation. *Neuron* 1992; **8**: 821–9.
5 Collins FS. Cystic fibrosis: molecular biology and therapeutic implications. *Science* 1992; **256**: 774–9.
6 Riordan JR. The cystic fibrosis transmembrane conductance regulator. *Annu Rev Physiol* 1993; **55**: 609–30.
7 Lin M, Nairn AC, Guggino SE. cGMP-dependent protein kinase regulation of a chloride channel in T84 cells. *Am J Physiol* 1992; **262**: C1304–12.
8 Housley PR. Aluminum fluoride inhibition of glucocorticoid receptor inactivation and transformation. *Biochemistry* 1990; **29**: 3578–85.
9 Cohn JA, Nairn AC, Marino CR, et al. Characterization of the cystic fibrosis transmembrane conductance regulator in a colonocyte cell line. *Proc Natl Acad Sci USA* 1992; **89**: 2340–4.

10 Picciotto MR, Cohn JA, Bertuzzi G, et al. Phosphorylation of the cystic fibrosis transmembrane conductance regulator. *J Biol Chem* 1992; **267**: 12742–52.
11 Berger HA, Travis SM, Welsh MJ. Regulation of the cystic fibrosis transmembrane conductance regulator $Cl^-$ channel by specific protein kinases and protein phosphatases. *J Biol Chem* 1993; **268**: 2037–47.
12 Chang XB, Tabcharani JA, Hou YX, et al. Protein kinase A (PKA) still activates CFTR chloride channel after mutagenesis of all 10 PKA consensus phosphorylation sites. *J Biol Chem* 1993; **268**: 11304–11.
13 Hyde SC, Emsley P, Hartshorn MJ, et al. Structural model of ATP-binding proteins associated with cystic fibrosis, multidrug resistance and bacterial transport. *Nature* 1990; **346**: 362–5.
14 Ames GF, Lecar H. ATP-dependent bacterial transporters and cystic fibrosis: analogy between channels and transporters. *FASEB J* 1992; **6**: 2660–6.
15 Kennelly PJ, Krebs EG. Consensus sequences as substrate specificity derminants for protein kinases and protein phosphatases. *J Biol Chem* 1991; **266**: 15555–8.
16 Gregory RJ, Cheng SH, Rich DP, et al. Expression and characterization of the cystic fibrosis transmembrane conductance regulator. *Nature* 1990; **347**: 382–6.
17 Rich DP, Anderson MP, Gregory RJ, et al. Expression of cystic fibrosis transmembrane conductance regulator corrects defective chloride channel regulation in cystic fibrosis airway epithelial cells. *Nature* 1990; **347**: 358–63.
18 Drumm ML, Pope HA, Cliff WH, et al. Correction of the cystic fibrosis defect in vitro by retrovirus-mediated gene transfer. *Cell* 1990; **62**: 1227–33.
19 Kartner N, Hanrahan JW, Jensen TJ, et al. Expression of the cystic fibrosis gene in non-epithelial invertebrate cells produces a regulated anion conductance. *Cell* 1991; **64**: 681–91.
20 Berger HA, Anderson MP, Gregory RJ, et al. Identification and regulation of the cystic fibrosis transmembrane conductance regulator-generated chloride channel. *J Clin Invest* 1991; **88**: 1422–31.
21 Tabcharani JA, Chang X-B, Riordan JR, Hanrahan JW. Phosphorylation-regulated $Cl^-$ channel in CHO cells stably expressing the cystic fibrosis gene. *Nature* 1991; **352**: 628–31.
22 Nagel G, Hwang T-C, Nastiuk KL, et al. The protein kinase A-regulated cardiac $Cl^-$ channel resembles the cystic fibrosis transmembrane conductance regulator. *Nature* 1992; **360**: 81–4.
23 Shenolikar S, Nairn AC. Protein phosphatases: recent progress. *Adv Second Messenger Phosphoprotein Res* 1991; **23**: 1–121.
24 Cheng SH, Rich DP, Marshall J, et al. Phosphorylation of the R domain by cAMP-dependent protein kinase regulates the CFTR chloride channel. *Cell* 1991; **66**: 1027–36.
25 Rich DP, Berger HA, Cheng SH, et al. Regulation of the cystic fibrosis transmembrane conductance regulator $Cl^-$ channel by negative charge in the R domain. *J Biol Chem* 1993; **268**: 20259–67.
26 Casanova JE, Breitfeld PP, Ross SA, Mostov KE. Phosphorylation of the polymeric imunoglobulin receptor required for its efficient transcytosis. *Science* 1990; **248**: 742–5.
27 Thorsness PE, Koshland DE Jr. Inactivation of isocitrate dehydrogenase by phosphorylation is mediated by the negative charge of the phosphate. *J Biol Chem* 1987; **262**: 10422–5.
28 Fong YL, Taylor WL, Means AR, Soderlin TR. Studies of the regulatory mechanism of $Ca^{2+}$/calmodulin-dependent protein kinase II: mutation of threonine 286 to alanine and aspartate. *J Biol Chem* 1989; **264**: 16759–63.

29 Rich DP, Gregory RJ, Anderson MP, et al. Effect of deleting the R domain on CFTR-generated chloride channels. *Science* 1991; **253**: 205–7.
30 Rich DP, Gregory RJ, Cheng SH, et al. Effect of deletion mutations on the function of CFTR chloride channels. *Recept Chan* 1993; **1**: 221–32.
31 Hoshi T, Zagotta WN, Aldrich RW. Biophysical and molecular mechanisms of Shaker potassium channel inactivation. *Science* 1990; **250**: 533–8.
32 Zagotta WN, Hoshi T, Aldrich RW. Restoration of inactivation in mutants of Shaker potassium channels by a peptide derived from ShB. *Science* 1990; **250**: 568–71.
33 Granell R, Solera J, Carrasco S, Molano J. Identification of a nonframeshift 84-bp deletion in exon 13 of the cystic fibrosis gene. *Am J Hum Genet* 1992; **50**: 1022–6.

# Part III

## Clinical Aspects

## Chapter Eleven

# Respiratory Viral Infections in Cystic Fibrosis

Peter W. Hiatt
*Baylor College of Medicine, Department of Pediatrics, Pulmonology Section, Houston, Texas, USA*

## INTRODUCTION

Although significant improvement has been made in the therapy of cystic fibrosis (CF), chronic obstructive airway disease continues to develop in patients with CF and is the major cause of death. Life expectancy has improved remarkably over the last 20 years with the advent of new antimicrobial agents. However, progressive deterioration of pulmonary function occurs in spite of their routine use in the treatment of pulmonary exacerbations. Although bacteria play an important role in producing airway damage and altered pulmonary function the mechanisms remain controversial in CF patients[1]. Initially, airway infection typically occurs with *Staphylococcus aureus* and *Haemophilus influenzae*[2,3]. Chronic colonization and infection develops with *Pseudomonas aeruginosa*[4]. Once colonization with *Ps. aeruginosa* is established, progressive deterioration in lung function is observed. A pathogenic role for bacteria is suggested by the presence of immune complexes in the lungs of CF children, the improvement clinically following treatment with antibiotics, and the increased survival observed since the introduction of antibiotics in treating these patients. However, during

*Cystic Fibrosis—Current Topics, Volume 2.* Edited by J. A. Dodge, D. J. H. Brock and J. H. Widdicombe

pulmonary exacerbations, the absence of fever, leucocytosis, or apparent systemic toxicity suggest the role of non-bacterial factors in their initiation.

Most patients become colonized during the first decade of life with *Ps. aeruginosa*, yet little information exists defining when this colonization begins and the cofactors which facilitate its early adherence to the respiratory epithelium. Host immune response, bacterial virulence characteristics, abnormal respiratory mucins and airway injury following viral respiratory infection have all been thought to influence colonization and progressive lung disease[5]. It is very important to define the role of these early cofactors of lung injury if we are to be effective in reducing pulmonary disease. Prevention of early lung disease should enhance growth and development of the lungs. New therapeutic interventions, with prophylactic antibiotics, vaccines and immunotherapy, will be dependent on our understanding of the pathophysiology of lung disease in CF. Proposed modalities for gene therapy[6] involve replacement therapy using various forms of aerosol administration. Limiting the inflammatory disease in the airway, maintenance of airway patency and minimizing early lung insult will be of considerable importance for effective delivery of the gene vector to the smaller airways of the lung. This chapter will review the role of viral respiratory infections in the development of early pulmonary dysfunction in infants and children with CF and explore how these infections may influence the predisposition for *Ps. aeruginosa* colonization, and the occurrence of pulmonary exacerbations in children and adults with CF.

## VIRAL RESPIRATORY INFECTIONS IN CYSTIC FIBROSIS

### WRIGHT ET AL. (1976)[7]

Wright et al. were the first investigators to evaluate the effects of respiratory viral infections in children with CF. The study was conducted at the Children's Hospital Medical Center, Boston, Massachusetts. The study was designed to evaluate the effectiveness of amantidine, an oral antiviral drug, against influenza A virus infection in children with CF. Influenza failed to reach epidemic proportions in the New England area during the study, so that the effectiveness of amantidine could not be assessed in the CF subjects enrolled. One hundred and fifty-three children with CF were recruited for the study with a mean age of 12 years and followed for a period of two months. Paired samples of serum from each child in the study were examined for haemagglutination inhibition antibodies to influenza viruses. In addition, serum samples from all patients with exacerbations of respiratory illness were also tested for complement fixation antibodies to other respiratory viruses. Only three viral cultures were attempted in acutely ill children. Minor and major respiratory infections were determined with a respiratory questionnaire designed to assess the incidence and severity of illness. Serological evidence of viral infection was documented in 33% of patients experiencing a respiratory illness (28 minor and 18 major episodes). Of the 18 subjects with a major pulmonary exacerbation, seven (39%) had serological evidence of viral infection. Influenza and respiratory syncytial virus (RSV) accounted for 12 of 13 viral infections identified in the study. These results did not include a method of identifying rhinoviruses and corona viruses—agents well documented to be important causes of respiratory disease.

## PETERSEN ET AL. (1981)[8]

In 1981 Petersen et al. enrolled 116 CF patients in Copenhagen, Denmark, to investigate the importance of non-bacterial agents in exacerbations of the pulmonary disease observed in children with CF. The children ranged in age from six months to 29 years (mean age not provided) and were followed for eight months. A serum sample was taken from each patient at the beginning of the study and two to four weeks following a pulmonary exacerbation. Acute infections were reported by the enrolled subjects or their parents to the investigators. No weekly determination of respiratory disease was made by the investigators nor were viral cultures obtained during acute illnesses. Serum samples were used to measure antibodies to respiratory viruses, *Mycoplasma pneumoniae* and precipitating antibodies against *Ps. aeruginosa*. Three hundred and thirty-three exacerbations were recorded during the eight-month study, 20% of which were attributed to non-bacterial causes. The investigators noted a greater number of exacerbations in the CF patients with chronic *Pseudomonas* colonization compared to non-colonized *Pseudomonas* CF patients. RSV was the most commonly identified respiratory virus triggering acute pulmonary illness in the study, followed by parainfluenza and influenza viruses. The investigators found seven of 116 subjects developed the onset of chronic *Pseudomonas* colonization following infection with RSV and that RSV infection was associated with an increase—although sometimes temporary—in the number of precipitins against *Ps. aeruginosa*. No attempt was made to isolate rhinoviruses or coronaviruses in this study, probably causing an underestimation of respiratory virus disease.

## WANG ET AL. (1984)[9]

At the Hospital for Sick Children in Toronto, Wang et al. examined the role of viral infections in the pulmonary deterioration of patients with CF. The study was conducted from May 1981 to May 1983. Patients with CF and their siblings were assessed in the CF clinic at the time of enrolment, and at routinely scheduled visits. History, physical examination, chest radiograph,

Shwachman scores, and height and weight measurements were made routinely. A weekly telephone surveillance was administered by a study nurse to identify the first signs or symptoms of respiratory illness. Once an illness was identified either a clinic appointment or a home visit was arranged to evaluate each patient. Serum for viral antibodies, nasopharyngeal washings for viral isolation and sputum samples for quantitative bacteriological studies were then obtained. Forty-nine patients with CF and 19 sibling controls were enrolled and followed for two years. The mean age of study subjects with CF was 13.7 years, all having the ability to perform pulmonary function tests. All viral infections were identified by seroconversions. No viruses were isolated by culture. A total of 105 infections were identified in CF patients, of which 42 were asymptomatic. Parainfluenza viruses and adenoviruses caused the majority of infections in their study. Significant correlations were found between the annual incidence of viral infections and every measure of pulmonary disease progression during the two-year study. These parameters included the Shwachman score, weight for height, forced vital capacity, forced expiratory volume in 1 s ($FEV_1$) and the frequency and duration of hospitalization. Sixteen of 41 hospitalizations (39%) were associated with a seroconversion to a respiratory virus. No correlation was found between the annual incidence of viral infections and colonization with *Ps. aeruginosa*. The inability to isolate respiratory viruses in this study was attributed to: (1) frequently culturing asymptomatic patients; (2) assessing a group of older children (age is inversely associated with respiratory viral isolation); (3) freezing specimens prior to attempted growth in tissue culture; and (4) postulating the presence of an unidentified substance in the secretions of CF patients which inhibits viral growth in tissue culture.

## EFTHIMIOU ET AL. (1984)[10]

From January to April 1980, Efthimiou and co-workers enrolled 46 young adult CF subjects to investigate the role of viruses and *Legionella pneumophila* in acute respiratory exacerbations. The study was conducted at the Brompton Hospital, London, England. The mean age of the CF group was 22.2 years; however, the information for the control group was not given. Patients were classified as either 'deteriorated' or 'stable' based on a reduction in their $FEV_1$ one month prior to the start of the study and an increase in cough, sputum production or breathlessness. Twenty-four subjects were in the deteriorated group and 22 patients were considered clinically stable. Nose and throat swabs and samples of sputum and serum were collected from the patients and controls at entry, one month and one year following enrolment. A four-fold rise in complement-fixing antibody titre to respiratory viruses was observed in paired sera from five of 24 patients in the deteriorated group and in only one of 22 in the stable group. Significantly fewer patients in the stable group experienced seroconversion to respiratory viruses compared to the deteriorated group. No difference was demonstrated between groups in terms of their principal sputum pathogens. These findings led the authors to suggest that severely affected CF patients may be more susceptible to non-bacterial infections. The study did not perform routine surveillance for acute respiratory disease nor obtain frequent serum or culture samples.

STROOBANT (1986)[11]

In a study conducted at the Hospital for Sick Children, Great Ormond Street, London, two groups of children with CF were followed for 12 months. The children ranged in age from 5 to 16 years. Group 1 consisted of 17 children chronically colonized with *Ps. aeruginosa* and group 2 consisted of children without *Pseudomonas*. Culture and serological techniques were used to investigate 41 of 65 (63%) upper respiratory tract infections in group 1 and 22 of 32 (69%) in group 2. A respiratory virus was identified in 21 of 42 chest infections in group 1 and three of 16 in group 2. In every case where a virus was identified pulmonary deterioration occurred. The authors suggested that viral respiratory infections were frequent triggers of pulmonary deterioration in CF children especially if chronic colonization with *Ps. aeruginosa* existed. Viruses were recovered by culture in 13% of identified cases. No pulmonary function results or clinical scores were mentioned in the paper.

ABMAN ET AL. (1988)[12]

In the first study to assess the effects of viral infection in young CF infants, Abman et al. enrolled 48 children with CF identified by newborn screening. The study was conducted at the University of Colorado School of Medicine, Denver. The study protocol consisted of history, physical examination, chest radiograph and throat cultures at the time of diagnosis, at six and 12 months of age, and yearly thereafter. In addition to the above visits children were seen for their routine clinic visits. When hospitalization for respiratory distress was required, culture specimens were obtained for viral pathogens. No sera for respiratory virus antibody titres were obtained for subjects enrolled in this study. Viral cultures were not routinely acquired with the onset of acute respiratory infections unless the CF infants required hospitalization. At a mean follow-up age of 28 months, 18 infants had been hospitalized a total of 30 times for acute respiratory distress. Respiratory viruses were identified for 12 of the hospitalizations, with RSV accounting for seven of 12 isolates. Hospitalization was prolonged (mean 22 days) for CF infants hospitalized with proven RSV infection. Of the seven infants, three required mechanical ventilation for respiratory failure. At discharge, five of the seven infants required supplemental oxygen at home for an average of almost three months. As serological evaluation for RSV and other respiratory viruses were not routinely undertaken, the true incidence of RSV related illness was probably underestimated. Nevertheless, the impact of RSV infection cannot be overstated in their study. The authors speculated that early viral infection predisposes infants with CF to earlier onset of chronic *Ps. aeruginosa* colonization.

## PRZYKLENK ET AL. (1988)[13]

The role of respiratory viruses in the development of acute bronchopulmonary exacerbations of patients with CF was investigated in Munich, Germany, by Przyklenk et al. Seventy-five patients were enrolled with a mean age of 15 years (range 4–28 years) and evaluated from November 1984 to April 1987. Sera for antibody measurements were collected intermittently, ranging from 1 to 18 samples from each patient. Fifty-two per cent of samples were collected as outpatients and 48% during hospitalizations. No viral cultures were obtained. Bacterial specimens from sputum were obtained and analysed at the same time as serology. The sputum was used to measure sputum antibodies against different lipopolysaccharide antigens of *Ps. aeruginosa*. Twenty-nine viral respiratory infections were identified in this study by serology. Influenza A and B viruses accounted for 16 of 29 viral infections. Other respiratory viruses isolated included adenovirus, parainfluenza virus, and RSV. The authors did not find any correlation between colonization with *Ps. aeruginosa* and viral infection.

Respiratory viral infections in CF patients were associated with more frequent admissions and longer hospitalizations compared to CF patients without serological conversion to respiratory viruses. Pulmonary deterioration occurred in 78% of CF subjects during their viral infections, with 93% demonstrating a three-fold increase in bacterial colony-forming units per millilitre of sputum. In addition an increase in immunoglobin A (IgA)-specific antibodies to the O-antigens of *Ps. aeruginosa* was noted in 62% of viral respiratory tract infections. The authors concluded that there was a strong ‘microbial synergism’ between the bacterial flora of the sputum and infection with respiratory viruses. The study did not assess the true incidence of viral respiratory infections as serum and viral cultures were not measured in a systematic fashion for all subjects enrolled in the study.

## ONG ET AL. (1989)[14]

Thirty-six adult patients with CF were followed for one year at Monsall Hospital, University of Manchester School of Medicine. The mean age of the subjects was 23.6 years (range 17–32 years). Patients consisted of two groups. Nineteen subjects in group 1 entered the study with an acute exacerbation of respiratory symptoms and a fall in $FEV_1$. Group 2 consisted of 17 patients who were stable clinically with regard to pulmonary function. Eighteen healthy adults from the hospital were used as controls. Nasopharyngeal aspirates, throat swabs and samples of sputum were collected when patients experienced an exacerbation. A second serum sample was obtained two weeks later. Healthy controls contributed only one sample for throat culture and serum for respiratory viral antibody measurement. Seroconversion occurred in five patients of group 1 and six of group 2. *Pseudomonas* was isolated more frequently in group 1 patients and only one patient with viral seroconversion did not have *Pseudomonas* colonization. There was a mean of 2.6 infective exacerbations in group 1 subjects and 1.1 in group 2. A weak association was noticed between viral seroconversion and isolation of *Ps. aeruginosa* from sputum. The study again demonstrated the low rates of viral infection in adults with CF and the importance of chronic *Ps. aeruginosa* infection.

## RAMSEY ET AL. (1989)[15]

A two-year prospective study at Children's Hospital and Medical Center, Seattle, prospectively assessed the incidence and effect of viral infections on pulmonary function and clinical score in CF children and sibling controls. Enrolment age ranged from 5 to 22 years. Sibling pairs were seen every two months when asymptomatic. At two-monthly intervals throughout the study pulmonary function tests, throat cultures and serology for respiratory viruses were obtained. The same laboratory specimens were collected at the time of an acute respiratory illness.

The frequency of culture and seropositive viral infections was not significantly different for CF patients compared to their sibling controls. The CF subjects with the highest rates of infection were younger and had the lowest rates of decline in pulmonary function during the two-year study. The authors concluded that the rates of infection were similar in CF patients and their sibling controls. In addition, they did not observe any correlation between the decline in pulmonary function and rate of viral infection.

## HORDVIK ET AL. (1989)[16]

Hordvik and associates examined the role of acute respiratory infections in precipitating acute pulmonary exacerbations in patients with CF. The study was carried out over a 20-month period from September 1985 through April 1987. Sixteen subjects were enrolled initially into the study; however, only 10 completed the protocol. The mean age of the subjects was 14 years, with a range of 5 to 32 years. Study patients kept daily diary cards on which specific upper and lower respiratory tract symptoms, peak flow measurements and antibiotic use were recorded. Spirometry was performed during routine clinic visits and twice weekly during hospital admission. Specimens for viral isolation were obtained at home at the onset of a respiratory illness, then mailed to the state virology laboratory. Blood for viral serology was drawn at the beginning of an illness and two weeks after the onset of viral infection.

A total of 35 acute respiratory infections were identified during the study (annual rate of 1.75 infections per patient). The infections were identified by virus isolation, seroconversion, or within three days of illness in the CF patient if a similar infection occurred in a household member. Thirteen of 35 (31%) acute respiratory infections were identified by either viral culture or a four-fold rise in antibody titre. Influenza virus was the most common respiratory virus identified. There was a significant correlation between the severity of baseline pulmonary disease and the magnitude of the fall in peak flow during an acute respiratory viral infection. Initial pulmonary severity was found to correlate with the number of days for peak flow measurements to return to pre-illness levels. The authors concluded that CF children with more advanced pulmonary disease were at enhanced risk for acute pulmonary deterioration due to viral respiratory illness. The long-term effects of acute respiratory infections were not discussed in the paper. The results of the above studies are summarized in Table 1[101].

The majority of the above clinical studies demonstrate a clear correlation between respiratory viral infection and exacerbations of lung disease in CF. The studies have focused on school-aged and adult patients with CF. This group has a lower incidence of childhood respiratory infection compared to infants and toddlers. The impact of viral infection is probably even greater in younger children. The only study assessing infants was by Abman, where RSV infection was found to correlate with a very poor early clinical course. The majority of the above studies did not use weekly respiratory viral surveillance methods to determine viral illness and therefore probably underestimate the true incidence of viral respiratory disease. Few studies were controlled and many were unable to identify viral infections by tissue culture. Seroconversions were used to establish infections. When convalescent serum is collected weeks to months after a clinical illness a direct relationship between the illness and viral infection is less well defined.

The interrelationship with *Pseudomonas* colonization and viral infection remains unclear. Petersen and Ong reported more severe exacerbations with viral disease in the presence of *Pseudomonas* colonization, yet Przyklenk found no correlation. Przyklenk did demonstrate an increase in bacterial colony-forming units in sputum following viral infection, suggesting synergism between bacteria and respiratory viruses. Hordvik and Efthimiou found CF patients with severe pulmonary disease recovered slowly from viral infection, suggesting the underlying condition of the patient was critical in response to viral respiratory infection. Although it appears from the above studies that respiratory viral infections play an important role in exacerbations and

**Table 1** Studies addressing the impact of respiritory viral infection in patients with CF

| Author | No. of patients | No. of controls | Study duration (months) | Age range (years) | Diagnostic methods: Serology | Diagnostic methods: Cultures | PFT[a] reported | No. of culture and seropositive infections in patients | Illness per 100 child years | Percentage of exacerbations attributed to respiratory viral infection |
|---|---|---|---|---|---|---|---|---|---|---|
| Wright | 153 | 0 | 2 | 1–32 | + | – | – | 13 | 47.1 | 39% |
| Petersen | 116 | 0 | 8 | 0.5–29 | + | – | – | 65 | 84.1 | 20% |
| Wang | 49 | 19 | 24 | NR[a] | + | + | + | 105 | 107.1 | 39% |
| Efthimiou | 46 | 30 | 4 | 16–41 | + | + | + | 6 | 32.6 | See text |
| Stroobant | 30 | 0 | 12 | 5–16 | + | + | – | 24 | 80.0 | See text |
| Abman | 48 | 0 | 28 | 0.5–5 | – | + | – | 21 | 18.8 | See text |
| Przyklenk | 75 | 0 | 30 | 4–28 | + | – | – | 29 | 15.5 | 78% |
| Ong | 36 | 0 | 12 | 17–32 | + | + | + | 12 | 33.3 | See text |
| Ramsey | 19 | 19 | 24 | 5–22 | + | + | + | 41 | 107.9 | See text |
| Hordvik | 10 | 0 | 20 | 5–32 | + | + | + | 13 | 78.0 | See text |

[a] PFT = pulmonary function tests; NR = not reported.
Adapted from Prober[101], by permission of Humana Press.

progression of lung disease in older patients with CF, little data exist describing the early pathophysiology of viral infection, bacterial colonization, nutrition and host immune response in the infant.

## EPIDEMIOLOGY OF NON-BACTERIAL PNEUMONIAS

Non-bacterial pneumonias are the most frequently encountered lower respiratory infections in paediatrics. The epidemiology of these respiratory infections consists primarily of RSV, parainfluenza viruses, influenza viruses and adenoviruses, and *Mycoplasma pneumoniae*. Because of the ease of transmission of these agents, spread through communities occurs rapidly and usually in well-defined epidemic patterns. Annual rates of childhood pneumonia show a general inverse relation with age, ranging from 40 per 1000 in children under age 5 years, to seven per 1000 in children aged 12–15 years[17]. The majority of studies demonstrate a male predominance in paediatric lower respiratory tract infections and increased rates in lower socioeconomic groups[17].

Viral infections are responsible for yearly epidemics of lower respiratory tract diseases in both normal and compromised hosts. RSV is now generally accepted as the most common agent in paediatric pneumonias. The incidence of lower respiratory tract involvement with primary infection with RSV is approximately 20–30%, although the rate of hospitalization of these children is much lower. Infants have the highest rates of hospitalization with RSV infection, ranging from one in 50, to one in 100[18]. Parainfluenza virus type 3 closely mimics RSV with respect to the amount of lower respiratory tract disease it produces. It is second only to RSV as a cause of pneumonia and bronchiolitis in infants. Between 10% and 50% of primary infections with parainfluenza virus type 3 affect the lower respiratory tract[19]. Parainfluenza virus types 1 and 2 generally occur in epidemics and usually cause laryngotracheobronchitis. Toddlers and preschool-aged children have the highest rates of hospitalization when parainfluenza viruses circulate in the community. Although not nearly as prevalent as RSV and parainfluenza, involvement of the lungs following infection with influenza A and B viruses occurs in 5–10% of children. It primarily accounts for hospitalization in preschool to school-aged children[20].

Although most children recover clinically from viral lower respiratory infections in a short period of time, histological and physiological changes in the lower airways may remain and take weeks to resolve[21,22]. Until recently, lung function abnormalities were not felt to persist into later childhood; however, a number of investigators are now reporting persistent airway abnormalities and reductions in arterial oxygenation 5–10 years following hospitalization for bronchiolitis[23–25]. In addition to these findings, a strong association between hospitalization for RSV bronchiolitis and asthma has been observed. Studies have reported recurrent wheezing episodes in 30–50% of hospitalized RSV infants[25–26]. These studies suggest that acute viral respiratory illnesses produce lower airway obstruction and may alter airway reactivity. The mechanism of airway obstruction is not well defined but existing information will be reviewed in the following section.

A brief review of the impact of lower respiratory viral infections on the airways is best undertaken by considering first the differences between lung physiology in children and adults. These differences are important because they may partially explain the greater morbidity observed with viral infections in infants and young children compared to adults. In addition, because a tremendous amount of alveolar growth occurs within the first three to four years of life, any insult to the lung during that period can potentially have a detrimental impact on lung growth and development.

The airways are established by the 17th week of gestation and subsequently grow principally by enlargement[27]. In contrast, the alveoli develop late in gestation and are incompletely formed at birth. New alveoli continue to develop in significant numbers for three to four years after birth, with growth continuing primarily by alveolar enlargement throughout childhood. During infancy the lungs have less elastic recoil and the chest wall is more compliant compared to adults[28]. This allows airway closure to occur at a higher lung volume in infants and children and accentuates gas trapping and ventilation–perfusion mismatch in diseases affecting the lower airways. Flow limitation in the airways is directly proportional to their cross-sectional area. Resistance is inversely proportional to the airway radius to the fourth power. Therefore small increases in the thickness of the airway wall, changes in luminal contents or increases in bronchial smooth muscle tone can drastically reduce airflow. For infants this problem is compounded because the peripheral airways account for a larger proportion of total airway resistance compared to adults, predisposing them to more severe symptoms with small airway obstruction[29]. Animal data suggest that the airway epithelium in young animals contains higher numbers of mucus-secreting cells and decreased mucociliary clearance, further increasing the risk for airway obstruction[30]. Lack of collateral ventilation, increased airway resistance and a greater number of mucus-secreting cells may all combine to predispose the infant to more severe disease following infection with respiratory viruses compared to older children and adults[28].

The higher incidence of lower respiratory tract disease seen in infants compared to older children is a not only physiological in nature but also a function of an immature and naive immune system. Both cell-mediated immunity and humoral immunity are altered during infancy[31]. Diminished neonatal T lymphocyte cytotoxic ability, decreased production of certain lymphokines and altered antibody production to certain antigens can all inhibit the lysis of virus-infected cells and elimination of the virus from the respiratory tract[32]. Antibacterial defences may be altered in infancy as manifested by decreased chemotaxis of neutrophils and blood monocytes, a diminished neutrophil storage pool and an altered ability of tissue macrophages to process antigen[33-35]. Most of these abnormalities resolve in the normal infant by one year of age; however, their importance in the early lung disease of infants with CF is unknown.

## MECHANISMS OF VIRAL-INDUCED LOWER AIRWAY OBSTRUCTION IN CHILDREN

There are three potential mechanisms for viral-induced lower airway obstruction: (1) increased thickness of the airway wall; (2) increased luminal content of secretions or cellular debris; and (3) airway smooth muscle contraction (Table 2)[36]. Increased thickness of the airway wall can result from vascular engorgement, cellular infiltration and mucosal oedema. Leukotriene B4 released from virally infected epithelial cells may initiate the inflammatory process[37]. Many cells have been implicated in the inflammatory process; however the neutrophil and eosinophil appear to be very prominent[38-40]. Once the inflammatory cascade begins, chemical mediators cause disruption of cellular junctions, increased endothelial permeability and attraction of more inflammatory cells[41,42]. These changes lead to oedema and airway obstruction.

**Table 2** Potential mechanisms in viral induced lower airway obstruction

| Increased thickness of the airway wall | Increased luminal content | Airway smooth muscle contraction |
|---|---|---|
| Vascular engorgement | Increased secretions | Autonomic nervous system dysfunction |
| Celular infiltration | Rheological changes in mucus | Chemical mediator release from recruited cells |
| Mucosal and submucosal edema | Epithelial sloughing | Impairment of epithelial-mediated muscle relaxation |
| | Impaired ciliokinesis | Altered activation characteristics of airway smooth muscle |
| | Cellular inflammation | |

Adapted from Smith et al.[36], by permission.

Viruses and viral immune complexes can enhance the inflammatory response by increasing chemotatic activity, activating oxidative and arachidonic pathways and facilitating mediator release[43-45]. One mechanism proposed for viral-induced inflammation is the degranulation of mast cells via cell-bound IgE. Increased levels of viral-specific IgE and histamine have been found in nasopharyngeal secretions of children hospitalized with RSV infection[46]. Elevated levels of serum IgE anti-RSV antibodies have also been associated with airway obstruction[47]. A reduction in suppressor T lymphocytes has been reported to correlate inversely with specific RSV IgE[48], suggesting a direct role of suppressor T lymphocytes in the regulation and/or production of RSV IgE antibodies. An imbalance of T suppressor to T helper cells may allow increased production of RSV IgE or IgE to other viral antigens and allergens. In a prospective study of hospitalized infants, Welliver found that the initial RSV IgE response positively correlated with recurrent wheezing episodes[47]. Similar data were observed with parainfluenza infection[49]. These studies suggest that RSV and other respiratory viruses may influence T lymphocyte function and in turn host response for the development and severity of airway obstruction.

Viral infections can alter granulocyte function and play a role in airway hyperreactivity[50-52]. Transient airway hyperresponsiveness can develop in normal individuals following a viral respiratory infection and may in part be mediated by the neutrophil[53,54]. Respiratory epithelial cells infected by respiratory viruses can release leukotriene B4, precipitating an influx of neutrophils[36]. Animal models of airway hyperreactivity induced by ozone or antigens require neutrophils[55,56]. Ozone-induced airway hyperreactivity in humans correlates with the number of neutrophils in bronchoalveolar lavage fluids[57]. If neutrophils are depleted in a similar ozone animal model, no increase in reactivity is observed[38]. Once activated, neutrophils can preferentially release leukotrienes C4 and D4, causing airway smooth muscle constriction[58]. In addition, leukotrienes C4 and D4 could indirectly modulate production of prostacyclin (exacerbations) and thromboxane A2 (bronchoconstrictor) via the cyclooxygenase pathway[59,60]. These pathways can facilitate the persistent heightened responsive state observed in individuals following viral respiratory infection.

Specific molecular mechanisms of virus-induced changes in cell-mediated immune responses are now receiving attention. Adhesion molecules are receptors located on cell membranes of vascular endothelium and respiratory epithelium, as well as antigen-presenting cells, which mediate leucocyte recruitment. The corresponding ligand for these adhesion molecules is located on circulating leucocytes. Cultured human airway epithelial cells are known to express adhesion molecules *in vitro* in response to viral pathogens and support increased adhesion by eosinophils and neutrophils[61-63]. By blocking ICAM-1 or its corresponding ligand Mac-1 with antibody, this response can be decreased. Grove et al. have demonstrated that ICAM-1 is the major receptor for human rhinovirus[64]. By binding to ICAM-1, rhinovirus could potentially block leucocyte attachment and alter or prevent leucocyte migration. Alternatively, rhinovirus attachment to ICAM-1 could stimulate the initial steps in antigen recognition for the T lymphocyte and proliferation of antigen-specific T cell clones. Thus, *in vitro* studies suggest that upregulation of adhesion molecules on vascular endothelium or airway epithelium following viral infection may be part of the mechanism by which leucocyte attachment and migration are initially mediated.

The second mechanism by which airway obstruction can occur following viral infection is by increased luminal contents. Injury to lining epithelial and mucus-secreting cells can alter mucociliary clearance by alterations in ciliokinesis, epithelial sloughing and changes in the consistency of the mucus itself[65–67]. Inflammatory cells can cause both an increase in the quantity of mucus and the viscosity and elasticity of the mucus produced. Leukotrienes C4 and D4 are potent stimulators of mucous secretions, as are macrophages and metabolites of arachidonic acid[68,69]. Cholinergic and $\alpha$-adrenergic stimulation of submucosal glands can also increase secretions[70]. A direct ciliotoxic effect is observed with viral infection and ciliary movement is further impaired by ciliated epithelial cell injury and destruction[66]. Altered fluid transport by cellular infection or disruption of cellular junctions can further alter the sol layer of respiratory secretions. Thus, altered mucociliary clearance by changes in the rheological properties of the mucus, destruction of the lining respiratory epithelial cells and direct ciliotoxic effects all lead to increased luminal contents and airway obstruction.

Finally airway obstruction mediated by bronchial smooth muscle contraction is another potential mechanism of virally induced airway disease. Airway smooth muscle contraction is mediated by both cholinergic and adrenergic stimulation of the autonomic nervous system. Both enhanced response to cholinergic stimulation or blunted $\beta$-adrenergic function have been reported in asthmatic patients. $\beta$-adrenergic receptors are located on both airway smooth muscle and granulocyte cell membranes[71]. $\beta$-adrenergic stimulation by agonists produces smooth muscle relaxation as well as inhibition of mediator release from granulocytes. Busse et al. have isolated leucocytes from subjects with asthma following upper respiratory infection, after incubation with rhinovirus or live-attenuated influenza vaccine[72–74]. These investigators found enhanced mediator release in all three circumstances, indicating diminished $\beta$-adrenergic function. In murine lung, virus-induced inhibition of $\beta$-adrenergic function is mediated by attenuation in adenylate cyclase activity rather than altered $\beta$-receptor cell numbers[75]. These studies suggest that respiratory virus infection decreases $\beta$-adrenergic regulation of granulocyte mediator release. Because catecholamines are important in inhibiting the leucocyte inflammatory response, alterations in $\beta$-adrenergic regulation could result in leucocytes with enhanced inflammatory potential, affecting mucus production, airway tone and reactivity.

Cholinergic stimulation results in bronchial smooth muscle constriction and is increased both during and following viral infection. Cholinergic-mediated bronchoconstriction can be mediated by both the afferent and efferent limb of the vagal reflex arc. There is evidence that both the afferent and efferent limbs of the cholinergic reflex may be affected following viral infection, altering airway tone. Bruckner et al. have demonstrated that electrical field stimulation of distal ends of the vagus nerve in virus infected, vagotomized guinea-pigs resulted in greater bronchoconstriction to histamine compared to uninfected controls[76]. This suggests greater sensitivity of the afferent limb of the vagus nerve following viral infection. Cholinergic M2 receptors are located on post-synaptic ganglia of pulmonary postsynaptic nerves. When stimulated they inhibit neural activity and produce bronchodilation. Fryer et al. have found that these M2 receptors are damaged following Sendai viral infection in a guinea-pig model and thereby enhance bronchoconstriction[77,78].

Airway hyperresponsiveness can be blocked with atropine and this has led to speculation that injury to the respiratory epithelium has a modulating effect on airway reactivity via the cholinergic pathway. Airway epithelial cells produce substances such as neutral endopeptidase and cyclooxygenase which modulate airway responsiveness and smooth muscle tone. Neutral endopeptidase is an enzyme which helps degrade substance P and other tachykinins, mediators that can cause bronchoconstriction and promote inflammation. Several studies using animal models have demonstrated diminished neutral endopeptidase activity, epithelial desquamation and greater hyperresponsiveness to substance P following viral infection[79–81]. It appears therefore that the airway epithelium is important in maintaining normal smooth muscle tone and if injured during respiratory virus infection can lead to a loss of several enzymes, including neutral endopeptidase and cyclooxygenase.

## BACTERIAL AND VIRAL INTERACTION IN CYSTIC FIBROSIS

The exact interaction between respiratory virus infection and bacterial colonization in children with CF is unclear. Early respiratory findings in infants with CF include chronic cough, pneumonia and wheezing. Two studies have reported prolonged bronchiolitis-like syndromes in CF infants[82,83]. Both involved CF infants under six months of age. These infants required aggressive respiratory therapy including mechanical ventilation in some instances. Abman et al.[12] were the first to report the effects of specific virus infections in CF children less than three years of age. In a prospective study they identified viral pathogens in 12 of 30 hospitalizations among CF children hospitalized for respiratory difficulties. Seven of the 12 isolates were RSV. CF children infected with RSV experienced prolonged hospitalizations, three of seven required mechanical ventilation and 75% were discharged home with supplemental oxygen. When evaluated longitudinally at a mean of 28 months following hospitalization, CF children hospitalized with RSV had more chronic respiratory symptoms and worse radiograph scores than CF children who did not require hospitalization for RSV. In our study assessing the effects of respiratory viral infection in CF infants, we also found that RSV resulted in hospitalization in about one-half of the CF infants infected during a six-month respiratory viral season[84,85]. Although severe sequelae consisting of prolonged hospitalization and supplemental oxygen were not observed in our study, lower pulmonary function was noted in the RSV-infected CF infants. These studies suggest that viral respiratory infection, especially RSV, has a significant and detrimental impact on the early respiratory course of CF infants.

*Staph. aureus* is the most common bacterial organism isolated in CF infants and children and usually precedes *Ps. aeruginosa* colonization[28]. *Staph. aureus* colonization may increase adherence of *Ps. aeruginosa* by contributing to airway inflammation, neutrophil activation and epithelial cell injury. Increased bacterial adherence to pharyngeal cells has been reported during viral infections. Fainstein et al.[86] measured bacterial adherence to pharyngeal cells from patients with naturally acquired respiratory viral infection and experimentally infected volunteers with live attenuated influenza vaccine. Increased adherence was found for *Staph. aureus*, *Haemophilus influenzae* and *Streptococcus pneumoniae*. Similar findings have been reported following viral respiratory infection in normal adults and patients with chronic bronchitis[87,88]. *Ps. aeruginosa* does not bind to normal respiratory epithelium unless the cell membrane is somehow injured. Increased adherence of *Ps. aeruginosa* to epithelial cells is observed if cells are pretreated with mild acid, trypsin or influenza virus[89]. Niedrerman et al. have further shown that *Ps. aeruginosa* adherence to tracheal cells correlated with increased elastase levels in sputum—a condition commonly found with inflamed airways in CF[90]. Studies have suggested that actual receptor for *Ps. aeruginosa* is *N*-acetylneuraminic acid[89]. Johansen and Høiby retrospectively reviewed the onset of chronic colonization with *Ps. aeruginosa* in 300 CF patients from 1965 to 1990[91]. Despite changes in treatment and antibiotics over the 25-year period, 68% of their patients developed chronic colonization with *Ps. aeruginosa* during the winter months. This prompted the investigators to suggest that 'respiratory viral infection paves the way for *Ps. aeruginosa* infection'.

The role of nutrition and viral infection in CF children remains unclear. Secretory IgA can be diminished in non-CF malnourished subjects and is generally the first line of defence against respiratory viruses[92]. Malnutrition in non-CF individuals affects cellular immune function but not humoral immunity or phagocytes[92]. T lymphocyte depletion has been noted in malnourished hosts and impaired macrophage function has been reported with influenza virus infection. Investigators have suggested that the defect in T lymphocytes is secondary to a lack of T cell maturation[92]. Animal studies using underfed and fasted animals have reported that these animals are surprisingly more resistant to infection compared to normal animals[93–95]. Yet studies by Woodruff et al. using protein calorie malnutrition in mice demonstrated increased severity of infection with Coxsackie virus[96,97]. The severity of infection in mice correlated with the degree of malnutrition. If refed a balanced diet the mice were protected from further infections and deterioration.

Tupasi et al. assessed the effects of malnutrition with respiratory viral infection in Filipino children[98]. Malnutrition was measured by weight-for-age *Z* scores. Both acute upper and lower respiratory tract viral disease was associated with greater morbidity and mortality in malnourished children under five years of age. These differences remained significant when gender, age, crowded living conditions and parental smoking were accounted for. CF infants with protein calorie deficiency are reported to have a greater risk for severe respiratory disease compared to their well-nourished counterparts. Abman et al. reported that CF infants with early low albumin levels identified by newborn screening experienced increased rates of hospitalization for respiratory distress, a persistent need for supplemental oxygen and maintained a chronic cough[99,100]. In our prospective study of CF infants, viral lower respiratory tract infection occurred predominantly in infants with lower weight-for-height percentiles[84,85]. Both infection with RSV and lower weight-for-height percentiles were associated with worse pulmonary function at the conclusion of the study. The incidence of viral infection in our CF infants was less than normal controls; however, the severity of viral disease and involvement of the lower respiratory tract were more pronounced in the CF group.

## SUMMARY

In summary, normal airway clearance is altered in CF with respiratory secretions that are highly viscous. These abnormalities exist because of the dysfunctional CF transmembrane regulator protein located in respiratory epithelial and mucous cells of the airway. Although the lungs are normal at birth, airway plugging, inflammation and increased bronchial tone begin to appear at an early age. The pathophysiological mechanisms by which viral infections, bacterial colonization, and immune and non-immune-mediated inflammatory responses interrelate remain ill defined. It would seem that viral respiratory infection would likely play an important role in the early injury of the airway in CF because of the high rates of viral infection in children during the first five years of life. How these viral infections lead to colonization with *Staph. aureus* and subsequently *Ps. aeruginosa* remains undefined. Certainly rapid identification of respiratory viral infection in children of all ages with CF should impact on clinical care. Initiation of antiviral therapy, use of vaccines, aggressive antimicrobial therapy and anti-inflammatory agents for airway hyperreactivity should all be considered.

At a time when we are rapidly approaching gene therapy trials using adenoviral vectors, liposomes and direct inoculation of gene vectors into the airway, it will be crucial for us as clinicians to assist families in maintaining their children in an optimal state of health. By understanding the multiple variables that influence lung growth and development in CF, we can improve the level of care they receive until the full benefits of gene therapy can be realized.

## REFERENCES


1 Beaudry PH, Marks MI, McDougall D, et al. Is anti-*Pseudomonas* therapy warranted in acute respiratory exacerbation in children with cystic fibrosis? *J Pediatr* 1980; **97**: 144–7.

2 Mearns MB. Natural history of pulmonary infection in cystic fibrosis. In: *Perspectives in Cystic Fibrosis* (ed JM Sturgess), Canadian Cystic Fibrosis Foundation, Toronto, pp 325–35.

3 Abman SH, Ogle JW, Harbeck RJ, et al. Early bacteriologic, immunologic, and clinical courses of young infants with cystic fibrosis identified by neonatal screening. *J Pediatr* 1991; **119**: 211–17.

4 Smith AL, Ramsey B, Redding G, et al. Endobronchial infection in cystic fibrosis. *Acta Paediatr Scand Suppl* 1989; **363**: 31–6.

5 Accurso FJ, Sokol RJ, Hammond KB, Abman SH. Early respiratory course in infants with cystic fibrosis: relevance to newborn screening. *Pediatr Pulmonol* 1991; **7**: 42–5. (Suppl).

6 Rosenfeld MA, Yoshimura K, Trapnell BC, et al. In vivo transfer of the human cystic fibrosis transmembrane conductance regulator gene to the airway epithelium. *Cell* 1992; **68**: 143–55.

7 Wright PF, Khaw KT, Oxman MN, Shwachman H. Evaluation of the safety of amantadine-HCl and the role of respiratory viral infections in children with cystic fibrosis. *J Infect Dis* 1976; **134**: 144–9.

8 Petersen NT, Høiby N, Mordhorst CH, et al. Respiratory infections in cystic fibrosis patients caused by virus, chlamydia and mycoplasma: possible synergism with *Pseudomonas aeruginosa*. *Acta Paediat Scand* 1981; **70**: 623–8.

9 Wang EE, Prober CG, Manson B, et al. Association of respiratory viral infections with pulmonary deterioration in patients with cystic fibrosis. *N Engl J Med* 1984; **311**: 1653–8.

10 Efthimiou J, Hodson ME, Taylor P, et al. Importance of viruses and *Legionella pneumophila* in respiratory exacerbations of young adults with cystic fibrosis. *Thorax* 1984; **39**: 150–4.
11 Stroobant J. Viral infection in cystic fibrosis. *J R Soc Med* 1986; **79**: 19–22.
12 Abman SH, Ogle JW, Butler SN, et al. Role of respiratory syncytial virus in early hospitalizations for respiratory distress of young infants with cystic fibrosis. *J Pediatr* 1988; **113**: 826–30.
13 Przyklenk B, Bauernfeind A, Bertele RM, et al. Viral infections of the respiratory tract in patients with cystic fibrosis. *Serodiagn Immunother Infect Dis* 1988; **2**: 217–25.
14 Ong EL, Ellis ME, Webb AK, et al. Infective respiratory exacerbations in young adults with cystic fibrosis: role of viruses and atypical microorganisms. *Thorax*, 1989; **44**: 739–42.
15 Ramsey BW, Gore EJ, Smith AL, et al. The effect of respiratory viral infections on patients with cystic fibrosis. *Am J Dis Child* 1989; **143**: 662–8.
16 Hordvik NL, Konig P, Hamory B, et al. Effects of acute viral respiratory tract infections in patients with cystic fibrosis. *Pediatr Pulmonol* 1989; **7**: 217–22.
17 Boyer KM, Cherry JD. Nonbacterial pneumonia. In; *Textbook of Pediatric Infectious Diseases*, eds. Feigin RD, Cherry JD, 2nd edn, Vol 1. Saunders, Philadelphia, 1987, pp 288–300.
18 Hall CB. Respiratory syncytial virus. In; *Textbook of Pediatric Infectious Diseases*, eds. Feigin RD, Cherry JD, 2nd edn, Vol 2. Saunders, Philadelphia, 1987, pp 1653–75.
19 Hall CB. Parainfluenza viruses. In: *Textbook of Pediatric Infectious Diseases*, eds. Feigin RD, Cherry JD, 2nd edn, Vol 2. Saunders, Philadelphia, 1987; pp 1632–45.
20 Zahradnik JM, Cherry JD: Influenza viruses. In: *Textbook of Pediatric Infectious Diseases*, eds. Feigin RD, Cherry JD, 2nd edn, Vol 2. Saunders, Philadelphia, 1987, 1709–28.
21 Reid L. Influence of the pattern of structural growth of lung on susceptibility to specific infectious diseases in infants and children. *Pediatr Res* 1977; **11**: 210–15.
22 Hiatt P, Sellers C, Taber L. Longitudinal pulmonary function (PF) in infants following hospitalization for RSV bronchiolitis. *Am Rev Respir Dis* 1990; **141**: A688.
23 Kattan M, Keens TG, Lapierre J, et al. Pulmonary function abnormalities in symptom free children after bronchiolitis. *Pediatrics* 1977; **59**: 683.
24 Pullan CR, Hey EN. Wheezing, asthma, and pulmonary dysfunction 10 years after infection with respiratory syncytial virus in infancy. *Br Med J* 1982; **284**: 1665.
25 Gurwitz D, Mindorff C, Levison H. Increased incidence of bronchial reactivity in children with a history of bronchiolitis. *J Pediatr* 1981; **98**: 551.
26 Rooney JC, Williams HE. The relationship between proven viral bronchiolitis and subsequent wheezing. *J Pediatr* 1971; **79**; 744.
27 Bucher U, Reid L. Development of the intrasegmental bronchial tree: the pattern of branching and development of cartilage at various stages of intrauterine life. *Thorax* 1961; **16**: 207–18.
28 Rosenfeld M, Ramsey B. Evolution of airway, microbiology in the infant with cystic fibrosis: role of nonpseudomonal and pseudomonal pathogens. *Semin Respir Infect* 1992; **7**; 158–67.
29 Hogg JC, Williams J, Richardson JB, et al. Age as a factor in the distribution of

lower-airway conductance and in the pathogenic anatomy of obstructive lung disease. *N Engl J Med* 1970; **282**: 1283–7.
30 Whaley SL, Muggenberg BA, Seiler FA, et al. Effect of ageing on tracheal mucociliary clearance in beagle dogs. *J Appl Physiol* 1987; **62**: 1331–4.
31 Wilson CW. Developmental immunology and role of host defenses in neonatal susceptibility. In *Infectious Diseases of the Fetus and Newborn Infant* (eds JS Remington, JO Klein), Saunders, Philadelphia, 1990, pp 17–68.
32 Sullender WM, Miller JL, Yasukawa LL, et al. Humoral and cell-mediated immunity in neonates with herpes simplex virus infection. *J Infect Dis* 1987; **155**: 28–37.
33 Klein RB, Fischer TJ, Gerd SE, et al. Decreased mononuclear and polymorphonuclear chemotaxis in human newborns, infants and young children. *Pediatrics* 1977; **60**: 467–72.
34 Alenghat E, Esterley JR. Alveolar macrophages in perinatal infants. *Pediatrics* 1984; **74**: 221–4
35 Christensen RD, Rothstein G. Exhaustion of mature marrow neutrophils in neonates with sepsis. *J Pediatr* 1980; **96**: 316–18.
36 Smith JJ, Lemen RJ, Taussig LM. Mechanisms of viral-induced lower airway obstruction. *Pediatr Infect Dis* 1987; **6**: 837–42.
37 Holtzman MJ, Aizawa H, Nadel JA, et al. Selective generation of leukotriene $B_4$ by tracheal epithelial cells from dogs. *Biochem Biophys Res Commun* 1983; **114**: 1071–6.
38 O'Byrne PM, Walters H, Gold BD, et al. Neutrophil depletion inhibits airway hyperresponsiveness induced by ozone exposure. *Am Rev Respir Dis* 1984; **130**: 214–19.
39 Smith LW, Greenberger PA, Patterson R, et al. The effect of inhaled leukotriene $D_4$ in humans. *Am Rev Respir Dis* 1985; **131**: 368–72.
40 O'Byrne PM, Walters EH, Aizawa H, et al. Indomethacin inhibits the airway hyperresponsiveness but not the neutrophil influx induced by ozone in dogs. *Am Rev Respir Dis* 1984; **130**: 220–4.
41 Drazen J, Austen KF, Lewis RA, et al. Comparative airway and vascular activities of leukotrienes C-1 and D *in vivo* and *in vitro*. *Pro Natl Acad Sci USA* 1980; **77**: 4354–8.
42 Al-Bazzaz FJ, Yadava VP, Westenfelder C. Modification of Na and Cl transport in canine tracheal mucosa by prostaglandins. *Am J Physiol* 1981; **240**: F101–5.
43 Ida S, Hooks JJ, Siraganian RP, et al. Enhancement of IgE-mediated histamine release from human basophils by viruses: role of interferon. *J Exp Med* 1977; **145**: 892–906.
44 Roberts NJ Jr. Different effects of influenza virus, respiratory syncytial virus, and Sendai virus on human lymphocytes and macrophages. *Infect Immun* 1982; **35**: 1142–6.
45 Faden H, Kaul TN, Ogra P. Activation of oxidative and arachidonic acid complexes: possible role in disease. *J Infect Dis* 1983; **148**: 110–16.
46 Welliver RC, Wong DT, Sun M, et al. The development of respiratory syncytial virus-specific IgE and the release of histamine in nasopharyngeal secretions after infections. *N Engl J Med* 1981; **305**: 841–6.
47 Welliver RC, Sun M, Rinaldo D, et al. Predictive value of respiratory syncytial virus-specific IgE responses for recurrent wheezing following bronchiolitis. *J Pediatr* 1986; **109**: 776.
48 Welliver RC, Kaul TN, Sun M, et al. Defective regulation of immune responses in respiratory syncytial virus infection. *J Immunol* 1984; **133**: 1925–30.

49 Welliver RC, Wong DT, Middleton E Jr, et al. Role of parainfluenza virus-specific IgE in pathogenesis of croup and wheezing subsequent to infection. *J Pediatr* 1979; **94**: 370.

50 Busse WW, Anderson CL, Dick EC. Reduced granulocyte response to isoproterenol, histamine, prostaglandin E after incubation with rhinovirus 16. *Am Rev Respir Dis* 1980; **122**: 641.

51 Busse WW, Swenson CA, Borden EC, et al. The effect of influenza A virus on leukocyte histamine release. *J Allergy Clin Immunol* 1983; **71**: 382.

52 Busse WV, Vrtis RF, Steiner R, et al. In vitro incubation with influenza virus primes human polymorphonuclear leukocyte generation of superoxide. *Am J Respir Cell Mol Biol* 1991; **4**: 347.

53 Empey DW, Laitinen LA, Jacobs L, et al. Mechanisms of bronchial hyperreactivity in normal subjects after upper respiratory tract infection. *Am Rev Respir Dis* 1976; **113**: 131–9.

54 Aquilina AT, Hall WJ, Douglas RG Jr, et al. Airway reactivity in subjects with viral upper respiratory tract infection: the effects of exercise and cold air. *Am Rev Respir Dis* 1980; **122**: 3–10.

55 Chung KF, Aizawa H, Leikauf GD, et al. Airway hyperresponsiveness induced by platelet-activating factor: role of thromboxane generation. *J Pharmacol Exp Ther* 1986; **236**: 580–4.

56 O'Byrne PM, Leikauf GD, Aizawa H, et al. Leukotre $B_4$ induces airway hyperresponsiveness in dogs. *J Appl Physiol* 1985; **59**: 1941–6.

57 Seltzer J, Geoffroy B, Stulbarg M, et al. Association between airway inflammation and changes in bronchial reactivity induced by ozone exposure in human subjects. *Am Rev Respir Dis* 1984; **129**: A262.

58 Weichman BM, Muccitelli RM, Osborn RR, et al. *In vitro* and *in vivo* mechanisms of leukotriene-mediated bronchoconstriction in the guinea pig. *J Pharmacol Exp Ther* 1982; **222**: 202–8.

59 Omini C. Folco GC, Vigano T, et al. Leukotriene-$C_4$, induces generation of $PGI_2$ and $TXA_2$ in guinea pig *in vivo*. *Pharmacol Res Commun* 1981; **13**: 633–40.

60 Dahlen SE, Hedqvist P, Westlund P, et al. Mechanisms of leukotriene-induced contractions of guinea pig airways: leukotriene $C_4$ has a potent direct action whereas leukotriene $B_4$ acts indirectly. *Acta Physiol Scand* 1983; **118**: 393–403.

61 Stark JM, Tosi MF. Use of a microtiter assay to demonstrate enhanced neutrophil adhesion to human airway epithelial cells. *Am Rev Respir Dis* 1991; **143**: A43.

62 Stark JM, Smith CW, Gruenert DC, et al. Neutrophil adhesion to parainfluenza virus-infected human airway epithelial cells: possible contributions of ICAM-1 dependent and ICAM-1 independent mechanisms. *Chest* 1992; **101**: 405.

63 Tosi MF, Stark, JM, Hamedani A, et al. Neutrophil adhesion to human airway epithelium: role of epithelial ICAM-1 in cells infected with respiratory viruses or treated with IL-1 or TNF. *Pediatr Pulmonol Suppl* 1991; **6**: 301.

64 Greve JM, Davis G, Meyer AM, et al. The major human rhinovirus receptor is ICAM-1. *Cell* 1989; **56**: 839.

65 Lourenco RV, Stanley ED, Gatmaitan B, et al. Abnormal deposition and clearance of inhaled particles during upper respiratory viral infections. *J Clin Invest* 1971; **50**: 62A.

66 Carson JL, Collier AM, Hu SS. Acquired ciliary defects in nasal epithelium with acute viral respiratory infections. *N Engl J Med* 1985; **312**: 463–8.

67 Charman J, Reid L. Sputum viscosity in chronic bronchitis, bronchiectasis, asthma and cystic fibrosis. *Biorheology* 1972; **9**: 185–99.

68 Coles SJ, Neill KH, Reid LM, et al. Effects of leukotrienes $C_4$ and $D_4$ on glycoprotein and lysozyme secretion by human bronchial mucosa. *Prostaglandins* 1983; **25**: 155–70.
69 Marom Z, Shelhamer JH Kaliner M. Human monocyte-derived mucus secretagogue. *J Clin Invest* 1985; **75**; 191–8.
70 Basebaum CB, Ueki I, Brezina J, et al. Tracheal submucosal gland serous cells stimulated *in vitro* with adrenergic and cholinergic agonists: a morphometric study. *Cell Tissue Res* 1981; **220**: 481–98.
71 Szentivanyi A. The beta-adrenergic theory of atopic abnormality in asthma. *J Allergy* 1968; **42**: 203.
72 Busse WW. Decreased granulocyte response to isoproterenol in asthma during upper respiratory infections. *Am Rev Respir Dis* 1977; **115**: 783.
73 Busse WW, Anderson CL, Dick EC. Reduced granulocyte response to isoproterenol, histamine, prostaglandin E, after in vitro incubation with rhinovirus 16. *Am Rev Respir Dis* 1980; **122**: 641.
74 Busse WW, Cooper W, Warshauer DM, et al. Impairment of isoproterenol, $H_2$ histamine, prostaglandin E, response of human granulocytes after incubation in vitro with live influenza vaccines. *Am Rev Respir Dis* 1979; **119**: 561.
75 Scarpace PJ, Bender BS. Viral pneumonia attenuates adenylate cyclase but not $\beta$-adrenergic receptors in murine lung. *Am Rev Respir Dis* 1989; **67**: 1504.
76 Buckner CK, Songsiriderj V, Dick EC, et al. In vivo and in vitro studies on the use of the guinea pig as a model for virus-provoked airway hyperreactivity. *Am Rev Respir Dis* 1985; **132**: 305.
77 Fryer AD, Jacoby DB. Parainfluenza virus infection damages inhibitory $M_2$ muscarinic receptors on pulmonary parasympathetic nerves in the guinea pig. *Br J Pharmacol* 1991; **102**: 267.
78 Fryer AD, El-Fakahany EE, Jacoby DB. Parainfluenza virus type 1 reduces the affinity of agonists for muscarinic receptors in guinea pig lung and heart. *Eur J Pharmacol* 1990; **181**: 51.
79 Drusser DJ, Jacoby DB, Djokic TD, et al. Virus induces airway hyperresponsiveness to tachykinins: role of neutral endopeptidase. *J Appl Physiol* 1989; **67**: 1504.
80 Jacoby DB, Tamaoki J, Borson DB, et al. Influenza infection causes airway hyperresponsiveness by decreasing enkephalinase. *J Appl Physiol* 1988; **64**: 2653.
81 Saban R, Dick EC, Fishleder RI, et al. Enhancement by parainfluenza 3 infection of contractile responses to substance P and capsaicin in airway smooth muscle from the guinea pig. *Am Rev Respir Dis* 1987; **136**: 586.
82 Lloyd-Still JD, Khaw KT, Shwachman H. Severe respiratory disease in infants with cystic fibrosis. *Pediatrics* 1974; **53**: 678–82.
83 Garland JS, Chan YM, Kelly KJ, Rice TB. Outcome of infants with cystic fibrosis requiring mechanical ventilation for respiratory failure. *Chest* 1989; **96**: 136–8.
84 Hiatt PW, Taber L, Raboud S, Treece D. Respiratory viral infection and pulmonary function in infants with cystic fibrosis. *Am Rev Respir Dis* 1992; **145**: 115A.
85 Hiatt PW, Piedra P, Raboudi S, Treece D. Respiratory viral infection in infants with cystic fibrosis. *Am Rev Respir Dis* 1993; **147**; A464.
86 Fainstein V, Musher DM, Cate TR. Bacterial adherences to pharyngeal cells during viral infection. *J Infect Dis* 1980; **141**: 172–6.
87 Ramirez-Ronda CH, Fuxench-Lopez Z, Nevarez M. Increased pharyngeal bacterial colonization during viral illness. *Arch Intern Med* 1981; **114**: 599–603.
88 Smith CB, Golden C, Kaluber MR, Kanner R, Renzetti A. Interactions between viruses and bacteria in patients with chronic bronchitis. *J Infect Dis* 1976; **134**: 552–61.

89 Fick RB, Sonoda F, Hornick DB. Emergence and persistence of *Pseudomonas aeruginosa* in the cystic fibrosis airway. *Semin Respir Infect* 1992; **7**: 168–78.
90 Niederman MS, Merrill WW, Feranti RD, et al. Nutrition status and bacterial binding in lower respiratory tract in patient with chronic tracheostomy. *Ann Intern Med* 1984; **100**: 795–800.
91 Johansen HK, Høiby N. Seasonal onset of initial colonisation and chronic infection with *Pseudomonas aeruginosa* in patients with cystic fibrosis in Denmark. *Thorax* 1992; **47**: 109–11.
92 Boyer KM, Cherry JD. Interaction of infection and nutrition. In: *Textbook of Pediatric Infectious Diseases*, 2nd edn, Vol 2. Saunders, Philadelphia, 1987, pp 17–27.
93 Rasmussen, AF Jr, Waisman HA, Elvehjem CA, et al. Influence of the level of thiamine intake of the susceptibility of mice to poliomyelitis virus. *J Infect Dis* 1944; **74**: 41–7.
94 Sprunt DH. Effect of undernourishment on the susceptibility of rabbit to infection with vaccinia. *J Exp Med* 1942; **75**: 297–304.
95 Squibb RL, Grun J. Effect of nutritional status on resistance to infection in the avian species. *Fed Proc* 1966; **25**: 1695–700.
96 Woodruff JF. The influence of quantitated post-weaning undernutrition on Coxsackie virus B3 infection of adult mice. II. Alteration of host defense mechanisms. *J Infect Dis* 1970; **121**: 164–81.
97 Woodruff JF, Kilbourne ED. The influence of quantitated post-weaning undernutrition on Coxsackie virus B3 infection of adult mice. I. Viral persistence and increased severity of lesions. *J Infect Dis* 1970; **121**: 137–63.
98 Tupasi TE, Mangubat NV, Sunico MES, et al. Malnutrition and acute respiratory tract infections in Filipino children. *Rev Infect Dis* 1990; **12**: S1047–54.
99 Abman SH, Reardon MC, Accurso FJ, et al. Hypoalbuminemia at diagnosis as a marker for severe respiratory course infants with cystic fibrosis identified by newborn screening. *J Pediatr* 1985; **107**; 933–5.
100 Abman SH, Accurso FJ, Sokol RJ. Hypoalbuminemia in young infants with cystic fibrosis. *J Pediatr* 1990; **116**: 841–2 (letter).
101 Prober CG. The impact of respiratory viral infections in patients with cystic fibrosis. In: *Clinical Reviews in Allergy, Vol 9: Cystic Fibrosis* (ed ME Gershwin) Humana, Totowa NJ, 1991, pp 87–102.

Chapter Twelve

# Energy Requirements in Cystic Fibrosis

John A. Dodge and Angela M. O'Rawe
*Queen's University of Belfast, Nuffield Department of Child Health, Belfast, UK*

## INTRODUCTION

Cystic fibrosis (CF) is frequently accompanied by refractory malnutrition. The onset of nutritional compromise is as variable as its severity and reflects an imbalance between energy intake and output. Although a greater proportion of the increased energy requirement in most patients may be explained by the increased work of breathing consequent upon lung damage, the effect of infection and persisting maldigestion and/or malabsorption, other influencing factors have been suggested and will be considered in this review.

Adverse effects of CF on growth and nutrition have been recorded since its earliest descriptions. Were the evidence for energy imbalance in CF patients and the significance of the resultant deficit in body mass in any doubt, the nutritional management of CF patients would have ceased long ago to be a central issue in patient care. Deficits in body composition are identified even in presymptomatic infants[1]. The degree of underweight correlates inversely with survival[2] and nutritional status has been shown to influence the course of pulmonary disease[3].

*Cystic Fibrosis—Current Topics, Volume 2.* Edited by J. A. Dodge, D. J. H. Brock and J. H. Widdicombe

In recent years, programmes of nutritional intervention have been devised based on calculated nutrient losses and 'precise' estimates of energy requirements both in the resting and physically active state, from which prescriptions of energy intake for the individual may be derived. Nevertheless, modern CF management, particularly the advances in pulmonary and nutritional care which aim to improve lung function and longevity, simply postpone the inevitable decline, and nutrient imbalance eventually supervenes. Digestibility of macronutrients often remains suboptimal, notwithstanding improved microsphere preparations of pancreatic enzymes. The evolving natural history of CF as it becomes increasingly a condition of adulthood provides a further source of variation, and most new clinical observations in CF are the result of increased longevity and iatrogenic complications. The clinical implications of genetic heterogeneity also continue to be defined. A comprehensive understanding of the molecular defect in cells expressing a CF mutation will ultimately provide the rationale for full correction of the biochemical and nutritional manifestations of the disease in the patient.

## THE ONSET OF NUTRITIONAL COMPROMISE

Nutrient and energy imbalance may begin early in the course of the disease, even before birth. Several groups have reported a mean birth weight in CF infants approximately 0.5 SD below the population mean[4,5]. Important early nutritional deficits have been documented following neonatal screening[1], with subclinical nutritional disturbances indicating an energy deficit prior to the onset of symptoms. Inadequate accretion of total body potassium and thus body cell mass (BCM) has been shown in some presymptomatic screened infants[6]. There is also evidence that early deficits in body cell mass are largely correctable with supplementation. This has important implications for the outcome and management in the early phases of CF. Deficits in serum vitamins A and E, and low serum albumin levels, have also been identified in CF infants[7] in whom the clinical syndrome of protein energy malnutrition may occur in up to 5%[8].

Subsequent growth depends on the interaction of multiple factors, which include severity of pulmonary disease, frequency of respiratory infections, degree of malabsorption and maldigestion and the extent to which treatment modifies these factors. Final heights and weights are greater in those who have been relatively free of respiratory symptoms, and there is marked stunting of growth and wasting in those with a long history of lung disease in childhood[9]. Survival is worse in patients markedly underweight for their height, and this parameter depends more on respiratory than digestive disease[2]. Despite this, growth retardation in CF may be largely preventable, and CF and healthy control subjects have been shown to have similar growth potential[60]. More recent reports, however, suggest a more complex phenotype, with different growth potential in CF related to genes at specific loci close to the CF gene[55,59].

Thirty years ago less than 10% of affected children were above the 25th centile for weight and height, but nowadays steady increases in both weight and height can be expected in the first 10 years of life (although the medians run roughly along the 25th centile)[61]. Normal growth and weight velocity are now possible achievements, but gastrointestinal problems occur in most patients with CF and produce significant morbidity. Malabsorption is largely attributable to pancreatic insufficiency, but despite improved pancreatic microsphere supplements which enable up to 90% fat absorption, the response is highly variable[39]. Growth retardation of affected children and wasting of CF adults remain a clinical problem.

The number of CF children showing significant growth retardation appears to vary widely between centres, from 10% to 40%[10], which may be partly explained by differences in policies for nutritional supplementation. The conclusions from studies of supplementary nutrition, as with other clinical trials in CF, have to date been based on results from a genetically heterogeneous group, which may make it more difficult to detect significant differences[11].

Ideally, the child with CF adhering to dietary guidelines should be growing at a normal velocity along his or her own genetically determined growth centiles, while CF adults should be maintaining their body weight. The effect of active nutritional intervention and improved chemotherapy is to postpone the fall-off in growth to later adolescence, with a more marked decline in weight than height[61]. Later faltering of growth or weight loss is generally

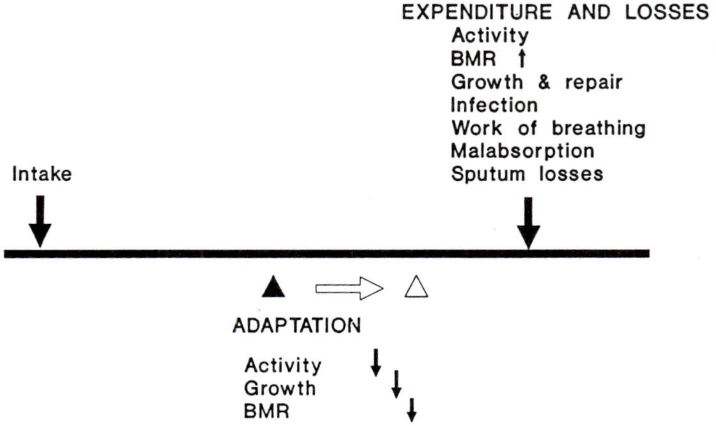


**Figure 1** Energy balance in cystic fibrosis

associated with deteriorating pulmonary disease, although the relationship between various contributory factors is complex. Clinical and other factors determining energy balance in CF are indicated in Figure 1.

## EXPENDITURE AND LOSSES

### THE ENERGY DEFICIT IN CYSTIC FIBROSIS

To determine the nature of the *energy deficit*, and to provide an important reference for comparison of rates of energy expenditure among individuals, accurate measurements of body composition *in vivo* are necessary. Animal studies of body composition have shown that the percentage of fat is the most variable component, followed by water content; protein and mineral content change very little, and carbohydrate and glucogen stores are the most constant[12]. Such measurements enable the establishment of an optimal feeding regimen to ensure appropriate reconstitution of body fat and lean body mass (LBM). Autopsy studies on infants dying of CF show findings similar to those of malnourished infants dying from other causes, infants dying from meconium ileus showing more profound changes than the others[13].

Comparison of methods used to measure body composition *in vivo* in CF has demonstrated the inappropriateness of prediction equations for body fat from skinfold thickness[14]. The use of either total body potassium measurements or of the deuterium dilution method have been preferred[15]. Widespread use of these methods is limited either by cost or availability; however, reported studies[1,6] demonstrate a decrease in both body fat and LBM. Protein/energy supplementation in CF patients has been shown to produce catch-up weight gain with evidence of accretion of LBM in the process[16]

The calculation of *energy requirement* is based on the principle of meeting the demands of expenditure and losses (Figure 1). The relative importance of the various potential influences on CF energy balance (including pulmonary and gastrointestinal factors, cellular events, bacterial pathogens and inflammatory mediators) is unclear. Wherever possible energy expenditure data should be used in preference to using intake data to estimate energy needs. The general practice of estimating energy intake from an exact knowledge of the quantity and type of food eaten, using food tables, is of limited accuracy[17] because it assumes fixed levels of digestibility for foods, and it is subject to significant under-reporting of dietary intake.

### TOTAL ENERGY EXPENDITURE

In tailoring appropriate nutrition in CF patients, a reliable estimate of total energy expenditure (TEE) is important. TEE includes the energy cost of basal metabolism (which comprises the largest part), physical activity, thermogenesis and the cost of synthesizing new tissue. In order to reliably estimate TEE of individuals it is necessary to have a measurement of basal metabolic rate (BMR), and a detailed description of time use and activity. Recommended equations for estimating BMR are those of Schofield et al. [18] (incorporating the largest and widest data group); however, these are subject to a wide error margin in a healthy population and cannot be extrapolated to an unwell population. BMR is measured by indirect respirometry and is expressed in terms of body mass and composition.

Until recently, techniques to directly measure TEE in the free-living subject have been either cost prohibitive or of poor predictive value. Simultaneous measurement of free-living energy expenditure by the doubly labelled water (DLW) method and heart rate (HR) monitoring in adults and children have shown a good level of agreement, and the latter provides a technique demonstrating good predictive power for group estimates of TEE[19]. Both these methods have been used to assess TEE in CF patients[20,21].

## The doubly labelled water method

The (DLW) method is the most widely accepted method for accurate determination of TEE in free-living subjects. It does not, however, give day-to-day variations in activity and it is expensive. The method assesses the rate of production of carbon dioxide by measuring the differential disappearance of the stable isotopes deuterium and $^{18}O_2$ after subjects have been given an oral loading dose of labelled water[22]. TEE is calculated from carbon dioxide production using classic respirometry formulae in which turnover is estimated from individually determined values for sedentary energy expenditure (EE), calculated as the average EE during lying, sitting and standing at rest. In four CF patients studied by DLW and HR methods, we found good agreement (Table 1). All were monitored for seven days, which took adequate account of the intra-individual and day-to-day variability in TEE. In view of the high coefficient of variation (CV) an increased number of days would be more representative of habitual daily energy expenditure.

**Table 1** Comparative values for mean TEE by the DLW and HR methods (MJ/day)

| Patient No. | Age (years) | DLW TEE (MJ/day) | HRTEE (MJ/day) | % Difference (HR − DLW) |
|---|---|---|---|---|
| 1 | 17 | 13.9 | 13 (CV = 13.5%) | −7.0 |
| 2 | 13 | 15.2 | 15.3 (CV = 20.1%) | +0.07 |
| 3 | 10 | 7.1 | 7.6 (CV = 13.6%) | +7.2 |
| 4 | 19 | 9.8 | 10.8 (CV = 9.8%) | +10.2 |

**The heart rate method**

The HR method is based on the simple physiological correlate between oxygen consumption and HR during exercise. The relationship between HR and $\dot{V}O_2$ is unique to the individual[23,24] and is linear at expenditures above basal and below maximal activity (Figure 2).

TEE is estimated from HR using the equation TEE = sleep EE + sedentary EE + activity EE[23]. Values for BMR are determined by calorimetry and substituted for sleep EE. For estimation of EE in the low-HR range an average value for sedentary EE is used. The success of the method lies in the definition of a 'flex' HR. Flex HR is defined as the mean of the highest HR during rest and the lowest HR during exercise. Minute-by-minute HR is converted into energy expenditure using individual calibration curves. Above flex HR the slope of the calibration curve obtained is used to calculate $\dot{V}O_2$. Ambulatory HR monitors record minute-by-minute throughout the day allowing a different EE to be assigned to each minute's activity, according to the individual's calibration profile.

Thirteen CF subjects studied by this method were found to demonstrate levels of energy expenditure and physical activity in the free-living condition similar to that of healthy control subjects, despite a significant elevation in their mean resting energy expenditure[21]. We have also studied TEE and physical activity level (PAL) in a group of 30 mild and moderately affected CF patients aged 6–26 years (M : F = 2 : 1). PAL is calculated as TEE/BMR. TEE

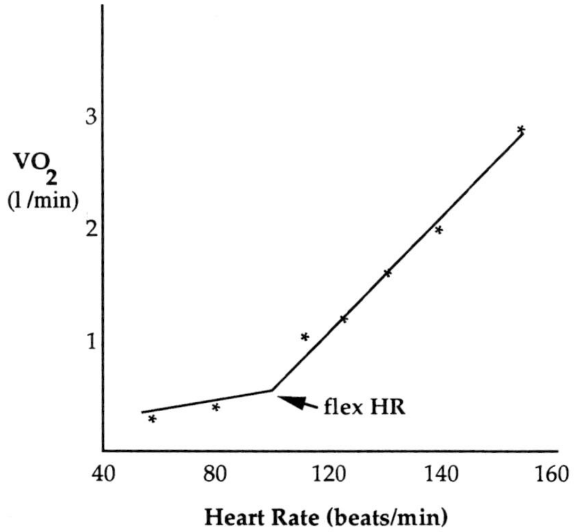


**Figure 2** Calibration profile for 15-year-old CF male. Calibration points shown below flex HR are for sitting and standing; above are for grades 1–5 Bruce treadmill protocol

was measured in free-living individually calibrated subjects, using the minute-by-minute HR method (HR TEE) over three days. All subjects were free of acute infection for four weeks or more and were in a stable clinical condition with respect to body weight and stool frequency. Patients taking medication known to alter energy expenditure were excluded from the study. The results are shown in Table 2.

## ACTIVITY LEVELS

As a group male CF patients performed to consistently higher levels of exertion than females; 16/20 males achieved grade 5 or better, compared with 4/10 females reaching a comparable level. There was no significant difference in pulmonary function, ventilation rate or chest radiological score between the two groups to explain the difference. Both groups had similar LBM as indicated by mid arm circumference (Table 2), although females had significantly higher body fat content, biceps skin fold 9.5 mm (sd 4.4) compared with males 3.9 (1.0), $p < 0.01$. Examining the time spent at a given percentage of predicted maximum heart rate, both sexes spent approximately equal times at >50% maximum HR. Girls expended less energy at high activity levels, $p < 0.001$. The within-sex differences are consistent with those observed in healthy controls[19,26].

On the basis of physical activity level, CF patients were expending levels comparable to FAO/WHO/UNU estimates[27] (Table 3). Patients were further subdivided to examine the effect of genotype on TEE and physical activity in view of a report of a possible genotype influence on the resting component of energy expenditure[28]. We found no significant effect of genotype on PAL: the

**Table 2** Physical activity level in CF subjects

| | Male ($n = 20$) | Female ($n = 10$) |
|---|---|---|
| Age (years) | 15.3 (4) | 13.3 (4) |
| Mean heart rate (b.p.m,) | 98 (11) | 101 (10) |
| BMP | 95.8 (9.4) | 102.9 (14.7) |
| Mid-arm circumference (mm) | 23.4 (3.8) | 23.3 (3.5) |
| CN score | 7 (3) | 5 (3) |
| $FEV_1$ (% predicted) | 86 (19.6) | 88 (20.1) |
| FVC (% predicted) | 97.6 (19.9) | 90.7 (12.6) |
| PAL (TEE/BMR) | 1.79 (0.21) | 1.64 (0.34) |
| >50% max HR (min) | 37.6 (24.6) | 39.8 (25.1) |
| >70% max HR (min) | 17.4 (21.1)* | 5.2 (5.6) |
| >85% max HR (min) | 5.8 ($n = 17$) | 1.5 ($n = 2$) |

*$p<0.001$
Results are average values over three days and are given as mean (s.d.).

**Table 3** CF: variation in PAL with age

| Age (years) | $n$ | PAL | Predicted PAL[a] |
|---|---|---|---|
| 6–9 | 3 | 1.58 (0.26) | 1.53–1.60 |
| 10–13 | 11 | 1.88 (0.28) | 1.63–1.73 |
| 14–17 | 8 | 1.63 (0.2) | 1.55–1.62 |
| ⩾17 | 8 | 1.70 (0.022) | 1.52–1.60 |

[a]Predicted values for age-matched controls from FAO/WHO/UNU (1985)[27]; values are mean (SD).

mean value for DF508 homozygotes was 1.70, DF508 heterozygotes 1.69, and patients without the DF508 mutation 1.82.

In the study of CF patients by HR methods, selection of a relatively fit subgroup is necessary for several reasons. In a subject with severe pulmonary disease, or in the presence of infection, there will not only be a reduced level of motor activity with an increased overlap in resting and activity HR, but the 'usual' difficulties in defining a discrete flex point, i.e. threshold HR, will be compounded by a complex interaction of additional factors influencing HR, including the potential effects of chemical mediators, and of declining cardiopulmonary function. This will potentially exaggerate the normal cardiovascular responses to a number of confounding physiological variables (e.g. fatigue, posture, prandial status), particularly in the terminal and preterminal stages of CF.

Validation studies using whole-body calorimetry[23,24] and the DLW method[29] as standards have demonstrated that the flex HR method provides a close estimation of the TEE of population groups. In theory the method should be of higher predictive value in children[29], in whom HR more closely follows changes in physical activity.

Clearly there was no evidence for the alteration in PAL often attributed to CF children. However, CF girls with comparable pulmonary function were less likely to participate in physical activity than boys—a pattern observed to a lesser extent in healthy age-matched control populations. Using similar HR criteria Riddoch et al. found that healthy Northern Ireland schoolboys spent on average 20 and 13 min, respectively, at HR ⩾70% maximum, compared with CF boys and girls who spent 17 and 5 min, respectively[26]. Whether the reduced time spent by CF females at moderately vigorous activity levels during childhood has any long- or short-term significance on health remains to be seen. However, whilst for males the duration of increased activity may be sufficient to produce a training effect[27], the time spent by female patients at HR ⩾70% maximum is insufficient to do so. This may be a factor influencing longevity in male patients, promoting improved cardiorespiratory well-being, not least as an adjunct to chest physiotherapy.

## EFFECTS OF PULMONARY DISEASE AND INFECTION

An association between severe chronic lung disease (of whatever cause) and weight loss has been well recognized, but is not well understood. Progressive weight loss in chronic obstructive pulmonary disease (COPD) is invariably associated with a poor prognosis, but the contribution of malnutrition cannot easily be separated from that of pulmonary disease. Studies in CF have shown a stepped decline in both pulmonary function and in weight related to an acute respiratory infection, but the relationship is not linear[30]. Both the increased resistive load and the reduced respiratory muscle efficiency (defined as the energy required to accomplish a given work output) contribute to the increased cost of breathing. However, whilst recognizing an important contribution from declining lung function to increases in oxygen consumption, the exact relationship between nutritional and pulmonary parameters in CF remains unclear.

It has been suggested that if the stepped decline model applies to CF, it should be possible for nutritional intervention to return pulmonary function to premorbid levels. Data are conflicting. Results of one study concluded that respiratory muscle strength was not related to nutritional status in patients with CF and asthma[31], but on the other hand improved nutrition has been associated with a slower deterioration in lung function[3]. Further studies are necessary to confirm unequivocally the beneficial influence of increased energy intake on the progression of lung disease in CF.

A further consideration in any programme of nutritional intervention is to ensure that the additional metabolic load does not place excessive strain on pulmonary gas exchange. The major function of the respiratory system is to meet the body's demand for oxygen and to eliminate carbon dioxide, and in patients with chronic lung disease the effect of various nutrients on oxygen consumption and carbon dioxide consumption must be monitored. In a study administering a variety of formula feeds varying in carbohydrate content to a group of stable CF patients with moderate to advanced COPD (given as nocturnal supplements) there was no significant alteration in respiratory gas exchange, despite increased metabolic expenditure, although carbon dioxide retention was proportional to the carbohydrate content of the feed[32].

As with some other aspects of CF, there is some uncertainty about the onset of the pulmonary component of the disease. Histological studies do not all agree that the lungs are normal at birth. Fetal abnormalities in CF have included abnormalities of the tight junctions and intracellular organelles of respiratory epithelial cells[33]. Although it has been presumed that at birth the lungs are functionally normal, and that the progression of lung disease in CF can be controlled if detected and treated early[34], most CF infants have respiratory symptoms documented during the first year of life. In one study of 13 newly diagnosed CF infants who were asymptomatic at the time of diagnosis, with no overt pulmonary involvement at the time of study, approximately 50% of the infants demonstrated nutritional deficits, with average weight below the 10th centile. These infants also exhibited a significant response to physio- and bronchodilator therapy, indicating increased resistive respiratory loads[35].

Malnourished patients have an increased incidence of infections in general. In one series nutritional status appeared to relate to both tracheal cell adherence and colonization patterns in the lower airway, suggesting that the airway was susceptible to colonization in response to nutritional variables[36]. The catabolic response to infection is similar from illness to illness despite differing aetiologies. Pyrexia, impaired dietary intake and duration of illness are the key factors determining the magnitude of the catabolic losses. Alterations in patterns of host protein metabolism are the most important nutritional consequences of infection. The evolution and resolution of an inflammatory response, as well as the repair of cellular and tissue damage, are all dependent on protein-synthesizing mechanisms. The complexity of factors involved makes any meaningful assessment of the contribution of chronic sepsis in CF patients difficult.

The presence of infection may also induce nutritional deficits, not least by the associated anorexia. The role of tumour necrosis factor (TNF) and other cytokines mediating the inflammatory process in producing anorexia and weight loss is becoming apparent. Plasma TNF is increased during infective exacerbations of CF due to *Pseudomonas aeruginosa* and does not return to normal following therapy[37]. TNF has been shown to induce increased protein and fat catabolism, to decrease their synthesis, to increase gluconeogenesis and is associated with glucose intolerance[38]. It would seem probable therefore that raised levels of TNF in CF will exert some effect on host intermediary metabolism.

## STOOL ENERGY LOSSES

The availability of ingested energy depends on the efficiency of digestion, absorption and metabolism of nutrients. 'Absorbed' energy is not, however, equivalent to its true digestibility, the difference arising because faecal analysis does not distinguish food residues from similar endogenously derived substances such as desquamated cells and various nitrogenous compounds and fatty acids derived from gut bacteria.

The complex pathophysiology of gastrointestinal disease in CF appears to be related not only to exocrine pancreatic insufficiency but also to defects in absorption and motility changes. The response to exogenous pancreatic enzyme is variable, with a maximum of 85–90% fat absorption demonstrated. Excess faecal fat and nitrogen losses were noted in all patients in one study[39] despite pancreatic supplementation bearing little relation to existing intestinal symptoms and stool energy losses. In a similar group, losses were as much as 20% of the gross energy intake[40]. Adjuncts to enzyme therapy, such as the $PGE_1$ analogue misoprostol, may further improve apparent fat absorption[41]. In addition, a variety of associated intestinal pathology has been described in CF, including chronic giardiasis, coeliac disease and Crohn's disease[42], all of which may compromise nutrition. Refractory digestive symptoms in CF apparently requiring excessive pancreatin dosage merit further investigation.

Stool energy content more closely relates to stool weight than to its lipid content, and either wet weight or dry weight of stool can be taken as a reasonable indication of stool energy, both in controls and in CF patients[40]. Monitoring of stool weight is therefore a more appropriate means of estimating total energy than repeated fat balances, and it should be borne in mind that there is a very poor correlation between faecal fat and faecal protein in individual patients (personal observations). As others have pointed out, it should not be assumed that stool energy is simply maldigested and malabsorbed dietary residue, because bacterial microflora may account for approximately 30% of total stool dry weight, and a similar proportion of its energy content[40].

## AN INTRINSIC METABOLIC DEFECT?

The earliest suggestion of a basic defect increasing metabolic demand in CF was based on the observation that mean birth weight in a group of CF infants was significantly reduced, suggesting *in utero* nutrient insufficiency, at least in some patients[4,5]. Later metabolic balance studies demonstrated an elevation in resting metabolic rate (RMR) in CF patients compared to controls, although this is subject to wide variability[20,21,43,58]. Others reported similar findings attributing this largely to deteriorating lung functions[44].

There are two clinical subgroups of CF patients: those with increased RMR and those whose RMR is normal. The observation is not easily explained; for example, RMR does not always correlate with pulmonary function. Although patients with severe pulmonary disease tend to have higher energy expenditure this is not invariable. Increased levels of energy expenditure are also seen in those with normal pulmonary function and in patients with above average weight for expected age[45]. This suggests that a more complex paradigm accounts for individual differences in resting metabolism and inherited variation must be considered as a potential component of such a model. Heritability is believed to account for between 11% and 40% of the total variance in RMR between healthy subjects[46]. Family studies[47] and studies on identical twins suggest the presence of as yet 'undetermined genetic elements affecting metabolic rate as well as the tendency to oxidize preferentially lipid or carbohydrate substrates' under certain conditions[48].

The concept of an influence of genetic variables on metabolism is not new. There have been many attempts over the years to analyse the various factors involved in the regulation of metabolic rate in both health and disease. Investigation has involved the use of human calorimetry and studies of oxygen consumption in isolated cell culture. Observations have supported the idea that it is appropriate to extrapolate results from the cell culture system to the *in vivo* situation[12]. Mutations of many kinds can eliminate particular reaction pathways and the perturbed cell reacts so as to restore its initial state. In states of starvation or disease, the cell can adapt and continue to function provided that certain minimum requirements for energy and nutrients are met, surviving as a result of an elaborate network of control mechanisms. Cells achieve such biological order through energy-requiring processes. Among the many reactions driven by this energy are those involved in the synthesis of biological molecules, and in the active transport of molecules across cell membranes.

Although the details of ion-transporting abnormalities in CF epithelium are now known, this does not explain observed increases in essential fatty acid turnover[49,50]. Interactions between membrane phospholipids and membrane proteins are recognized. How they interact (in processes which may be energy requiring), and the connection between these and other functional abnormalities in CF and the genetic defect are not known. Lipids have been shown to have a regulatory effect on ion pumps, specifically the $Na^+/K^+$-ATPase pump[51]

There is also experimental evidence for protein participation in transmembrane movement of lipids[52], itself an ATP-dependent process, and membrane phospholipids are involved in the regulation of membrane protein function[51]. *In vivo* cell-specific expression of CFTR provides a new perspective from which to consider the normal function of this protein, and may in the future help clarify the situation. Whilst it functions as a regulated chloride channel (in lung and testis, for example), CFTR expression is not restricted to surface epithelia and it may perform other functions, e.g. actively transporting some other unidentified substrate[53,54]. The observations reported in the course of studies of energy requirement in CF have suggested that the CF genotype may exert some influence on energy needs. This gives rise to a number of interesting possibilities, including: (a) that the CF carrier state may be a factor in the genetic contribution to variation in RMR in the normal population; (b) CFTR may help determine body composition variation and energy intake or energy expenditure phenotypes; and (c) it has been suggested that other genes adjacent to the CF locus may have a major impact on growth, even in patients with the same genotype[55]. The possibility that the CF gene, or a linked locus, may influence nutrient partitioning or cellular metabolism would provide an exciting hypothesis to explain observed differences in the primary components of body composition and in resting energy expenditure in presymptomatic CF infants[20,43]. Such a finding would also represent the first major gene effect for these measures of nutritional assessment.

## ENERGY INTAKE

Early studies of total energy intake in CF usually revealed a serious deficit, which was largely explained by the unpalatable nature of the low-fat diets then in vogue[56] and by the anorexia accompanying serious illness. The typical picture was of poor weight gain in infancy prior to diagnosis, and improvement when pancreatin therapy and supplementary nutrition was instituted, with an average weight about 1 SD below the mean during the preadolescent years. During adolescence the weight tended to fall off again, with simultaneous deterioration in the pulmonary condition[57]. For more than 20 years the literature documented a relentless decline of CF patients on a low-fat diet, to the extent that growth failure was assumed to be an inevitable consequence of the disease. By 1980 it had become clear that growth failure was preventable at least in the short term, and that near-normal growth was achievable. Growth failure was attributed to adherence to a low-fat, energy-deficient diet[56]. From the first challenge to this dietary misconception, it had taken at least 20 years to accept that CF subjects required a normal fat diet, 'covered' by adequate pancreatin supplements.

The contribution of dietary intake to nutrient and energy deficiency in CF patients is not completely clear, partly because of a lack of uniformity in the methods used to assess intake, and partly due to inherent bias in the diet intake methodology itself. One study used a control group with other gastrointestinal conditions and found CF patients to have significantly higher energy intakes, whereas previous studies recorded decreased food intake in CF subjects. These, however, compared values to what was termed the 'recommended daily allowance' (RDA) and not to actual controls. RDA values were derived for healthy population groups and established to exceed average requirements of most people in order to be sure that the recommendations will be adequate for almost the entire population. They may not be appropriate for populations of individuals who do not fit into the 'normal healthy' category.

### ASSESSMENT OF DIETARY INTAKE

There are a variety of methods for estimating energy requirements, including seven-day weighed intake, diet history, three-day weighed food record and 24 h recall[17]. Each assumes that the individual is in state of energy balance over the time of measurement, although the day-to-day variation in level of food consumption is considerable. All of these methods are subject to systematic error and none is indisputably valid in routine use, although there is some indication that under-reporting is less of a problem when using a method which does not require the subject to weigh the food[25]. There are also a number of assumptions and imperfections inherent in the food composition tables used to determine nutrient intake from dietary records.

Until recently the seven-day weighed dietary record was accepted as the 'gold standard' for assessing habitual dietary intake. The results of a recent study measuring energy intake using simultaneous measurement by the DLW method and seven-day weighed food intakes have indicated some serious discrepancies[29]. Average recorded energy intakes were significantly lower than measured expenditure in the group overall, suggesting a serious bias in reporting habitual energy intake. At the very least these data emphasize the need for caution in reliance on any one method of assessment. It is therefore recommended that wherever possible energy expenditure data rather than intake data should be used in determining energy requirements[27].

Various methods are available to identify non-physiological results[17], including a 24 h urinary nitrogen output. BMR may be used as an approximate check of underestimation of intake, either from actual values for the individual or in the case of groups of healthy controls using equations estimating BMR[18]. Reports of habitual intakes of $<1.4$ BMR are thus almost certainly underestimates[59].

In a recent study of 30 CF patients aged 5–25 years, and 30 healthy age-matched controls, we used the seven-day weighed recording method with careful checking by research personnel on alternate days.

Table 4 shows the mean ($\pm$s.e.) intakes for energy and macronutrients. Individual values for energy intake were expressed as multiples of BMR. Individual values for BMR were estimated by indirect respirometry under standardized conditions. Energy intake for the CF group ranged from 71% to 141% RDA. Eighty per cent of patients had an energy intake of $\geqslant 1.4$ BMR, with a group mean of 1.87 BMR. In the control group the mean energy intake was 81.8% (2.8) RDA, with less than half of the subjects recording energy intakes above the cut-off point. The group mean was 1.3 BMR.

The subject groups studied were both highly motivated, but the impression in feedback sessions was that the healthy controls tended to under-report and the CF patients, all of whom receive dietary advice as part of their management, were anxious to impress with high calorie intakes in compliance with the nutritional advice they were currently receiving. Thus the bias in the healthy control group is likely to be an underestimate and that of the patient group possibly an overestimate in a number of cases.

**Table 4**

| | Intake (% RDA) | % Fat | % Protein |
|---|---|---|---|
| Patients[a] | $100.1 \pm 3.8$* | $34.7 \pm 0.9$ | $13.1 \pm 0.4$ |
| Controls | $81.8 \pm 2.8$ | $37.5 \pm 1.4$ | $11.8 \pm 0.5$ |

[a] $n = 26$ energy intake $> 1.5 \times$ BMR; in $n = 1$ energy intake $< 1.35 \times$ BMR.
*$p < 0.01$ v controls.

A difficult problem, which occurred in our study in one case, is the occasional coexistence in the same family of a child with CF and a parent with heart disease. The CF child was being encouraged to take a high-fat, high-calorie diet, while the opposite recommendations were being given to the father. This exemplifies that the need for frequent nutrition counselling is essential to support the CF family, in all circumstances.

## A STRATEGY FOR NUTRITIONAL MANAGEMENT IN CYSTIC FIBROSIS

The result of a series of reports in the late 1980s demonstrating an increase in resting metabolic rate in CF patients[20,58,62] (values ranging from 95% to 153% of predicted) was that energy requirements in CF were set at 120–150% of the recommended daily allowance for age. It became increasingly apparent, however, that in many cases this was neither necessary nor practical[63]. It was also recognized that there would need to be both qualitative and quantitative control of nutrient intake, in view of the high incidence of glucose intolerance, and in recognition of the particular nutritional problems in CF infants[1,6–8]. As with many treatment regimes for CF, adequate, objective scientific assessment of programmes for nutritional intervention has been a problem. The inherent variability of CF has traditionally made it difficult to evaluate therapeutic regimens. Indeed it would be neither desirable nor appropriate to adhere rigidly to one set of guidelines for clinical management in the light of such heterogeneity. Current recommendations for nutritional management in CF necessitate a spectrum of dietary recommendations individually tailored[64].

It has been indirectly suggested (by ourselves, among others[65]) that CF patients who maintain normal growth and have well-controlled faecal fat losses have adequate levels of dietary intake. Unfortunately this assumption ignores the subgroup of patients with normal growth and near-normal pulmonary function[45], who have increased appetites and sustain high levels of intake to meet their increased metabolic need. By achieving and sustaining normal growth at least in the short term, these patients are not identified as a problem group, However, in the long term they constitute a potentially high-risk group in whom a rapid downward course may be pursued when intercurrent illness upsets their equilibrium. The evidence indicating the importance of energy balance in longevity in CF, despite an incomplete understanding of the factors causing the variable increase in energy needs, necessitated a rationalization of nutritional therapy in the disease.

In 1992, a consensus report from the United States CF Foundation outlined recommendations for the nutritional management of all CF patients[64]. This based nutritional requirements on an individualized, unrestricted eating pattern, with regular anthropometric assessment and early intervention. Determination of total energy requirements were to be calculated as multiples of

BMR, consistent with WHO[27] and COMA Panel guidelines[66], and with the individual's physical activity (i.e. lifestyle). Additional increments were to be added for declining pulmonary function and disease severity. The efficacy of these guidelines will be the subject of prospective studies based on their implementation over the next decade.

## FEEDING OR HYPERALIMENTATION?

The practical management of nutritional support will be dealt with in a later volume, but certain general principles should be kept in mind. The benefits of nutritional therapy must be evaluated in terms of tolerance, acceptability, complications and expense. Energy density is a critical factor in the translation of estimates of dietary needs into practical food intakes at any age. High-energy liquid supplements are not always well tolerated when given orally. If substances such as fat and carbohydrate are added to increase the energy density and palatability of food, care must be taken to ensure that the concentrations of protein and other nutrients are not reduced to unacceptably low levels, particularly with the use of glucose polymers. Whole milk may be the single most useful food for the provision of extra dietary fat and energy[67].

Elemental diets have been widely used in the management of CF. They tend to be unpalatable and expensive, and their prolonged use may lead to only marginal clinical benefit[68]. Newer products are greatly improved. In short-term studies, protein deposition is as good with protein-rich, calorie-dense non-elemental nutritional supplements as with more expensive elemental formulae[69]. Supplemental feeding with elemental diet during periods of hospital treatment for respiratory infections will enhance weight gain, but the increased weight is not maintained when patients return home[70]. When such children are maintained on nocturnal tube feeds at home, weight and height velocity can be sustained at an increased rate over several months, but the gains cease when the tube feeding is discontinued[71]. Placement of a gastrostomy, instead of a nasogastric tube, is usually preferred by the patient.

Parenteral nutrition is reserved for short-term treatment of those with severe malnutrition, with varied success. In a group of 19 severely affected patients[72] 10 died despite intervention. The group contained one previously diagnosed diabetic and two others developed diabetes during rehabilitation. None of the three survived more than 0.8 years after intervention. None of those receiving intravenous supplementation survived. This technique may therefore achieve an increased caloric intake, but at what cost to the individual?

Psychological factors need careful consideration when contemplating a programme of active nutritional intervention as it generally involves significant modification to the eating patterns and behaviour not only of the individual, but of the whole family, recognizing in addition that the individual patient and family may be functioning poorly due to depression. This area is of particular relevance in the adolescent and older patient. The short-term weight gain and the general improvement in well-being which often follows the introduction of aggressive nutritional rehabilitation, however, are usually accompanied by an improvement in mood and outlook.

Frequent and thorough nutritional surveillance is an essential component of CF care, and good dietary advice based on the CFF recommendations[64], coupled with optimum management of digestion and absorption, may be expected to postpone—often for many years—the stage at which more heroic measures may be needed.

## REFERENCES

1 Greer R, Shepherd R, Cleghorn G, et al. Evaluation of growth and changes in body composition following neonatal diagnosis of cystic fibrosis. *J Pediatr Gastroenterol Nutr* 1991; **13**: 52–8.

2 Kraemer R, Rudeberg A, Hadorn B, Rossi E. Relative underweight in cystic fibrosis and its prognostic value. *Acta Paediatr Scand* 1978; **67**: 33–7.

3 Luder E, Kattan M, Thornton JC, et al. Efficacy of a nonrestricted fat diet in patients with cystic fibrosis. *Am J Dis Child* 1989; **143**: 458–64.

4. Hsia DY. Birth weight in cystic fibrosis of the pancreas. *Ann Hum Genet* 1959; **23**: 239–99.

5 Dodge JA, Yassa JG. Food intakes and supplementary feeding programme. In: *Perspectives in Cystic Fibrosis* (ed JM Sturgess) Imperial Press, Toronto, 1980; pp 125–36.

6 Shepherd RW, Holt TL, Greer R, et al. Total body potassium in cystic fibrosis. *J Pediatr Gastroenterol Nutr* 1989; **9**: 200–5.

7 Sokol RJ, Reardon MC, Accurso FJ, et al. Fat-soluble vitamin status during the first year of life in infants with cystic fibrosis identified by screening of newborns. *Am J Clin Nutr* 1989; **50**: 1064–71.

8 Abman SH, Accurso FJ, Bowman CM. Persistent morbidity and mortality of protein calorie malnutrition in young infants with cystic fibrosis. *J Pediatr Gastroenterol Nutr* 1986; **5**: 393–6.

9 Corey M, McLaughlin FJ, Williams M, Levison H. A comparison of survival, growth and pulmonary function in patients with cystic fibrosis in Boston and Toronto. *J Clin Epidemiol* 1988; **41**: 588–91.

10 Editorial. Supplementary nutrition in cystic fibrosis. *Lancet* 1986; **i**: 249–51.

11 Pattishall EN. Negative clinical trials in cystic fibrosis research. *Pediatrics* 1990; **85**: 277–81.

12 Kleiber M. *The Fire of Life: An Introduction to Animal Energetics*, 2nd edn. Krieger, New York, 1975.

13 Lloyd-Still JD. Clinical studies on the effects of malnutrition during infancy on subsequent physical and intellectual development. In: *Malnutrition and Intellectual Development* (ed JD Lloyd-Still) MTP Press, Lancaster, 1976, pp 103–59.

14 Johnston JL, Leong MS, Checkland EG, et al. Body fat assessed from body density and estimated from skinfold thickness in normal children and children with cystic fibrosis. *Am J Clin Nutr* 1988; **48**: 1362–6.

15 Newby MJ, Keim NL, Brown DL. Body composition of adult cystic fibrosis patients and control subjects as determined by densitometry, bioelectric impedance, total-body electrical conductivity, skinfold measurements and deuterium oxide dilution. *Am J Clin Nutr* 1990; **52**: 209–13.
16 Shepherd RW, Thomas BJ, Bennett D, et al. Changes in body composition and muscle protein degradation during nutritional supplementation in nutritionally growth-retarded children with cystic fibrosis. *J Pediatr Gastroenterol Nutr* 1983; **2**: 439–46.
17 Bingham SA. The dietary assessment of individuals: methods, accuracy, new techniques and recommendations. *Nutr Abstr Rev (series A)* 1987; **57**: 705–42.
18 Schofield WN. Predicting basal metabolic rate, new standards, and review of previous work. *Hum Nutr Clin Nutr* 1985; **39C** (Suppl 1): 5–41.
19 Livingstone MBE, Coward WA, Prentice AM, et al. Daily energy expenditure in free-living children: comparison of heart-rate monitoring with the doubly labelled water method. *Am J Clin Nutr* 1992; **56**: 343–52.
20 Shepherd RW, Holt TL, Vasques-Velasquez L, et al. Increased energy expenditure in children with cystic fibrosis. *Lancet* 1988; **i**: 1300–3.
21 Spicher V, Roulet M, Schultz Y. Assessment of total energy expenditure in free-living patients with cystic fibrosis. *J Pediatr* 1991; **118**: 856–72.
22 Coward WA, Roberts SB, Cole TJ. Theoretical and practical considerations in the doubly-labelled water method for the measurement of carbon dioxide rate in man. *Eur J Clin Nutr* 1988; **42**: 207–12.
23 Ceesay SM, Prentice AM, Day KC, et al. The use of heart rate monitoring in the estimation of energy expenditure: a validation study using indirect whole-body calorimetry. *Br J Nutr* 1989; **61**: 175–86.
24 Spurr GB, Prentice AM, Murgatroyd PR, et al. Energy expenditure from minute-by-minute heart-rate recording: comparison with indirect calorimetry. *Am J Clin Nutr* 1988; **48**: 552–9.
25 Livingstone MBE, Prentice AM, Strain SJ, et al. Accuracy of weighed dietary records in studies of diet and health. *Br Med J* 1990; **300**: 708–12.
26 Riddoch C, Mahoney C, Murphy N, et al. The physical activity patterns of Northern Ireland school children, 11–16 years. *Paediatr Exerc Sci* 1991; **3**: 300–9.
27 FAO/WHO/UNU. Energy and protein requirements: report of a joint expert consultation 1985; Tech Rep. Series No. 724. WHO, Geneva.
28 O'Rawe A, McIntosh I, Dodge JAD, et al. Increased energy expenditure in cystic fibrosis is associated with specific mutations. *Clin Sci* 1992; **82**: 71–6.
29 Livingstone MBE, Prentice AM, Coward WA, et al. Simultaneous measurement of free-living energy expenditure by the doubly labelled water method and heart-rate monitoring. *Am J Clin Nutr* 1990; **52**: 59–65.
30 Fried MD, Durie PR, Tsui L-S, et al. The cystic fibrosis gene and energy expenditure *J Pediatr* 1991; **119**: 913–16.
31 Marks J, Pasterkamp H, Tal A, Leahy F. Relationship between respiratory muscle strength, nutritional status, and lung volume in cystic fibrosis and asthma. *Am Rev Respir Dis* 1986; **133**: 414–17.
32 Kane RE, Hobbs PJ, Black PG. Comparison of low, medium and high carbohydrate formulas for nighttime enteral feedings in cystic fibrosis patients. *J Parenter Enteral Nutr* 1990; **14**: 47–52.
33 Gosden CM, Gosden JR. Fetal abnormalities in cystic fibrosis suggest a deficiency in proteolysis of cholecystokinin. *Lancet* 1984; **ii**: 541–6.
34 Taussig LM, Kattwinkel J, Friedewald WT, di Sant 'Agnese PA. A new prognostic score and clinical evaluation system for cystic fibrosis. *J Pediatr* 1973; **83**: 380–6.

35 Hardy KA, Wolfson MR, Schidlow DV, Shaffer TH. Mechanics and energetics of breathing in newly diagnosed infants with cystic fibrosis: effect of combined bronchodilator and chest physical therapy. *Pediatr Pulmonol* 1989; **6**: 103–8.
36 Niederman MS, Merrill WW, Ferranti RD, et al. Nutritional status and bacterial binding in the lower respiratory tract in patients with chronic tracheostomy. *Ann Int Med* 1984; **100**: 795–800.
37 Norman D, Elborn JS, Cordon SM, et al. Plasma tumour necrosis factor-$\alpha$ in cystic fibrosis. *Pediatr Pulmonol* 1991; **10**: 86–91.
38 August DA. Nutrition and malignancy. *Curr Opin Gastroenterol* 1990; **6**: 226–31.
39 Lapey A, Kattwinkel J, di Sant 'Agnese PA, Laster L. Steatorrhoea and azotorrhea and their relation to growth and nutrition in adolescents and young adults with cystic fibrosis. *Pediatrics* 1974; **84**: 328–34.
40 Murphy JL, Wootton SA, Bond SA, Jackson AA. Energy content of stool in normal healthy controls and patients with cystic fibrosis. *Arch Dis Child* 1991; **66**: 495–500.
41 Robinson PJ, Sly PD, Smith AL. Effect of misoprostol on fat malabsorption in cystic fibrosis. *Arch Dis Child* 1988; **63**: 1081–3.
42 Baxter PS, Dickson JAS, Variend S, Taylor CJ. Intestinal disease in cystic fibrosis. *Arch Dis Child* 1988; **63**: 1496–7.
43 Girardet JP, Tounian P, Sardet A, et al. Resting energy expenditure in infants with cystic fibrosis. *J Pediatr Gastroenterol Nutr* 1994; **18**: 214–19.
44 Vaisman N, Pencharz PB, Corey M, et al. Energy expenditure of patients with cystic fibrosis. *J Pediatr* 1987; **111**: 496–500.
45 Durie PR, Pencharz PB. A rational approach to the nutritional care of patients with cystic fibrosis. *J R Soc Med* 1989; **82** (Suppl 16): 11–20.
46 Bogardus C, Lillioja S, Ravussin E, et al. Familial dependence of the resting metabolic rate. *N Engl J Med* 1986; **315**: 96–100.
47 Bouchard C, Tremblay A, Nadeau A, et al. Genetic effect in resting and exercise metabolic rates. *Metabolism* 1989; **38**: 364–70.
48 Bouchard C, Savard R, Despres JP, et al. Body composition in adopted and biological siblings. *Hum Biol* 1985; **57**: 61–75.
49 Rogiers V, Dab I, Michotte Y, et al. Abnormal fatty acid turnover in the phospholipids of the red blood cell membranes of cystic fibrosis patients (in vitro study). *Pediatr Res* 1984; **18**: 704–9.
50 Dodge JA, Custance JM, Goodchild MC, et al. Paradoxical effects of essential fatty acid supplementation on lipid profiles and sweat electrolytes in cystic fibrosis. *By J Nutr* 1990; **63**: 259–71.
51 Yeagle PL. Lipid regulation of cell membrane structure and function. *Fed Am Soc Exp Biol J* 1989; **3**: 1833–42.
52 Kawashima Y, Bell RM. Assembly of the endoplasmic reticulum phospholipid bilayer: transporters for phosphatidylcholine and metabolites. *J Biol Chem* 1987; **262**: 16495–502.
53 Higgins CF, Hyde SC. Channeling our thoughts (news and views). *Nature* 1991; **352**: 194–5.
54 Bradbury NA, Jilling T, Berta G, et al. Regulation of plasma membrane recycling by CFTR. *Science* 1992; **256**: 530–2.
55 Wulbrand U, Dork T, Tummler B, Krawczak M. Genetic determinants in cystic fibrosis. *Lancet* 1991; **337**: 623.
56 Pencharz PB. Energy intakes and low-fat diets in children with cystic fibrosis. *J Pediatr Gastroenterol Nutr* 1983; **2**: 400–1.

57 Berry HK, Kellogg FW, Hunt MM, et al. Dietary supplement and nutrition in children with cystic fibrosis. *Am J Dis Child* 1975; **129**: 165–71.
58 Buchdahl RM, Cox M, Fulleylove C, et al. Increased resting energy expenditure in cystic fibrosis. *J Appl Physiol* 1988; **64**: 1801–6.
59 Prentice AM, Coward WA, Davies HL, et al. Unexpectedly low levels of energy expenditure in healthy women. *Lancet* 1985; **i**: 1419–22.
60 Mearns MB. The heights of CF patients aged 2–9 years allowing for parental height and severity of pulmonary episodes from birth. In: *Perspectives in Cystic Fibrosis* (ed JM Sturgess) Imperial Press, Toronto, 1980; pp 262–5.
61 Soutter VL, Kristidis P, Gruca MA, Gaskin KJ. Chronic undernutrition/growth retardation in cystic fibrosis. *Clin Gastroenterol* 1986; **15**: 137–46.
62 Vaisman N, Pencharz PB, Corey M, et al. Energy expenditure of patients with cystic fibrosis. *J Paediatr* 1987; **111**: 496–500.
63 Marcus MS, Sondel SA, Farrell PM et al. Nutritional status of infants with cystic fibrosis associated with early diagnosis and intervention. *Am J Clin Nutr* 1991; **54**: 578–85.
64 Ramsey BW, Farrell PM, Pencharz P and the Consensus Committee. Nutritional assessment and management in cystic fibrosis: a consensus report. *Am J Clin Nutr* 1992; **55**: 108–16.
65 Dodge JA. Nutritional requirements in cystic fibrosis. *J Pediatr Gastroenterol Nutr* 1988, **7** (Suppl 1): S8–11.
66 Department of Health Report of the Panel on Dietary Reference Values of the Committee on Medical Aspects of Food Policy. *Dietary Reference Values for Food Energy and Nutrients for the United Kingdom* (41), 1991, HMSO, London.
67 Buchdahl RM, Fulleylove C, Marchant JL, et al. Energy and nutrient intakes in cystic fibrosis. *Arch Dis Child* 1989; **64**: 373–8.
68 Yassa JG, Prosser R, and Dodge JA. Effects of an artificial diet on growth of patients with cystic fibrosis. *Arch Dis Child* 1978; **53**: 777–83.
69 Pelekanos JT, Holt TL, Ward LC, et al. Protein turnover in malnourished patients with cystic fibrosis: effects of elemental and nonelemental nutritional supplements. *J Pediatr Gastroenterol Nutr* 1990; **10**: 339–43.
70 Daniels L, Davidson GP, Martin AJ, Pouras T. Supplemental nasogastric feeding in cystic fibrosis patients during treatment for acute exacerbation of chest disease. *Aust Paediatr J* 1989; **25**: 164–7.
71 Moore MC, Greene HL, Donald WD, Dunn GD. Enteral tube feeding as adjunct therapy in malnourished patients with cystic fibrosis: a clinical study and literature review. *Am J Clin Nutr* 1986; **44**: 33–41.
72 Levy L, Durie P, Pencharz P, Corey M. Prognostic factors associated with patient survival during nutritional rehabilitation in malnourished children and adolescents with cystic fibrosis. *J Pediatr Gastroenterol Nutr* 1986; **5**: 97–102.

Chapter Thirteen

# The Evolution of Pancreatic Disease in Cystic Fibrosis

Catherine Figarella and Jacqueline Carrère
*Groupe de Recherche sur les Glandes exocrines, Faculté de Médecine, Marseille, France*

## INTRODUCTION

Pancreatic insufficiency has long been recognized as a hallmark of patients with cystic fibrosis (CF) and has even given its name to the disease[1]. It appears sooner or later in infancy but it has been recognized since the 1950s that about 15% of older CF patients have a functional exocrine pancreas[2–4]. Since fortunately the survival of patients with CF is steadily improving each year, there is now uncertainty concerning the maintenance of pancreatic function throughout their life. A clear-cut difference between pancreatic 'sufficient' and pancreatic 'insufficient' CF patients has therefore to be considered with caution and underlines the usefulness of an attempt to pinpoint the evolution of the pancreatic disease in CF patients throughout the course of their life.

## PANCREATIC DYSFUNCTION BEGINS *IN UTERO* AND IS EVIDENT AT BIRTH

As reported by Boué et al.[5] a criterion giving evidence for CF in the fetus is the presence of a periodic–Schiff (PAS)-positive mucus-like material in some

*Cystic Fibrosis—Current Topics, Volume 2.* Edited by J. A. Dodge, D. J. H. Brock and J. H. Widdicombe

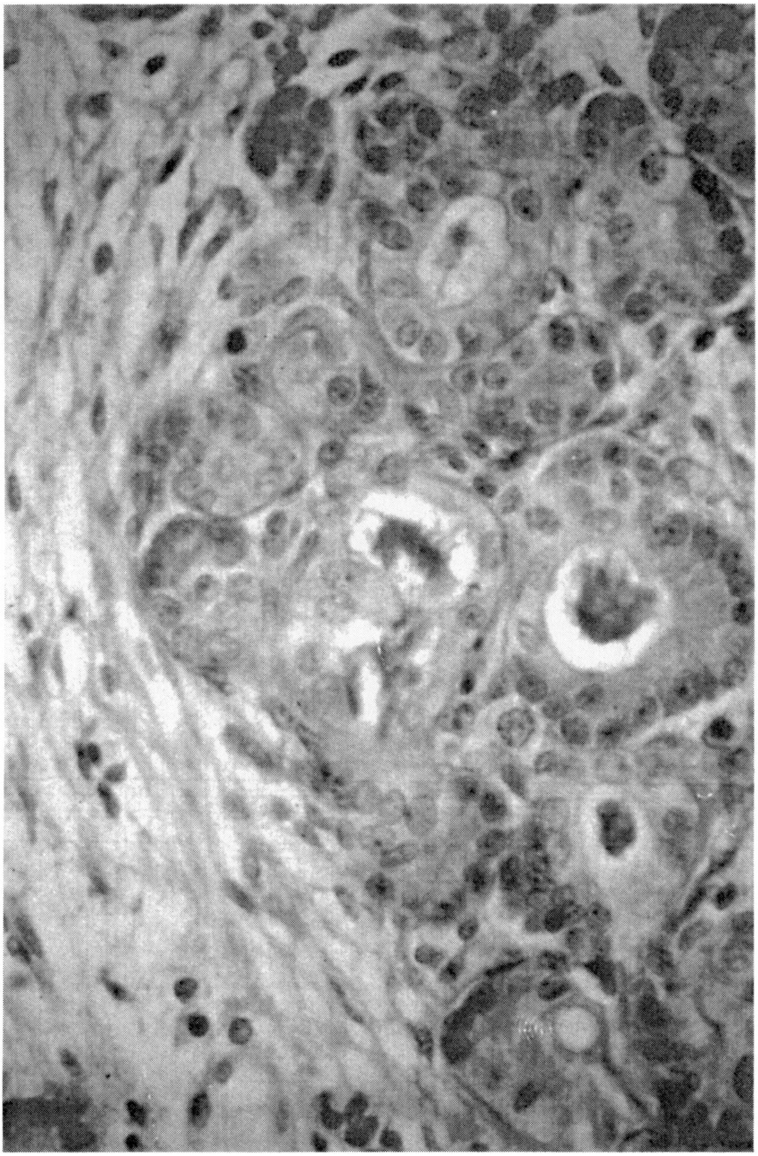

**Figure 1** Pancreatic acini of human fetus of 19 weeks' gestation with CF. Note the presence in acini of PAS-positive material (Courtesy of R. Gilly)

pancreatic acini. The distribution of these deposits was irregular and involved only a few of the peripheral acini of the fetal pancreatic lobules (Figure 1). Interestingly, the intra- and extralobular ducts were always empty, showing that the earliest CF lesions are not ductular but involve the glandular cells and their secretion[5].

The pancreatic secretion is probably already altered in the CF fetus. We studied two pancreatic enzymes: trypsin 1, and chymotrypsin A in amniotic fluids from mothers bearing a fetus with a one in four risk of CF[6]. The pancreatic enzymes were measured by non-competitive enzyme immunoassays[7,8] in fluids taken between 15 and 20 weeks of pregnancy, since it is well known that at this period the presence of these enzymes is due to a physiological transfer of fetal meconium into the amniotic fluid[9]. Our results have shown that the level of these enzymes was significantly decreased when the fetus had CF, obviously due to a hindered passage of fetal enzymes via the intestinal lumen into the amniotic fluid. We attributed this phenomenon to an already viscous consistency of intestinal mucus, as evidenced by the marked decrease in activity of several microvillar enzymes in these same fluids[10–14]. However, the possibility of early insipissation of pancreatic fluid cannot be ruled out, because the elevated blood immunoreative trypsin in CF newborns[15] is evidence of early pancreatic dysfunction. This elevated level of blood trypsin is used in neonatal screening for CF in several centres[16,17].

The phenomenon is not restricted to trypsin, and other serum pancreatic enzymes such as pancreatic lipase (reference 18 and unpublished data) are also increased at birth. These high values are probably due to a leakage of pancreatic proteins from the pancreas to the bloodstream, derived from functioning, but already ductally obstructed, pancreatic tissue. This obstruction was evident in the morphological studies performed by Sturgess and Imrie on autopsy specimens[19]. They showed that neonatal CF alterations are characterized by the presence of inspissated PAS-positive materials not only within acini but also within the intra- and extra-lobular ducts, accompanied by a loose interstitial fibrosis. A comparison of autopsy specimens of 31 CF infants (including 24 with a history of meconium ileus) with those of 29 control infants showed that there is a deficiency in normal acinar development in CF infants, resulting in a decrease in the ratio of acinar to connective tissue (Figure 2). Conversely, in control subjects, the volume of acinar to connective tissue increases linearly with age and as a result the ratio of acinar to connective tissue increases four-fold from birth to four months old. The authors found no difference in the exocrine pancreas from infants with or without meconium ileus, showing no relationship between pancreatic involvement and intestinal obstruction. Interestingly, these earlier findings are now clearly confirmed by the recent data obtained from transgenic mice who died of intestinal obstruction without signs of pancreatic disease[20,21].

Additional evidence for early pancreatic dysfunction in CF came from

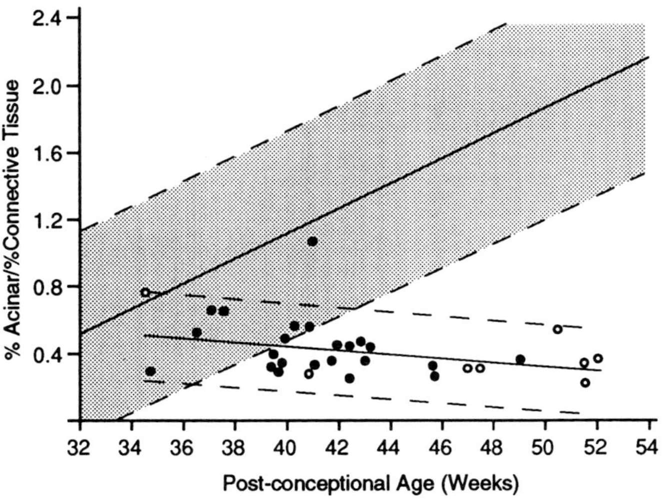


**Figure 2** Quantitative evaluation of the exocrine pancreas in control and CF infants. The solid lines represent the regression line calculated for the series of 30 cases in the control group; the shaded area within the broken lines represents the 95% confidence limits for the control group ($r = 0.81$; $p < 0.001$). The CF group is shown as individual points. Each point represents one case (open circle, no history of meconium ileus; closed circle, meconium ileus). The ratio of acinar/connective tissue is in the low percentiles of normal with or before birth and declines steadily with age. The deficiency in pancreatic development with age is statistically significant ($r = -0.47$; $p < 0.01$). There is no difference in the exocrine pancreas from infants with or without meconium ileus. (Reproduced from Sturgess and Imrie[19], with permission)

meconium studies. In 1958 a simple, rapid and cheap method of neonatal screening for CF was developed[22]. By means of a test strip the presence of undegraded albumin in the first passed meconium of newborns allowed the suspicion of CF. This phenomenon was thought to be due to a defect in pancreatic secretion leading to an absence of the normally secreted proteolytic enzymes. In fact, using the immunoreactive trypsin assay which enables the measurement of the protein by its mass rather than by its activity, it has been shown by different investigators that immunoreactive trypsin was present in the meconium of CF newborns at a concentration equal to or even higher than that of normal newborns[23,24]. However, this immunoreactive trypsin was devoid of catalytic activity, as shown by further gel filtration experiments whose results are shown in Figure 3. When filtered on a Sephadex G200 column, extracts of normal meconium gave only one peak of immunoreactive trypsin, which elutes with the proteins of a molecular weight of around 25 kDa. Trypsin catalytic activity elutes in parallel with the immunoreactive material. By contrast, two peaks of immunoreactive trypsin were obtained

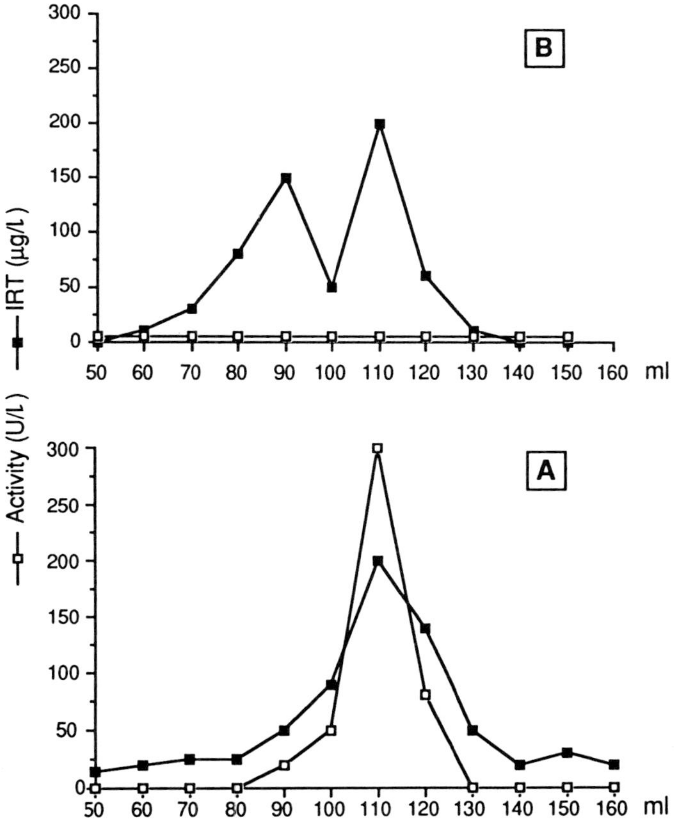


**Figure 3** Filtration of meconium extracts on Sephadex G-200. Filtration was carried out in a 50 mM Tris–HCl buffer pH 7.6 containing 0.5 M NaCl. (A) Meconium extract from a normal neonate. (B) Meconium extract from a CF neonate. (Reproduced from Lafont et al.[23], with permission of Walter de Gruyter, Berlin)

when the filtration was performed with the extracts of CF meconium. The first peak is eluted with the proteins of 75 kDa and represents a complex of trypsin with $\alpha_1$-proteinase inhibitor. The second one is eluted with the proteins of 25 kDa and corresponds to the peak observed with normal meconium but the fractions are devoid of catalytic activity. Therefore they correspond either to the zymogen or to an inactive form. Interestingly, this diagram closely corresponds to the diagram we obtained by gel filtration of amniotic fluids from a mother bearing a CF fetus and confirms an absence or a very low proteolytic activity in the duodenal fluid of CF newborns[6]. We have hypothesized that this absence of proteolytic activity in the intestine of CF newborns would contribute by an adaptative-like phenomenon to an increase of trypsin synthesis[25]. Taken together, all these data show that an early pancreatic dysfunction is a significant characteristic of the CF fetus and newborns and lead us to ask the following question: does the heterozygote have an altered pancreatic function?

## MILD PANCREATIC DYSFUNCTION IN HETEROZYGOTES?

It is now well established that a pitfall in the neonatal diagnosis of CF by the serum immunoreactive trypsin (IRT) assay is the relatively high percentage of false positives. This percentage varies from 0.3% to 0.7% between the different centres and according to the days when the sample is taken[16].

Thus, in any large sample of the healthy infant population, a small number will be found where blood IRT concentrations are elevated into the CF range. In these infants it is necessary to confirm the finding later on a second blood specimen before proceeding to confirm the diagnosis by clinical examination and sweat testing. These data prompted many investigators involved in neonatal screening to search for the deletion 508 mutation in dried blood spots as an additional test in IRT screening for CF.

It was then noticed by Laroche and Travert[26] and by Lucotte et al.[27] that an abnormal frequency of ΔF508 exists in the newborns showing a transient hypertrypsinaemia. A recent anonymous pilot study in Denmark on newborns was carried out with simultaneous analysis of IRT and ΔF508 on filtered blood specimens and has confirmed these first data[28]. The IRT concentration is slightly but significantly higher in heterozygotes than in controls ($p < 0.001$). These data strongly suggest that ΔF508 heterozygotes may have a predisposition to some mild biological abnormalities as early as the first days of life. We also observed a significant increase of blood IRT in older heterozygotes compared to controls (unpublished data). We used a protocol described by Vezzadini et al.[29] in alcoholic patients, where it has been established that the protein concentration in pancreatic juice was higher than in controls[30,31]. The experiment was as follows: 14 healthy volunteers aged 25–50 and 12 volunteer obligate heterozygotes (11 mothers, one father) aged 30–60 took part in the study. No subject used had a history of alcohol abuse and they were not long-term cigarette smokers. The secretin stimulation test was performed in the morning before breakfast and after a 12 h overnight fast. Blood samples were drawn from a peripheral vein and collected in test tubes 10 min before and 15, 30 and 45 min after the injection of secretin (75 clinical units in 10 ml of 0.9% NaCl injected intravenously over 2 min). After coagulation and centrifugation, about 3 ml of serum was collected from each tube and immediately frozen by aliquots. Blood IRT was measured in quadruplicate by a specific non-competitive enzyme immunoassay[7]. In control subjects, the mean concentration of blood IRT was 22.65 ± 1.67 μg/l before the secretin

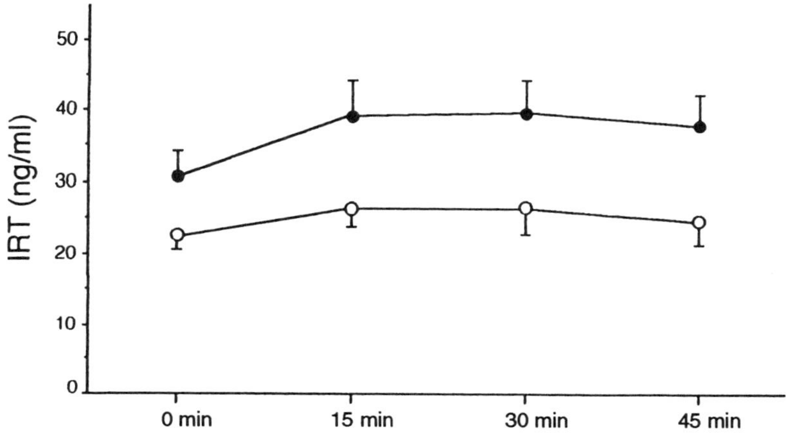


**Figure 4** Immunoreactive pancreatic trypsin in serum. Assays performed before and 15, 30 and 45 min after secretin stimulation. Mean ± s.e.m. Heterozygote (closed circle) and control (open circle) groups

injection, with a corresponding value in the heterozygote group of 31.11 ± 3.05 µg/l ($2p < 0.05$). As shown in Figure 4, there is a significant increase in the level of blood IRT 15 min after the secretin stimulation, but in this experiment we have observed a similar IRT increase in heterozygotes compared to controls.

As clearly seen in the figure, the values of IRT observed for heterozygotes are always significantly higher than for the controls. These data suggest that heterozygotes seem to have a greater reflux of secretory pancreatic protein into the blood and could indicate mild subclinical pancreatic damage with increased intraductal pressure.

## DEVELOPMENT OF PANCREATIC INSUFFICIENCY FROM THE FIRST YEARS OF LIFE

The evident pancreatic dysfunction of CF patients which appears as soon as the pancreas becomes functional (in intra-uterine life) is not necessarily accompanied by pancreatic insufficiency. This phenomenon may be easily understood by the fact that very little residual pancreatic function (10% or less) is required to prevent malabsorption[32,33]. Two studies from Gaskin and colleagues have shown that 50% of CF infants below four months of age have pancreatic sufficiency as assessed by measurement of fecal fat excretion and pancreatic stimulation tests[34,35]. As noticed by Waters et al.[34] this high proportion is in accordance with Andersen's original findings at autopsy[36], showing that half of the patients with CF who died in early life had less than 90% involvement of the exocrine pancreas on histological examination. For a better understanding of the development of pancreatic insufficiency in infants with CF, a careful follow-up study of pancreatic function would be worthwhile. Unfortunately, the complex and invasive nature of direct pancreatic function tests severely limits their utility for monitoring changes in pancreatic function among CF patients. A non-invasive test such as the measurement of blood immunoreactive trypsin level does not appear to be a sufficiently sensitive indicator of pancreatic dysfunction in the first years of life[37–39]. As shown in Figure 5 (drawn from two independent studies), below six[37] or seven[38] years of age, the values of IRT do not accurately reflect pancreatic function. If a low level of IRT is always correlated with pancreatic insufficiency, infants with a normal or elevated IRT also have, in the majority of cases, an insufficient pancreatic function. By contrast, above six to seven years a low level of IRT is nearly always synonymous with pancreatic insufficiency, whereas a normal or elevated level indicates a pancreatic sufficiency (in about 15% of older CF patients). A similar study on dried blood spots has confirmed these findings[39].

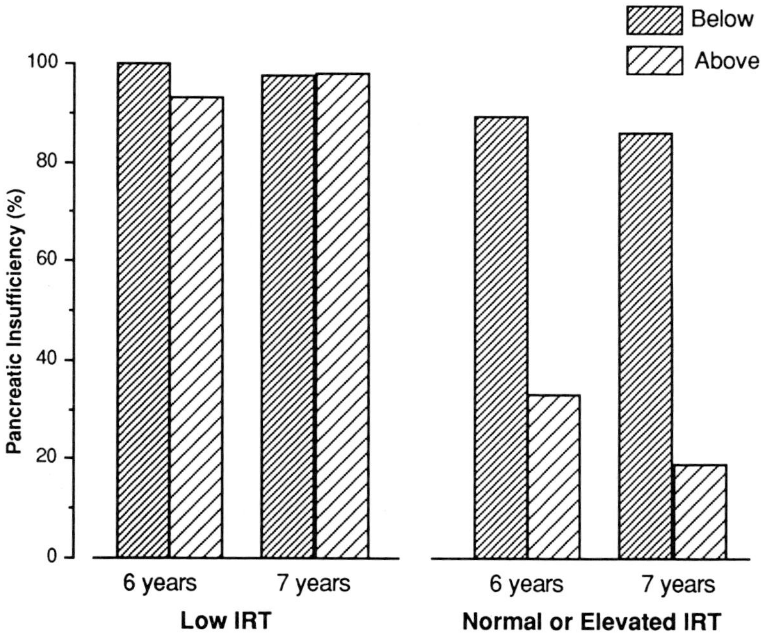


**Figure 5** Pancreatic insufficiency in relation to IRT levels in CF patients

## FUNCTIONAL FEATURES AND LONGITUDINAL STUDY OF EXOCRINE FUNCTION IN PANCREATIC 'SUFFICIENT' CYSTIC FIBROSIS PATIENTS

As observed above, persistence of an increased or normal trypsin level may be observed in 10–15% of older CF patients who have residual pancreatic function and who do not require pancreatic enzyme supplements with meals. Studies on the pancreatic function of these patients may help our knowledge of the pancreatic function of CF babies before the appearance of a pancreatic insufficiency.

An approach was made by Kopelman et al.[40] by comparing pancreatic proteins and water secretion of duodenal contents from patients with CF but who had normal pancreatic function as defined by the ability to secrete pancreatic trypsin. They found that secretions from the CF patients contained significantly higher concentrations of protein than those collected from the controls. These data are in keeping with the results obtained in the pioneer study of Hadorn and co-workers in 1968 on 10 patients with proven CF but without clinical symptoms of malabsorption[41]. In all 10 of the patients, the authors found lower bicarbonate and volume outputs than controls in response to a standardized dose of secretin (2 units/kg body weight). By contrast, enzyme output following pancreozymin stimulation was less severely affected and in three patients it was within the normal range. As a result of decreased volume responses in the presence of normal enzyme production, the duodenal contents of some patients were abnormally viscous and showed excessively high enzyme concentration.

We have repeated this study in collaboration with Dr J. P. Chazalette (Hôpital Renée Sabran, Giens) in eight CF patients who had no clinical pancreatic insufficiency[42]. As shown in Figure 6, we found a higher than normal response in enzyme concentration after secretin and pancreozymin stimulation. Bicarbonate concentration was markedly decreased in four cases, while in four other patients bicarbonate output and concentration were at the lower limit of the normal range. These results led Hadorn to reconsider his data and he noticed that some of his patients could also have nearly normal bicarbonate outputs and that bicarbonate secretion depended upon the dosage of secretin which was used for stimulation. When the secretin dose was increased to 12 units/kg per 30 min, bicarbonate concentration reached nearly normal levels, suggesting a higher than normal resistance of the ductular pancreatic cells to hormonal stimulation. (B. Hadorn, personal communication). The secretion of secretin-stimulated pancreatic fluid and bicarbonate occurs through a process mediated by cAMP[43] and it is quite possible that the defective response to secretin observed by Hadorn reflects the general defect in cAMP-mediated stimulation observed in CF[44].

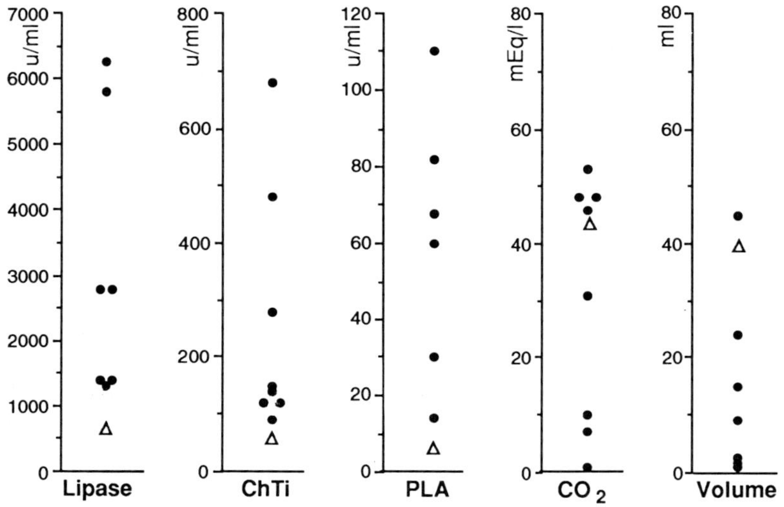


**Figure 6** Enzymatic and bicarbonate concentrations in duodenal contents of pancreatic sufficient CF patients. The assays were performed on eight patients (closed circles). Open triangle indicates the lower limit of normal values. ChTi, chymotrypsin; PLA, phospholipase $A_2$; $CO_2$, bicarbonate

From a clinical point of view, earlier studies by Gaskin et al.[45] have shown that pancreatic sufficient patients as a group have better pulmonary function, lower mean sweat chloride concentration and better survival rate in comparison with those with pancreatic insufficiency. We recently confirmed most of these findings by doing a statistical comparison of different parameters collected from 34 pancreatic sufficient CF patients (defined by a fat absorption coefficient of over 90% in the absence of enzyme therapy) and from the same number of pancreatic insufficient patients chosen at random out of 224 patients[46]. For each patient we recorded age at dignosis, sweat electrolyte levels, height and weight, age of *Pseudomonas aeruginosa* colonization, values of pulmonary function tests and Shwachman score. We found significant differences for pancreatic sufficient patients: an improved survival rate, a later diagnosis, a later incidence of *Pseudomonas* colonization, a lower sweat chloride concentration, a greater height, a better Shwachman score and a total absence of hepatobiliary disease. However, we found no difference between the two categories of patients for weight, and values of pulmonary function tests. The CF genotype, differences in early treatment with nutritional additives and/or pancreatic enzyme replacement or other environmental factors may explain the similarity in pulmonary function in our two groups of patients, but on the whole our results are similar to those previously observed.

On the other hand, quantitative data documenting the frequency and progression towards pancreatic insufficiency of the pancreatic sufficient patients are limited. A recent report by Cooper et al.[47] has shown that a subset of pancreatic sufficient patients developed pancreatic insufficiency over a variable period of time. We ran a longitudinal study of exocrine pancreatic function in the 34 previously studied pancreatic sufficient patients from 6 to 14 years. Blood immunoreactive pancreatic enzymes (trypsin/ogen[7] and lipase[48]) were studied in parallel with steatorrhoea. Three groups were observed: a major group ($n = 23$) with a constant level both of fat absorption and of blood pancreatic enzymes, a minor group ($n = 9$) with transitory elevated levels of the two serum enzymes probably indicating subclinical attacks of pancreatitis, and a few adult patients ($n = 2$) with a parallel fall of fat absorption coefficient and of levels of blood pancreatic enzymes. It would be interesting to see if a decline in pancreatic function could appear over time in the two other groups and if it would progress more rapidly in the patients of the minor group than in those of the major group.

## RELATION OF PANCREATIC DISEASE WITH GENETIC STATUS

Even before the cloning of the CF gene[49–51] Kerem et al.[52] suggested that pancreatic insufficient and sufficient patients could have different alleles[52]. They further developed the hypothesis that dominant 'mild' mutations exist and that their presence in conjunction with any other mutation would confer a pancreatic sufficient phenotype[51]. All further work has confirmed these early observations. An extensive study performed in 293 patients with CF who belonged to 233 families have shown that the pancreatic function status was strongly related to the presence of the ΔF508 mutation[53]. Among the 151 patients who were homozygous for ΔF508, only two patients (1%) had pancreatic sufficiency whereas 28 of those with the ΔF508/other genotype and 64 of those with the other/other genotype had pancreatic sufficiency at the time of their last examination. Similar results were reported in a series of 123 Italian patients[54]. Finally, a recent report from Kristidis et al. has completed and extended these findings[55]. The authors have analysed data from 394 of their patients for whom both CF gene mutant alleles were identified. Except for two cases, all given genotypes correlated with either pancreatic sufficiency or insufficiency but not with both. From their data the authors classified the mutations as severe or mild according to pancreatic function (Table 1). They concluded that pancreatic sufficiency occurs in patients who have one or two mild mutations whereas pancreatic insufficiency occurs in patients who are homozygous for or who are genetic compounds of two severe mutant alleles. Three of these mild mutations (R113H, R334W and R347P) affect arginine

**Table 1** Classification of CF gene mutations as severe or mild with respect to pancreatic function

| Type of mutation | Severe (location) | Mild (location) |
|---|---|---|
| Missense (point mutation) | I148T(exon 4) | R117H(exon 4) |
| | G480C(exon 9) | R334W(exon 7) |
| | V520F(exon 10) | |
| | G551D(exon 11) | R347P(exon 7) |
| | R560T(exon 11) | A455E(exon 9) |
| | N1303K(exon 21) | P574H(exon 12) |
| Single amino acid deletion | ΔF508(exon 10) | |
| | Δ1507(exon 10) | |
| Stop codon (nonsense) | Q493X(exon 10) | |
| | G542X(exon 11) | |
| | R553X(exon 11) | |
| | W1282X(exon 20) | |
| Splice junction | 621 + 1G → T(intron 4) | |
| | 1717 − 1G → T(intron 10) | |
| Frameshift | 556delA(exon 4) | |
| | 3659delC(exon 19) | |

Reproduced from Kristidis et al. Genetic determination of exocrine pancreatic function in cystic fibrosis, *American Journal of Human Genetics* 1992; **50**: 1178–84, by permission of Oxford University Press.

residues located in the first putative membrane-spanning domain. When expressed in heterologous epithelial cells these mutant CFTR are normally addressed and generate cAMP-regulated apical membrane $Cl^-$ currents[56]. It was therefore hypothesized that the dominant mild mutation provides sufficient CFTR $Cl^-$ channel function to confer pancreatic sufficiency[56]. Another hypothesis could be drawn from the recent data of Manavalan et al. showing a sequence and structural homology among membrane-associated domains of CFTR and certain transporter proteins[57]. From their data the authors suggested, as first hypothesized by Hyde et al.[58], that in addition to being a chloride channel CFTR may also transport larger molecules. Is this function less impaired in pancreatic sufficient patients? Further studies will be necessary to resolve this issue.

## EVOLUTION OF PANCREATIC ENDOCRINE FUNCTION

It has been known for a long time that approximately 50% of the CF patients have impaired glucose tolerance and that overt diabetes could occur in 6–15%

of CF patients[59-62]. The incidence and prevalence of impaired glucose tolerance and diabetes mellitus increase with age[63], so that the increase of life expectancy has led to a considerable increase in the prevalence of endocrine pancreas dysfunction in CF[64,65]. Fibrosis of the exocrine pancreas was essentially considered to be the main factor responsible for the impairment of endocrine function[66], but other factors may be involved[67,68]. A study by Lanng et al.[69] based on a relationship between the CF genotype, and endocrine and exocrine pancreatic function has shown that if, as is well known, the major mutation genotype in CF (ΔF508) affects the severity of the exocrine pancreatic insufficiency, the endocrine function is unrelated to this genotype. They therefore suggested that exocrine pancreatic insufficiency may be a primary genetic manifestation in CF, while glucose intolerance is a secondary non-genetic event. A recent study carefully carried out by Moran et al. has addressed these questions[70]. The authors examined the interrelationship among alterations in $\alpha$, $\beta$ and polypeptide cell functions in different CF patients and in controls. Patients with no exocrine insufficiency had normal fasting glucose and C-peptide levels, normal C-peptide response to oral glucose and normal responses to intravenous glucose and arginine, demonstrating a normal $\beta$ cell function. By contrast, a spectrum of abnormal $\beta$ cell activity was observed in pancreatic insufficient patients. Alpha cell function, as measured by the glucagon response to hypoglycaemia, was also abnormal in

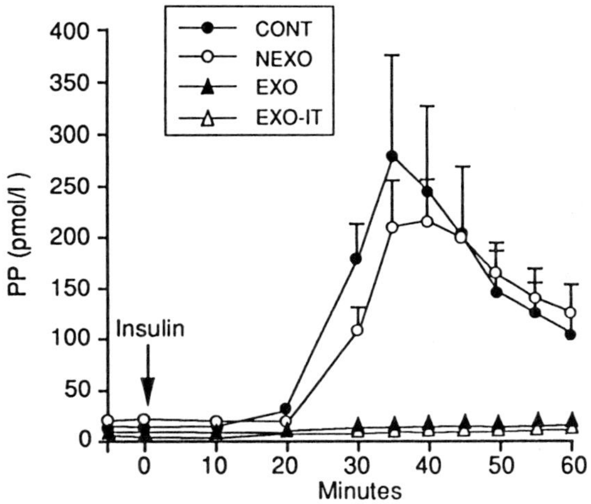


**Figure 7** Pancreatic polypeptide response to insulin-induced hypoglycaemia. Data are expressed as mean ± s.e.m. CONT, control subjects; NEXO, exocrine-sufficient patients with cystic fibrosis; EXO, exocrine-insufficient patients with cystic fibrosis; EXO-IT, insulin-treated, exocrine-insufficient patients with cystic fibrosis. (Reproduced from Moran et al.[70], Pancreatic endocrine function in cystic fibrosis, *Journal of Pediatrics* 1991; **118**: 715–23, by permission of C. V. Mosby Company)

patients with exocrine insufficiency. The most striking difference between these two groups of patients was the pancreatic polypeptide (PP) response to insulin-induced hypoglycaemia. Whereas the PP secretion is minimal in pancreatic insufficient patients, the response of pancreatic sufficient patients is not significantly different from that observed in controls (Figure 7). These findings raise the possibility of ongoing damage to entire islets in exocrine insufficient patients with CF different from type 1 diabetic patients who have a defect in glucagon secretion that is glucose specific. However, the 'all or nothing' PP response suggests a genetic difference rather than a progressive destructive progress. Finally an interesting observation from this study was the demonstration in two exocrine sufficient patients of an endocrine dysfunction suggesting that these patients may represent a transition from pancreatic sufficiency to insufficiency. They argue in favour of an impaired PP response to hypoglycaemia which could be an excellent indicator of exocrine pancreatic function in young adults with CF. They underline the usefulness of a prospective study of endocrine function in CF patients, particularly those who are currently exocrine sufficient.

## PATHOPHYSIOLOGY OF DETERIORATION OF PANCREATIC FUNCTION

From all the data reported above it may be assumed that the pancreatic tissue destruction is ongoing and its replacement by fibrosis and lipomatosis in CF patients is a progressive mechanism which begins *in utero* with the excessively high protein concentration of the pancreatic secretion. This protein hyperconcentration found by many investigators[40,41,71–75] is more likely to be due to an impaired secretion of fluid[40,41], but we cannot totally eliminate the possibility of an impaired protein secretion since we recently observed a constitutive protein hypersecretion from CF glandular tracheal cells in culture[76]. As a result, abnormally concentrated protein secretion becomes inspissated and precipitates within the acinar lumen and/or the ductular system, leading to secondary acinar lesions. Are these precipitates preceding or following an autoactivation of pancreatic zymogens, or both? Our previous studies on the pancreatic juice of patients suffering from chronic pancreatitis may help to answer this question. Indeed, an increase in pancreatic juice protein concentration after hormonal stimulation was also observed in chronic alcoholism[31,77] which is a well-recognized factor in the aetiology of pancreatitis[78]. We characterized several signs of premature zymogen activation in the juice of chronic pancreatitis patients: a high frequency of a detectable proteolytic activity[30], the presence of an $\alpha_1$-proteinase inhibitor–chymotrypsin complex[79] and a decrease in the potential activity of trypsinogens which could be due to a partial denaturation[80]. More importantly, we have demonstrated that the protein of 14 kDa isolated by Guy et al.[81] from protein precipitates present in the pancreatic juice of patients suffering from chronic pancreatitis was a proteolysis product[82]. This proteolysis product may be isolated from normal or slightly activated pathological juice and we called this protein, whose origin and function was unknown, protein X[82]. This protein, which precipitates at pH 8, is produced by the proteolytic cleavage of a soluble glycoprotein of 19 kDa with liberation of a small glycopeptide[83]. It is now well established that the pancreatic protein X is identical to the pancreatic thread protein isolated later from human pancreas by Gross et al.[84], to a form of pancreatic stone protein isolated from pancreatic calculi[85], and to a protein recently identified from regenerating islets and called 'reg' protein[86]. By studying duodenal secretions from subjects with and without cystic fibrosis, Forstner et al. have shown that the major proteins in precipitates from pancreatobiliary secretions are related to these proteins[87]. They found, as we previously showed, that their solubility was uniquely affected by concentration at neutral pH. They conclude that these proteins are therefore very susceptible to precipitation in CF concentrated ductal secretion where bicarbonate secretion is impaired and alkalinization of ductal fluid suboptimal. It is therefore highly probable that an activation phenomenon lies at the origin of the protein precipitates observed in cystic fibrosis. The detection of an abnormal $\alpha_1$-proteinase inhibitor–trypsin complex in the serum of about 25% of patients with CF supports this hypothesis[88]. In this context it should be pointed out that Shwachman et al.[89] were the first to describe attacks of acute pancreatitis occurring in patients with sufficient pancreatic function. The reasons why a premature zymogen activation may occur in CF remain an open question. As reported above, there is an impairment of proteolytic zymogen activation in the duodenum of CF fetus and newborns[6,23,90]. This impairment could be due to a defect in the accessibility of pancreatic zymogens to enterokinase, a non-secreted brush-border enzyme, caused by a thick intestinal mucus at the surface of enterocytes. An absent or lower duodenal proteolytic activity may lead to an increased synthesis of trypsinogen, as found in animals fed with trypsin inhibitors[91,92] and to an increased release of cholecystokinin, both conditions liable to provoke a premature activation[93]. Finally, it is difficult to know if this premature activation happens extracellularly into the pancreatic duct or intracellularly within the acinar cell. We have observed a full spontaneous activation of human cationic trypsinogen at pH 5.0 (which is a pH very close to lysosomal pH) without the addition of any activating enzyme or calcium and an increase of this phenomenon in the presence of cathepsin B[94,95]. These data and other morphological studies lead us to suggest that lysosomes might play a role in the premature activation of trypsinogen in pancreatitis and to propose the following hypothesis on the pathogenesis of chronic pancreatitis[96]. A deranged intracellular transport of secretory proteins in an over-stimulated pancreatic cell could lead to an abnormal admixture of digestive enzymes and lysosomal hydrolases and/or to a storage in acidic compartments which in turn could provoke an intracellular activation of trypsinogen. Such conditions are not improbable in CF.

## CONCLUSION AND PERSPECTIVES

The destruction of the exocrine pancreas in CF is an evolutive process more or less rapid according to individual cases and apparently the sole clinical manifestation of the disease clearly related to the genotype. However, as underlined by Dodge[97], all the genetic ingredients may be present but the rate of progress of the conditions of pancreatic insufficiency will depend on random, non-genetic factors within the organ itself and probably also on other environmental factors which remain to be determined. In this respect, the pursuit of the longitudinal study of the exocrine function of older pancreatic sufficient patients remains invaluable to afford additional indications on the evolution of pancreatic disease. In the same way, the study and follow-up of the atypical cases genetically diagnosed as having CF but apparently characterized by a unique clinical manifestation such as the congenital absence of vas deferens[98,99] or a chronic bronchial hypersecretion[100,101] would also be worthwhile. Finally, the fact that pancreatic insufficiency is an evolutive process should stimulate research attempting to slow down its progression. Data from ourselves and others showing a defect in the activation process of proteolytic zymogens in infancy leads us to tentatively suggest that supplementation by intestinal enzymes would be perhaps of interest.

## ACKNOWLEDGEMENTS

The authors would like to thank Dr J. P. Chazalette (Hôpital Renée Sabran, Giens) for his support and encouragement, and C. Galabert for her participation in the heterozygote study and her interest. They are deeply indebted to O. Guy-Crotte for stimulating discussions and for her help in reviewing the manuscript, and to C. Crotte for statistical analysis. The research in the authors' laboratory is supported by grants from INSERM (Institut National de la Santé et de la Recherche Médicale), from the Faculty of Medicine and from AFLM (Association Française de Lutte contre la Mucoviscidose).

## REFERENCES

1 Fanconi G, Uehlinger E, Knauer C. Das coeliakiesyndrom bel angeborener zystischer pancreasfibromatose und bronkiektasien. *Wein Med Wochenshr* 1936; **86**: 753–62.

2 Gibbs GE, Bostick WL. Incomplete pancreatic deficiency in cystic fibrosis of the pancreas. *J Pediatr* 1950; **37**: 320–5.

3 Di Sant'agnese PA. Fibrocystic disease of the pancreas with normal or partial pancreatic function. *Pediatrics* 1955; **15**: 683–97.

4 Shwachman H, Dooley R, Guilmett F, et al. Cystic fibrosis of the pancreas with varying degrees of pancreatic insufficiency. *Am J Dis Child* 1956; **92**: 347–68.

5 Boué A, Muller F, Nezeloff C, et al. Prenatal diagnosis in 200 pregnancies with a 1-in-4 risk of cystic fibrosis. *Hum Genet* 1986; **74**: 288–97.

6 Carrère J, Muller F, Boué A, et al. Levels and molecular forms of immunoreactive trypsin and chymotrypsin in amniotic fluids from normal and cystic fibrosis fetus: evidence for a lack of activation of proteolytic zymogens in cystic fibrosis fetus. *J Pediatr Gastroenterol Nutr* 1992; **14**: 198–203

7 Carrère J, Grataroli R, Martin J, et al. Non competitive immunoassay of human trypsin 1. *J Immunol Methods* 1983; **60**: 235–42.

8 Carrère J, Figarella C, Guy O, Thouvenot JP. Human pancreatic chymotrypsinogen A: a non-competitive enzyme immunoassay and molecular forms in serum and amniotic fluid. *Biochim Biophys Acta* 1986; **883**: 46–53.

9 Borgström A, Sveger T, Kullander S, et al. Determination and characterization of immunoreactive trypsin in amniotic fluid from normal and cystic fibrosis fetuses. *Pediatr Res* 1984; **18**: 957–9.

10 Carbarns NJB, Gosden C, Brock DJH. Microvillar peptidase activity in amniotic fluid: possible use in the prenatal diagnosis of cystic fibrosis. *Lancet* 1983; *i*: 329–31.

11 Baker S, Dann LG. Peptidases in amniotic fluid: low values in cystic fibrosis. *Lancet* 1983; **i**: 716–17.

12 Brock DJH. Amniotic fluid alkaline phosphatase isoenzymes in early prenatal diagnosis. *Lancet* 1983; **ii**: 941–3.

13 Van Diggelen OP, Janse HC, Kleijer WJ. Disaccharidases in amniotic fluid as possible markers for cystic fibrosis. *Lancet* 1983; **i**: 817.

14 Muller F, Berg S, Frott JF, et al. Alkaline phosphatase isoenzymes assays for prenatal diagnosis of cystic fibrosis. *Lancet* 1984; **ii**: 572.

15 Crossley JR, Elliot RP, Smith PA. Dried blood spot screening for cystic fibrosis in the newborn. *Lancet* 1979; **i**: 472–4.

16 Heeley AF, Bangert SK. The neonatal detection of cystic fibrosis by measurement of immunoreactive trypsin in blood. *Ann Clin Biochem* 1992; **29**: 361–76.

17 Figarella C. Quelle approche pour le dépistage néonatal de la mucoviscidose? *Immunoanal Biol Spec* 1992; **33**: 77–81.

18 Hammond KB, Ask CG, Watts DC. Immunoreactive pancreatic lipase test for neonatal detection of cystic fibrosis. *Lancet* 1984; **i**: 42.

19 Sturgess JM, Imrie JR. The development of the exocrine pancreas in cystic fibrosis. In: Approaches to cystic fibrosis (ed D Kaiser) Berlin, 1981, pp 175–88.

20 Snouwaert JN, Brigman KK, Latour AM, et al. An animal model for cystic fibrosis made by gene targeting. *Science* 1992; **257**: 1083–8.

21 Dorin JR, Dickinson P, Alton EWFW, et al. Cystic fibrosis in the mouse by targeted insertional mutagenesis. *Nature* 1992; **359**: 211–14.

22 Green MN, Clarke JT, Shwachman H. Studies in CF: protein pattern in meconium ileus. *Pediatrics* 1958; **21**: 635–42.

23 Lafont P, Barbier Y, Mathian J, et al. a1-proteinase inhibitor in meconium from healthy infants and infants with cystic fibrosis. In: *Marker Proteins in Inflammation* (eds P Arnaud, J Bienvenu, P Laurent) Walter de Gruyter, Berlin, 1984, pp 251–4.

24 Hsieh M, Berry HK. Proteinase inhibitor and defective proteolysis in cystic fibrosis. *Dig Dis Sci* 1988; **33**: 282–8.
25 Carrère J, Estevenon JP, Guy-Crotte O, et al. Physiologically elevated concentration of serum trypsin-like immunoreactivity in newborns. *Biol Neonate* 1986; **49**: 113–20.
26 Laroche D, Travert G. Abnormal frequency of ΔF 508 mutation in neonatal transitory hypertrypsinaemia. *Lancet* 1991; **337**: 55.
27 Lucotte G, Perignon JL, Lenoir G. Transient neonatal hypertrypsinemia as test for ΔF 508 heterozygosity. *Lancet* 1991; **337**: 988.
28 Norgaard-Petersen B, Hogdall E, Iitia A, et al. Immunoreactive trypsin and a comparison of two ΔF 508 mutation analyses in newborn screening for cystic fibrosis: an anonymous pilot study in Denmark. *Screening* 1993; **2**: 1–11.
29 Vezzadini P, Ferri GL, Bonora G, et al. Secretin-stimulated trypsin-like immunoreactivity in alcoholics. *Clin Chim Acta* 1981; **111**: 163–7.
30 Figarella C, Guy-Crotte O, Barthe C, Amouric M. Les protéines pancréatiques humaines à l'état normal et pathologique. *Gastroenterol Clin Biol* 1987; **11**: 891–7.
31 Renner IG, Rinderknecht H, Valenzuelas E, Douglas AP. Studies of pancreatic secretion in chronic alcoholic subjects without pancreatic insufficiency. *Scand J Gastroenterol* 1980; **15**: 241–4.
32 DiMagno EP, Go VLW, Summerskill WH. Relations between pancreatic enzyme outputs and malabsorption in severe pancreatic insufficiency. *N Engl J Med* 1973; **288**: 813–15.
33 Gaskin KJ, Durie PR, Lee L, et al. Colipase and lipase secretion in childhood onset pancreatic insufficiency: delineation of patients with steatorrhea secondary to relative colipase deficiency. *Gastroenterology* 1984; **86**: 1–7.
34 Waters DL, Dorney S, Gaskin KJ, et al. Pancreatic function in infants identified as having cystic fibrosis in a neonatal screening program. *N Engl J Med* 1990; **322**: 303–8.
35 Gaskin K, Waters D, Dorney S, et al. Assessment of pancreatic function in screened infants with cystic fibrosis. *Pediatr Pulmonol* 1991; Suppl 7: 69–71.
36 Andersen DH. Cystic fibrosis of the pancreas and its relation to celiac desease: a clinical and pathologic study. *Am J Dis Child* 1938; **56**: 344–99.
37 Masoero G, Andriulli A, Santini B, et al. Serum trypsinlike immunoreactivity in cystic fibrosis. *Am J Dis Child* 1983; **137**: 167–70.
38 Durie PR, Forstner GG, Gaskin KJ, et al. Age-related alterations of immunoreactive pancreatic cationic trypsinogen in sera from cystic fibrosis patients with and without pancreatic insufficiency. *Pediatr Res* 1986; **20**: 209–13.
39 Barbier Y, Lafont P, Galvain D, et al. Place de la trypsine immunoréactive (TIR) dans l'évaluation de la fonction pancréatique chez l'enfant atteint de mucoviscidose. *Immunoanal Biol Spec* 1991; **28**: 33–7.
40 Kopelman H, Durie P, Gaskin K, et al. Pancreatic fluid secretion and protein hyperconcentration in cystic fibrosis. *N Engl J Med* 1985; **312**: 329–34.
41 Hadorn B, Johansen PG, Anderson CM. Pancreozymin secretin test of exocrine pancreatic function in cystic fibrosis. *Can Med Assoc J* 1968; **98**: 377–85.
42 Guy-Crotte O, Carrère J, Figarella C. Physiopathologie de l'atteinte pancréatique dans la mucoviscidose. *Pathol Biol* 1991; **6**: 631–5.
43 Case RM, Johnson M, Scratcherd T, Sherratt HSA. Cyclic adenosine 3′5′ monophosphate concentration in the pancreas following stimulation by secretin, CCK-PZ and acetylcholine. *J Physiol* (London) 1972; **223**: 669–84.
44 Collins F. Cystic fibrosis: molecular biology and therapeutic implications. *Science* 1992; **256**: 774–9.

45 Gaskin K, Gurwitz D, Durie P, et al. Improved respiratory prognosis in CF patients with normal fat absorption. *J Pediatr* 1982; **100**: 857–62.
46 Graffin B, Carrère J, Boutin JP, et al. Clinical and biological features of pancreatic sufficient CF patients. *Pediatr Pulmonol* 1991; Suppl 6: 267–8.
47 Cooper RTL, Corey M, Moore DJ, et al. Decline of exocrine pancreatic function in cystic fibrosis patients with pancreatic sufficiency. *Pediatr Res* 1992; **32**: 179–82.
48 Carrère J, Galabert C, Thouvenot JP, Figarella C. Assay of human pancreatic lipase in biological fluids using a non-competitive enzyme immunoassay. *Clin Chim Acta* 1986; **161**: 209–19.
49 Rommens JM, Iannuzzi MC, Kerem BS, et al. Identification of the cystic fibrosis gene: chromosome walking and jumping. *Science* 1989; **245**: 1059–65.
50 Riordan JR, Rommens JM, Kerem BS, et al. Identification of the cystic fibrosis gene: cloning and characterization of complementary DNA. *Science* 1989; **245**: 1066–72.
51 Kerem BS, Rommens JM, Buchanan JA, et al. Identification of the cystic fibrosis gene: genetic analysis. *Science* 1989; **245**: 1073–80.
52 Kerem BS, Buchanan JA, Durie P, et al. DNA marker haplotype association with pancreatic sufficiency in cystic fibrosis. *Am J Hum Genet* 1989; **44**: 827–34.
53 Kerem E, Corey M, Kerem BS, et al. The relation between genotype and phenotype in cystic fibrosis: analysis of the most common mutation ($\Delta$F 508). *N Engl J Med* 1990; **323**: 1517–22.
54 Ferrari M, Antonelli M, Bellini F, et al. Genetic differences in cystic fibrosis patients with and without pancreatic insufficiency. *Hum Genet* 1990; **84**: 435–8.
55 Kristidis P, Bozon D, Corey M, et al. Genetic determination of exocrine pancreatic function in cystic fibrosis. *Am J Hum Genet* 1992; **50**: 1178–84.
56 Welsh MJ, Smith AE. Molecular mechanisms of CFTR chloride channel dysfunction in cystic fibrosis. *Cell* 1993; **73**: 1251–4.
57 Manavalan P, Smith AE, McPherson JM. Sequence and structural homology among membrane-associated domains of CFTR and certain transporter proteins. *J Prot Chem* 1993; **12**: 279–90.
58 Hyde SC, Emsley P, Hartshorn MJ, et al. Structural model of ATP-binding proteins associated with cystic fibrosis, multidrug resistance and bacterial transport. *Nature* 1990; **346**: 362–5.
59 Handwerger S, Roth J, Gorden P, et al. Glucose intolerance in cystic fibrosis. *N Engl J Med* 1969; **281**: 451–61.
60 DiSant'Agnese P, Davis PB. Cystic fibrosis in adults: seventy-five cases and a review of 232 cases in the literature. *Am J Med* 1979; **66**: 121–32.
61 Rodman HM, Matthews LW. Hyperglycemia in cystic fibrosis: a review of the literature and our own patient experience. In: *1,000 years of Cystic Fibrosis: Collected Papers* (ed WJ Warwick) St Paul, University of Minnesota Press, 1981, pp 67–76.
62 Finkelstein SM, Wielinski CL, Elliott GR, et al. Diabetes mellitus associated with cystic fibrosis. *J Pediatr* 1988; **112**: 373–7.
63 Lanng S, Thorsteinsson B, Erichsen G, et al. Glucose tolerance in cystic fibrosis. *Arch Dis Child* 1991; **66**: 612–16.
64 De Scheper J, Dah I, Derde MP, Loeb H. Oral glucose tolerance testing in cystic fibrosis: correlations with clinical parameters and glycosylated haemoglobin determinations. *Eur J Pediatr* 1991; **150**: 403–6.
65 Dodge JA, Morrison G. Diabetes mellitus in cystic fibrosis: a review. *J R Soc Med* 1992; **85** (Suppl 19): 25–8.

66 Löhr M, Goertchen P, Nizze H, et al. Cystic fibrosis associated islet changes may provide a basis for diabetes: an immunocytochemical and morphometrical study. *Virchows Archiv A Pathol Anat* 1989; **414**: 179–85.
67 Krueger LJ, Lerner A, Katz SM, et al. Cystic fibrosis and diabetes mellitus: interactive or idiopathic? *J Pediatr Gastroenter Nutr* 1991; **13**: 209–19.
68 Lanng S, Thorsteinsson B, Pociot F, et al. Diabetes mellitus in cystic fibrosis: genetic and immunological markers. *Acta Paediatr* 1993; **82**: 150–4.
69 Lanng S, Schwartz M, Thorsteinsson B, Koch C. Endocrine and exocrine pancreatic function and the ΔF508 mutation in cystic fibrosis. *Clin Genet* 1991; **40**: 345–8.
70 Moran A, Diem P, Klein DJ, et al. Pancreatic endocrine function in cystic fibrosis. *J Pediatr* 1991; **118**: 715–23.
71 Maddock CL, Farber S, Shwachman H. Pancreatic function and disease in early life. II. Effect of secretin on pancreatic function of infants and children. *Am J Dis Child* 1943; **66**: 370–5.
72 Gibbs GE. Secretin tests with bilumen gastroduodenal drainage in infants and children. *Pediatrics* 1950; **5**: 941–6.
73 Knauff RE, Adams JA. Proteins and mucoproteins in the duodenal fluids of cystic fibrosis and control subjects. *Clin Chim Acta* 1968; **19**: 245–8.
74 Lebenthal E, Lee PC. Effect of pancreozymin and secretin on intraluminal enterokinase, trypsin and chymotrypsin activities of cystic fibrosis and control children. *Digestion* 1982; **23**: 39–47.
75 Zoppi G, Hitzig WH, Shmerling DH, et al. Protein content and pancreatic enzyme activities of duodenal juice in normal children with exocrine pancreatic insufficiency. *Helv Pediatr Acta* 1958; **23**: 577–90.
76 Merten M, Figarella C. Constitutive hypersecretion and insensitivity to neurotransmitters by cystic fibrosis tracheal gland cells. *Am J Physiol (Lung Mol Physiol 8)* 1993; **264**: L93–9.
77 Sahel J, Sarles H. Modifications of pure human pancreatic juice induced by chronic alcohol consumption. *Dig Dis Sci* 1979; **24**: 897–905.
78 Sarles H, Figarella C, Tiscornia O. Alcoholic pancreatitis. *Mount Sinai J Med* 1975; **42**: 540–51.
79 Misczuk-Jamska B, Guy O, Figarella C. a1-Proteinase inhibitor in pure human pancreatic juice: characterization of a complexed form in patients with chronic calcifying pancreatitis and its significance. *Hoppe Seyler's Z Physiol Chem* 1983; **364**: 1597–601.
80 Colomb E, Guy O, Sarles H, Figarella C. Activités enzymatiques du suc pancréatique de malades atteints de pancréatite chronique calcifiante. *Gastroenterol Clin Biol* 1979; **3**: 763–8.
81 Guy O, Robles-Diaz G, Adrich Z, et al. Protein content of precipitates present in pancreatic juice of alcoholic subjects and patients with chronic calcifying pancreatitis. *Gastroenterology* 1983; **84**: 102–7.
82 Guy-Crotte O, Amouric M, Figarella C. Characterization and N-terminal sequence of a degradation product of 14000 molecular weight isolated from human pancreatic juice. *Biochem Biophys Res Commun* 1984; **125**: 516–23.
83 Figarella C, Amouric M, Guy-Crotte O. Enzyme activation and liberation: intracellular/extracellular events. In: *Acute Pancreatitis* (eds HG Beger, M Büchler) Springer-Verlag, Berlin, 1987, pp 53–60.
84 Gross J, Brauer AW, Bringhurst RF, et al. An unusual bovine pancreatic protein exhibiting pH-dependent globule–fibril transformation and unique amino acid sequence. *Proc Natl Acad Sci USA* 1985; **82**: 5627–31.

85 Montalto G, Bonicel J, Multignier L, et al. Partial amino acid sequence of human pancreatic stone protein, a novel pancreatic secretory protein. *Biochem J* 1986; **238**: 227–32.
86 Watanabe T, Yonekura H, Terazono K, et al. Complete nucleotide sequence of human reg gene and its expression in normal and tumoral tissues: the reg protein, pancreatic stone protein and pancreatic thread protein are one and the same product of the gene. *J Biol Chem* 1990; **265**: 7432–8.
87 Forstner GG, Vesely SM, Durie PR. Selective precipitation of 14 kDa stone/thread proteins by concentration of pancreaticobiliary secretions: relevance to pancreatic ductal obstruction, pancreatic failure and CF. *J Pediatr Gastroenterol Nutr* 1989; **8**: 313–20.
88 Carrère J, Chazalette JP, Figarella C. Behaviour of serum immunoreactive trypsin after serum activation by enterokinase in normal and cystic fibrosis patients: evidence of a trypsin-a1-proteinase inhibitor complex in some cystic fibrosis patients. *Biochim Biophys Acta* 1989; **993**: 137–42.
89 Shwachman H, Lebenthal E, Shaw K. Recurrent acute pancreatitis in patients with cystic fibrosis with normal pancreatic enzymes. *Paediatrics* 1975; **55**: 86–95.
90 Sips HJ, Class HW, Van Dongen JM, et al. Sucrase–isomaltase and cystic fibrosis. *J Inherited Metab Dis* 1985; **8**: 163–8.
91 MacLeod EP, Derbenwick JP, Snook JT. Comparison of pancreatic changes induced in rats by soybean and egg-white trypsin inhibitors fed with different levels of nitrogen. *J Nutr* 1972; **112**: 469–78.
92 Temler RS, Dormond CA, Simon E, Morel B. The effect on rat pancreas of feeding Kunitz soy bean trypsin inhibitor or a repeated injection of purified cholecystokinin. *Int J Vitam Nutr Res* 1982; **52**: 223.
93 Leach SD, Modlin IM, Scheele GA, Gorelick FS. Intracellular activation of digestive zymogens in rat pancreatic acini: stimulation by high doses of cholecystokinin. *J Clin Invest* 1991; **87**: 362–6.
94 Figarella C, Miszczuk-Jamskab, Barrett AJ. Possible lysosomal activation of pancreatic zymogens: activation of both human trypsinogens by cathepsin B and spontaneous acid activation of human trypsinogen 1. *Biol Chem Hoppe-Seyler* 1988; **369** (suppl): 293–8.
95 Figarella C, Basso D, Guy-Crotte O. Lysosomal enzyme activation of digestive enzymes during chronic pancreatitis? In: *Chronic Pancreatitis* (eds HG Beger, M Büchler, H Ditschuneit, P Malfertheiner) Springer-Verlag, Berlin, 1990, pp 134–9.
96 Steer M, Meldolesi J, Figarella C. Pancreatitis: the role of lysosomes. *Dig Dis Sci* 1984; **29**: 934–8.
97 Dodge JA. Determination of pancreatic and pulmonary status of cystic fibrosis. *Lancet* 1991; **337**: 54–5.
98 Dumur V, Gervais R, Rigot JM, et al. Abnormal distribution of CF delta F 508 allele in azoospermic men with congenital aplasia of epididymis and vas deferens. *Lancet* 1990; **336**: 512.
99 Gervais R, Dumur V, Rigot JM, et al. High frequency of the R117H cystic fibrosis mutation in patients with congenital absence of the vas deferens. *N Engl J Med* 1993; **328**: 446–7.
100 Dumur V, Lafitte JJ, Gervais R, et al. Abnormal distribution of cystic fibrosis delta F 508 allele in adults with chronic bronchial hypersecretion. *Lancet* 1990; **335**: 1340.
101 Gervais R, Lafitte JJ, Dumur V, et al. Sweat chloride and ΔF508 mutation in chronic bronchitis or bronchiectasis. *Lancet* 1993; **342**: 997.

## Chapter Fourteen

# Cytokines in Cystic Fibrosis

Dennis J. Shale
*Section of Respiratory Medicine, University of Wales College of Medicine, Llandough Hospital, Penarth, UK*

## INTRODUCTION

The inflammatory response is essentially protective to the host and comprises two major elements: the antigen-specific immune response mediated via the lymphoid system and the antigen-non-specific limb mediated by the macrophage system. The lungs are in a virtually unique situation, with a close association with the external environment, over a large surface area, and with a major vascular bed in close proximity. To cope with this potential for external assault the lung has developed a range of defence mechanisms in both the airways and the alveolar compartments.

The host response to short-term infection of the lungs, such as pneumonia, is extremely effective and usually leaves the lung undamaged. However, in more chronic conditions such as the adult respiratory distress syndrome (ARDS) and cystic fibrosis (CF), where there may be continued incitement to an inflammatory response, the lung may be injured as an 'innocent bystander'. Such infective–inflammatory injury affecting the lungs is a major factor determining survival in CF. In the UK, 85% of deaths in adults were due to lung disease[1].

Preservation of lung function by interventions that reduce the activity of the inflammatory response is a rational approach, whilst awaiting gene therapy, but to have an impact on injury requires a deeper knowledge of inflammatory

*Cystic Fibrosis—Current Topics, Volume 2.* Edited by J. A. Dodge, D. J. H. Brock and J. H. Widdicombe

mechanisms and their regulation. Cytokines are an expanding family of peptides which may act as autocrine, paracrine and endocrine intercellular signals. They are particularly important in regulating the host immune–inflammatory response to infection and cytokines such as the interleukins 1$\alpha$, 1$\beta$, 6 and 8 (IL-1$\alpha$, IL-1$\beta$, IL-6, IL-8), interferon $\gamma$ (IFN$\gamma$) and tumour necrosis factor $\alpha$ (TNF$\alpha$) are likely to be the key to understanding the inflammatory mechanisms underlying pulmonary injury in CF.

## THE POTENTIAL ROLE OF CYTOKINES IN LUNG DISEASE ASSOCIATED WITH CYSTIC FIBROSIS

Cytokines may have a variety of potential roles but the most probable ones are:

(1) The regulation of the local inflammatory response to infection.
(2) Regulation of the antibody response to infection.
(3) Direct injury to the airways.
(4) Indirect injury to the host.

This chapter will review these likely effects in the context of known features of the host–bacterium interaction in CF, though much of the role of cytokines remains speculative.

## PATHOPHYSIOLOGY OF LUNG DISEASE IN CYSTIC FIBROSIS

Changes in the structure of the airways are apparent within the first few days of life[2]. This occurs before any proven infective episodes, and consists of submucosal gland hypertrophy, duct obstruction and mucous cell hyperplasia[3]. Such changes are probably related to the background genetic defect and lead to viscous secretions, airways casts and obstruction, which may enhance colonization of the respiratory tract by microorganisms. Pulmonary infection, particularly viral infections, occurring in this setting during the first year of life are likely to add to the problem of airways obstruction by inducing a bronchiolar inflammatory response. The combination of obstruction with viral infection may be the nidus allowing bacterial infection to occur, leading to a vicious cycle of local infection and injury in the bronchiolar region[4]. This leads to mucus impaction, cyst formation and ultimately bronchiectasis which has been observed in children in the first two months of life[2,3]. Once initiated the vicious cycle will become an attritional process leading to lung destruction (Figure 1).

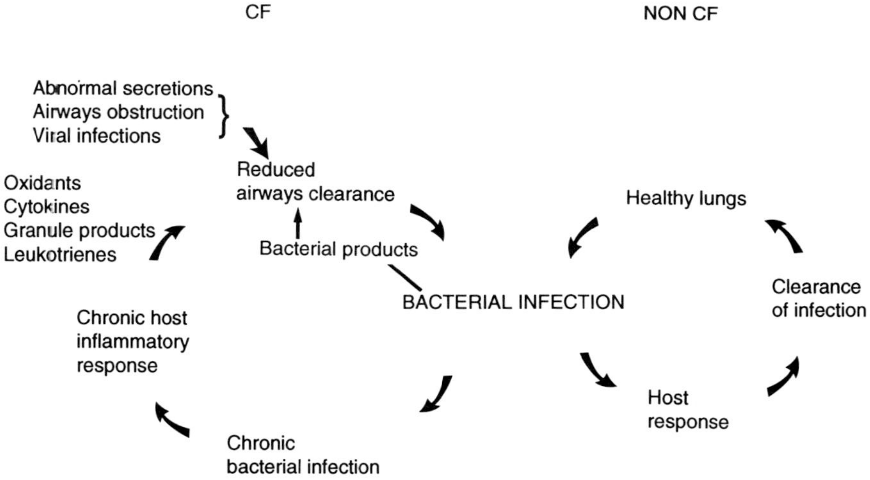


**Figure 1** The vicious cycle of infection and lung injury in cystic fibrosis

## BACTERIAL FACTORS

The main bacterial species causing chronic infection in the airways are generally of low virulence and mainly originate from the upper airways. They would not cause infection or colonize non-CF airways unless there were structural abnormalities causing reduced clearance or other impairment of local defence processes. The predominant bacteria in childhood are *Staphylococcus aureus*, *Haemophilus influenzae* and *Streptococcus pneumoniae*, with a steadily rising incidence of *Pseudomonas aeruginosa*[5].

It is likely that reduced clearance of lower respiratory tract secretions is a major factor in the colonization, with bacterial factors only being important at the time of the establishment of infection. Organisms such as *H. influenzae* and *Ps. aeruginosa* produce a range of so-called 'virulence factors' which probably enhance their likelihood of staying within the respiratory tract[6,7] (Table 1).

Specific products damaging to the airways include exotoxin A and exoenzyme S, leucocidin, phospholipase, lipase and alkaline phosphatase[8]. Proteolytic enzymes capable of degrading lung connective tissue may also act like virulence factors and these include proteinases, elastase, alkaline proteinase and the Las A fragment[9,10]. Other factors include alginate, which may physically block phagocytosis and lipopolysaccharide, a potent inducer of the host inflammatory response and regulator of the immune response. *Ps. aeruginosa* cells are somewhat distant from the respiratory tract cells, being largely bound to disaccharide sites in the mucin layer[11]. Hence, direct airways

**Table 1** Potential virulence factors of *Pseudomonas aeruginosa*

| | |
|---|---|
| Exotoxin A | Cytotoxin |
| Exoenzyme S | Pili |
| Alkaline proteinase | Lipopolysaccharide |
| Elastase | Exopolysaccharide |
| Las A fragment | Glycolipids |
| Phospholipase | Pigments |
| Lipase | Flagella |
| Alkaline phosphatase | Siderophore |

injury by bacterial products may be small, but they may activate inflammatory cells directly or secondarily via immune complex formation[12,13].

Supporting this notion is the characteristic switch to the mucoid phenotype by *Ps. aeruginosa* in the airways of patients with CF, which is often associated with a reduction in the secretion of other exoproducts. This ability to switch phenotype after relatively short periods of time may enhance retention, but suggests a minor role for bacterial exoproducts as virulence factors in the maintenance of colonization. In chronic infection there is production of antibodies to bacterial products[12–17], in particular, to alkaline proteinase, elastase, exotoxin A, phospholipase C, outer membrane proteins, lipopolysaccharide, alginate and exoenzyme S[12,13].

Specific antibodies for alkaline proteinase and elastase have neutralizing capacity *in vitro*[17]. Both enzymes occurred in bronchoalveolar lavage at the onset of *Ps. aeruginosa* infection, before antibodies have developed[18], but in chronic infection were undetectable by radioimmunoassay, suggesting either their absence or a concentration too low to have pathophysiological relevance[19,20] Immune complexes to these enzymes have been demonstrated, but their relevance to the pathophysiology of lung injury in CF remains unknown. This also supports the contention that bacterial factors have their major impact at the establishment of chronic infection.

## THE EFFECTS OF *PSEUDOMONAS AERUGINOSA* EXOPRODUCTS ON CYTOKINES (Figure 2)

Elastase and alkaline protease produced by *Ps. aeruginosa* may have a direct effect on the bioactivity of IL-2, IFN$\gamma$ and TNF$\alpha$. Most data relate to *in vitro* studies and the *in vivo* implications are largely unknown, though the potential for such effects remains to be disproved.

IL-2 is an important T cell growth factor which is inactivated by both elastase and alkaline protease[21], whilst the pigment pyocyanin inhibits both

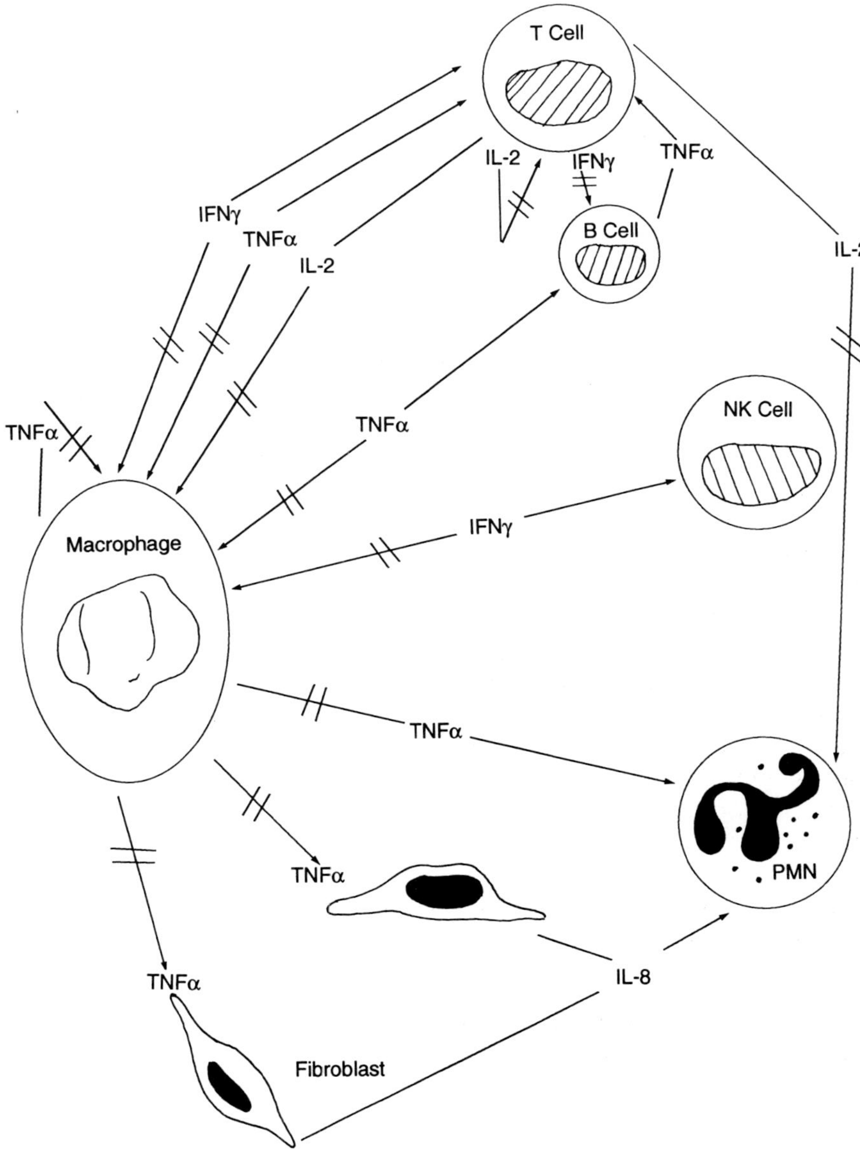


**Figure 2** All these interruptions may be circumvented by other parts of the cytokine network, e.g. IL – 1$\beta$ is still active in all the macrophage links to other cells

IL-2 production and its receptor expression by T cells[22,23]. Hence, there is potential for disruption of T cell-mediated immunity[24]. Several of the functions of IFN$\gamma$ may be impaired by proteolytic enzymes[24-27]. Destruction of IFN$\gamma$ may downregulate T cell function and in concert with the down-regulation of other pro-T cell cytokines this may have impact on the immune response[28]. Inhibition of IFN$\gamma$ activity might also affect bacterial killing by macrophages, as IFN$\gamma$ causes increased phago-lysosome fusion and triggers oxygen-independent killing and oxygen radical formation[29,30] This mechanism may or may not be important *in vivo* because IFN$\gamma$ has a reverse effect with inhibition of phagocytosis and killing of *Ps. aeruginosa* when the bacteria are extracellular[30]. Currently, the *in vivo* relevance of these observations is unknown in CF where the host develops a florid immunoinflammatory response.

Perhaps more important is the potential for the disruption of cytokine networks such as that leading to the influx of circulating neutrophils into the lung and their activation during the passage from the circulation to the air space[27]. Macrophage production of TNF$\alpha$ is important as a direct activator of neutrophils and secondarily as a co-stimulator with IL-1$\beta$ of the production and release of IL-8 by lung epithelial type II cells and fibroblasts[31]. Again, the potential for this effect is suggested by various *in vitro* studies but it remains to be proved to be an effective mechanism *in vivo*.

In summary, the role of bacterial products in progressive lung injury in CF remains unclear, but the current consensus is that direct injury is unlikely to be a major factor. However, the possibility remains that the low-level production of such bacterial products may drive the inflammatory response leading to indirect injury. The importance of bacterial interaction with specific cytokines and the potential impact of this on the host inflammatory response is currently unknown.

## HOST FACTORS

Lung injury and, ultimately, survival in CF are largely dependent on the host defence response to bacteria and other infective agents in the airways. The inability to clear airway infections leads to a sustained host response.

The neutrophil is considered a key mediator of injury[32], though other cells and humoral mediators, such as cytokines released from a variety of cells including macrophages, T lymphocytes, fibroblasts, endothelial and epithelial cells, may directly cause injury[33-35]. However, cytokines, functioning as autocrine and paracrine mediators, may have a subtle regulatory role on the inflammatory response by controlling neutrophil function[36,37]. The neutrophil produces over 30 injurious products from the cell membrane *de novo* and from preformed granules. There is no evidence of a functional defect in neutrophil function in CF and little evidence to support full activation of inflammatory cells in the circulation. Hence, the protective but potentially very injurious neutrophil only becomes fully activated in the close vicinity of the infected airway.

Phagocytosis of bacteria induces production of superoxide and its metabolites (hypochlorous acid, hydroxyl ion and hydrogen peroxide) which are capable of cellular destruction and the oxygenation of antiproteinases, such as $\alpha_1$-antitrypsin[38,39]. Preformed cationic proteins may damage cells, and proteolytic enzymes such as neutrophil elastase and cathepsins are particularly destructive to lung connective tissue, which is largely collagens, elastin and fibronectin[40,41]. Once the integrity of the overlying airways mucosa is breached, exposure of connective tissue to elastase activity, likely to be present in epithelial lining fluid or the sol phase of sputum, occurs with little or no antiproteinase activity in the vicinity.

## THE ROLE OF CYTOKINES IN ANTIBODY PRODUCTION

A network of cytokines regulates the function of T and B lymphocytes and antibody synthesis[42] (Table 2). In CF this process may follow traditional pathways or may be abnormal, probably secondary to continued bacterial stimulation. This latter possibility would explain the observations that lipopolysaccharide (LPS) from *Ps. aeruginosa* can downregulate the antibody response to pneumococcal antigen in the mouse. LPS is the most biologically active product of *Ps. aeruginosa*. It is a bacterial cell wall component and has distinct antigenic and immunomodulatory effects, making it responsible for the majority of the systemic and pathophysiological effects of infection.

Immunomodulation by LPS can occur via the whole molecule or the lipid A portion. Effects that have been described include B cell mutagenicity, induction of polyclonal antibody synthesis, immunogenicity, adjuvant activity, macrophage inhibition and IL-1$\beta$, IL-6 and TNF$\alpha$ secretion[43,44]. The precise balance of these various functions depends very much on the bacterial species; with LPS derived from *Ps. aeruginosa* there may be downregulation of antibody production in mice. However, other deficits may occur in what is clearly a complex interacting series of processes. However, there is no evidence of impairment of antibody production in CF, with most patients exhibiting a polyclonal hypergammaglobulinaemia directed at many bacterial antigens[12–20].

The antibody response seen in CF is the integrated outcome of a variety of interrelated factors, which include the concentration, the kinetics and temporal relationships of various cytokines (IFN$\gamma$, IL-2) which may lead to additive, antagonistic or synergistic effects. This is further complicated by the

**Table 2** Effects of cytokines likely to be involved in CF lung disease

| | |
|---|---|
| TNF$\alpha$ | Fever, tissue injury, anorexia, catabolic state<br>Increased acute-phase proteins, IL-1$\alpha$, IL-1$\beta$, IL-6, IL-8, IFN$\gamma$<br>Gluconeogenesis, lipolysis, adrenaline, cortisol release |
| IL-1$\alpha$ and $\beta$ | Fever, anorexia, activation of T and B cells<br>Increased acute-phase proteins, IL-2, IL-6, IL-8, ACTH<br>Increased hepatic protein synthesis |
| IL-2 | Clonal expansion of antigen specific T cells; augmentation of neutrophil and macrophage activity<br>Anorexia |
| IL-6 | Fever, anorexia, catabolic state<br>Increased acute-phase proteins, expression of TNF$\alpha$ and IL-1$\beta$<br>Increased IL-2 receptor expression<br>Stimulation of B cells to differentiate and secrete IgG |
| IL-8 | Increased expression of neutrophil adhesion molecules CD11c/CD18<br>Chemotactic for neutrophils |
| IL-10 | Reduced expression of TNF$\alpha$, IL-1$\beta$, IL-6 and IL-8<br>Increased production of IL-1RA |
| IFN$\gamma$ | Increased toxicity of TNF$\alpha$, IL-1$\beta$ secretion<br>Catabolic state; T cell regulation |

autocrine and paracrine induction of cytokine secretion and receptor expression, and also the maturation state of B cells. The presence of resting or previously activated cells is essential for a continued and effective antibody response.

In CF some of these processes may be out of balance, leading to the inappropriate antibody isotype or subclass patterns reported in some patients with chronic *Ps. aeruginosa* infections[43]. The precise components and their relative importance in the cytokine network is unclear, largely because of the overlapping functions, but IFN$\gamma$ has a degree of specificity relating to antibody isotype expression, it regulates $IgG_{2A}$ synthesis; IL-4 regulates $IgG_1$ and IgE, whilst IL-5 and transforming growth factor $\beta$ have an effect on IgA and IgM synthesis.

## CYTOKINE ACTIVITY IN THE INFLAMMATORY RESPONSE IN CYSTIC FIBROSIS

IL-1$\alpha$, IL-1$\beta$, IL-6, IL-8 and TNF$\alpha$ are all associated with inflammatory activity. All are produced by cells of the monocyte macrophage series, though other cells may produce them, either in response to bacterial products or secondary to other cytokine stimulation. This allows for the amplification of the inflammatory response, e.g. TNF$\alpha$ induces IL-1$\beta$ synthesis and secretion; and acts synergistically with IFN$\gamma$ to induce MHC class I and II expression on T lymphocytes. TNF$\alpha$ has a range of overlapping biological functions with other cytokines, particularly IL-1$\beta$ (Table 2). In many respects TNF$\alpha$ and IL-1$\beta$ should be considered as proximal or primary cytokines as they are secreted early in response to infection and influence the pattern of later cytokine secretion in the inflammatory response.

## REGULATION OF NEUTROPHIL RECRUITMENT TO THE LUNG IN CYSTIC FIBROSIS

The neutrophil is considered the main effector cell of injury in the lung. Control of its recruitment from the vascular space into the interstitium and finally the airways is of considerable importance in understanding the injury process in CF. Full understanding of these events might indicate useful therapeutic interventions. The events involved in recruitment from the circulation to the lung compartment include: activation of endothelial cells and the expression of neutrophil adhesion molecule receptors; activation of neutrophils and the expression of endothelium adhesion molecule receptors; neutrophil–endothelial cell adhesion; neutrophil diapedesis and migration within the extravascular space.

There is considerable evidence that much of this process is controlled by a network of interacting cytokines and that this may be a common mechanism active in many forms of lung disease.

## NEUTROPHIL ADHESION MOLECULES

Adhesion molecules expressed on the cell membrane of the neutrophil belong to two interacting groups, the $\beta$-integrins and the selectins (Table 3). $\beta$-integrin adhesion molecules are a family of heterodimeric glycoproteins only expressed in the plasma membrane of leucocytes. Each molecule consists of two chains: a variable amino acid sequence $\alpha$-chain and a constant sequence $\beta$-chain. They form clusters with the following designations: CD11a/CD18, CD11b/CD18 and CD11c/CD18. CD11b/CD18 is the major $\beta$-integrin associated with neutrophils and is expressed in a sequestered form in secondary and tertiary granules[45,46]. CD11a/CD18 is expressed by all leucocytes and may be less important for neutrophil adhesion than CD11b/CD18. When activated by factors such as IL-1$\beta$, TNF$\alpha$ and IL-8 there is rapid translocation of the CD11b/CD18 molecule to the cell surface[45,46]. The natural ligand or receptor for this complex is the split product of complement iC3b and the adhesion

**Table 3** Adhesion molecules active in neutrophil recruitment

| Neutrophils | Endothelial cells |
|---|---|
| β-Integrins | ICAM-1[a] |
| CD11a/CD18<br>CD11b/CD18[a] | |
| Selectins (LEC-CAMs) | Selectins |
| L selectin | |
| E selectin[a] | E selectin[a] |
| P selectin | P selectin |

[a]Adhesion factors that are upregulated by cytokine activity.

molecule 1 (ICAM-1), which is constitutively expressed on endothelial cells. Specific antibodies to either the CD11b or the CD18 component reduce neutrophil-dependent vascular permeability and haemorrhage and neutrophil accumulation in animal models[47–49].

The selectins, also known as LEC-CAMs (lectin, epidermal growth factor, complement, cellular adhesion molecules), are also important in neutrophil–endothelial adhesion[50]. Three members of the selectin family appear to be important: L selectin, E selectin and P selectin. L selectin is expressed on the surface of leucocytes constitutively, whilst E selectin expression can be induced by the presence of endotoxin, TNFα or IL-1β. P selectin is expressed on the surface after release either from platelets or endothelial cells[51]. It appears that the binding of neutrophils to the endothelium is dependent on both selectin and integrin molecules. It has been proposed that neutrophil-expressed L selectin interacts with activated endothelium as a primary event leading to margination or rolling when there are high shear force conditions in the capillary circulation. Neutrophil-expressed β-integrins appear to have no effect during this early phase of margination but are essential to ensure stable intravascular adhesion, leading then to transendothelial migration[52].

## ENDOTHELIAL CELL-DERIVED ADHESION MOLECULES

The major counter-receptor for the CD11b/CD18 and the CD11a/CD18 β-integrins expressed on the neutrophil is ICAM-1. This receptor is constitutively expressed by endothelial cells on their surface and increases in response to

LPS, TNF$\alpha$ and IL-1$\beta$[45,46]. It also occurs on the surface of mononuclear phagocytes, fibroblasts and epithelial cells, which is of potential interest in the setting of the chronic inflammatory state in CF. Neutralizing antibodies to the ICAM-1 molecule in animal models have been shown to be as effective as anti-$\beta$-integrin monoclonal antibodies in attenuating neutrophil-dependent lung injury.

Selectin E in particular is also expressed by surface endothelial cells in response to LPS, TNF$\alpha$ or IL-1[50] (Table 3). This appears to be very rapid expression and occurs more quickly than the expression of ICAM-1. P selectin is also rapidly mobilized to the surface of the endothelial cells following exposure to a variety of factors. Both selectins will promote neutrophil adhesion, which is dependent upon recognition of elements of the Lewis X oligosaccharide associated with the L selectin molecule[53]. This further supports the suggestion that the selectins are most important in the early margination of neutrophils in the vascular beds of the lung and this provides a ligand–receptor relationship for this event.

Combination of what is known of neutrophil and endothelial cell adhesion molecules allows the development of a hypothesis that neutrophil migration into the lung is largely under the control of a network of cytokines which, therefore, regulates much of the inflammatory injury process in CF. The signal may progress from the ingestion of bacteria by pulmonary macrophages, probably in the airways, which synthesize and secrete TNF$\alpha$, IL-1$\beta$, IL-6 and IL-8. Other cells, such as epithelial cells and pulmonary fibroblasts, may also respond to the stimulation by TNF$\alpha$ and IL-1$\beta$ to produce more IL-8 and thus generate a chemotactic gradient which would attract neutrophils across the extravascular space. IL-8 would also induce the expression of CD11b/CD18 on the surface of neutrophils. Thus IL-8 in concert with TNF$\alpha$ and IL-1$\beta$ increases the expression of adhesion factors for neutrophils and endothelial cells. This sets up a process that enhances neutrophil adhesion, activation, margination, diapedesis and extravascular migration to sites of infection within the lung. This hypothesis is largely based on the concept that TNF$\alpha$ and IL-1$\beta$ are important proximal or early-response cytokines that regulate the generation of distal mediators and develop a complex or network which controls the influx of neutrophils into the lung. This is, perhaps, a simplified version of what happens but is a model supported by studies of neutrophil migration into the lung from the circulation using intravascular stimulation, such as LPS and alveolitis induced by the intratracheal administration of LPS or IL-1$\beta$.

TNF$\alpha$ and IL-1$\beta$ have multiple effects, many overlapping and some synergistic, on cellular function. These effects in the lung in CF are important mediators of the early response and thereby regulate the initiation, maintenance and severity of tissue injury, as well as localizing infection and initiating healing[54–57].

## FACTORS AFFECTING CYTOKINE ACTIVITY

The preceding paragraphs describe a purely positive impact of cytokines on the host response. It should be remembered that inhibiting factors may act either directly or by secondary inhibiting actions on other cytokines. For TNF$\alpha$, both the 55 and 75 kDa soluble receptors may act as neutralizing factors[58-60]. The kinetics of TNF$\alpha$ and its soluble receptors, and the distribution of TNF$\alpha$ molecules between these and cell-related receptors, are currently unknown. However, this may be an important regulatory mechanism and part of the process that allows an enormous burden of chronic bacterial infection to be so well localized within the lung in CF. Other cytokines, such as IL-8, appear to have receptor clearance mechanisms, with a low-affinity IL-1$\beta$ and IL-8 receptor on erythrocytes[61]. Both IL-8 and TNF$\alpha$ may also be bound by immunoglobulins present in the circulation of healthy individuals, with higher levels or acute increases during periods of infection[62,63]. IL-1 also has a receptor antagonist, IL-1RA, a 22 kDa polypeptide with a high degree of molecular homology with IL-1$\beta$[57]. This is produced by monocytes in a response to LPS and other stimuli. Its function appears to be that of a competitive receptor antagonist with no agonist activity. *In vitro*, it will inhibit IL-1-induced neutrophil adhesion to endothelial cells and in animal models of LPS-induced neutrophilic alveolitis it will attenuate injury[64-66]. Data supporting such a hypothesis is largely based on *in vitro* studies with some animal work involved, but can be supported partially by evidence obtained in patients with CF.

## EVIDENCE OF CYTOKINE ACTIVITY IN PATIENTS WITH CYSTIC FIBROSIS

IL-1$\alpha$, IL-1$\beta$, IFN$\alpha$ and TNF$\alpha$ were detected in plasma and compared with levels of neutrophil elastase–$\alpha_1$-antiproteinase complex (NEAPC) in 25 patients with CF with a mean age of 15 years (range 6–35 years)[67]. They had a spectrum of severity of disease with a mean 19% reduction from ideal weight (0–32%). The mean erythrocyte sedimentation rate was 41 mm/h (range 2–77) and the mean white blood cell count 14 100 (range 5600–38 700/$\mu$l). Three patients were studied twice: two with intervals of two and five months between sampling and the other with a 3.5-year interval. No real differences were demonstrated for cytokine levels in these paired samples but the group was small and the intervals too different to draw valid conclusions. Comparison of 22 patients studied prior to antibiotic treatment and six following antibiotics revealed no significant differences between circulating levels of IL-1$\alpha$, IL-1$\beta$ and TNF$\alpha$, which was supported by the lack of difference for plasma NEAPC, suggesting similar levels of inflammatory activity. This observation has little validity due to the small group size and non-paired observation. Whole group comparisons for the three cytokines showed significantly greater levels in CF than control subjects. Again, partly from design, there was no relationship to disease staging; the four groups compared comprised 17, seven, three and one subject each. For the whole group there was no relationship between TNFα and NEAPC or between any of the cytokines and the plasma IgG concentrations. Notwithstanding these limitations, there was evidence of immunoreactive cytokines relevant to the upregulation of the inflammatory response and the activation of cells, such as the neutrophil, in the circulation of patients with CF and chronic pulmonary infection. Furthermore, these particular cytokines might be metabolically active and have an impact on the cachexia associated with CF[67] (Tables 2, 4 and 5).

**Table 4** Cellular/organ responses to TNFα

| | |
|---|---|
| Myocyte | Increased lactate production<br>Loss of glycogen and protein<br>Reduction of membrane potential |
| Adipocyte | Reduced expression of lipoprotein lipase<br>Increased release of free fatty acids and glycerol |
| Hepatocyte | Increased lipogenesis<br>Increased synthesis of acute-phase proteins<br>Increased uptake of amino acids under glucagon medication |
| Endothelial cells | Increased water and albumin permeability<br>IL-1β release<br>IL-8 release<br>Increased adhesion molecule expression<br>Increased surface pro-coagulant activity |
| Pituitary | Increased release of ACTH and prolactin |

**Table 5** Secondary mediators of TNFα effects

| | |
|---|---|
| Cytokines | IL-1α, IL-1β, IL-6, IL-8, IFNγ |
| Eicosanoids | Prostaglandins and leukotrienes |
| Counter-regulatory hormones | Adrenaline, cortisol, glucagon, ACTH |
| Others | Platelet-activating factor<br>Nitric oxide<br>IL-1RA<br>TNFα receptors (55 and 75 kDa) |

Support for these findings came from a study in 14 adults with CF (aged 14–22 years) and chronically infected with *Ps. aeruginosa*. Immunoreactive TNF$\alpha$, CRP, a surrogate marker of IL-6, and NEAPC were measured prior to the start of a course of antibiotics for an exacerbation of respiratory symptoms and after two weeks of treatment[68]. Further observations were made over a 12–14-month period yielding 189 samples from the same patients. In 129 of these samples immunoreactive TNF$\alpha$ was greater than the upper 95% confidence interval for healthy subjects (65 pg/ml ≡ 2.6 U/ml). At the commencement of antibiotic treatment median concentrations of TNF$\alpha$, CRP and NEAPC in plasma were greater than in a control population of healthy subjects. At the end of treatment all three indicators of inflammatory activity were reduced, with a median TNF$\alpha$ concentration of 120 pg/ml ≡ 4.8 U/ml. In three patients TNF$\alpha$ concentrations fell to within the 95% confidence intervals of the healthy subjects and this was mirrored by a similar fall in NEAPC for three of the patients. Hence, at the end of an antibiotic course, though there was a reduction in two markers of the local inflammatory process in the lung and a systemic indicator of inflammatory activity, the former two markers remained elevated for the majority of patients. When clinically stable, similar numbers of patients showed further elevation of TNF$\alpha$ and of NEAPC, with smaller increases in CRP. These findings suggest that cytokine networks may be active in CF and remain so following currently accepted periods of antibiotic treatment. Failure to suppress the inflammatory response probably indicates continuous lung injury in chronically infected patients. This is supported by the finding that at some point during the study period all 14 patients had TNF$\alpha$ values greater than the 95% confidence intervals for normal subjects, and 11 had median values for a series of samples in excess of the upper 95% confidence interval for TNF$\alpha$, NEAPC and for CRP[68].

In contrast, in 12 patients aged 10–46 years compared with 12 age- and sex-matched controls less clear-cut results were found, suggesting that circulating cytokines may be found less frequently[69]. There were marked differences between the populations studied, with only nine having cultured *Ps. aeruginosa* in the previous six months; it was not stated if they were chronically colonized, and only five were in clinical exacerbation. Interestingly, immunoreactive TNF$\alpha$ was detected in the plasma of only one patient but in five of the 12 control subjects. In neither group was immunoreactive IL-1$\alpha$ or IL-1$\beta$ detected in contrast to the earlier report[67]. Recovery of added recombinant TNF$\alpha$ from the plasma was virtually 100%, suggesting that the assay was capable of detecting TNF$\alpha$ in plasma. However, there was no increase in the concentration of TNF$\alpha$ in heparinized blood, which has been reported to increase TNF$\alpha$ release directly by monocytes. It is unknown why these discrepancies have occurred and explanations, such as *Pseudomonas* LPS being relatively weak or not being present in large quantities in the lung, are speculative. Other suggestions include the raised $\alpha_1$-antiproteinase suppressing

TNF$\alpha$ secretion by leucocytes as demonstrated *in vitro*, differences in the selection of control groups and differences between the assays used.

Explanation of differences in the detection of various cytokines is complicated by theoretical considerations, such as in which body compartments individual cytokines should be sought and the temporal patterns of secretion in chronic infection. In 19 children with CF, mean age 1.87 years, bronchoalveolar lavage (BAL) content was compared with 13 disease controls of average age 1.4 years[70]. Ten of the 21 CF bronchoalveolar lavages yielded $> 10^5$ pathogenic organisms per millilitre. There was no difference in levels of IL-1$\beta$ or IL-1 activity (IL-1$\alpha$ and IL-1$\beta$ plus other factors non-specifically detected by the D10.G4.1 proliferation assay) compared with the disease control group. A significant difference occurred in the CF group when comparing infection with no infection on the basis of bacterial colony counts for both immunoreactive IL-1$\beta$ and IL-1 activity. Hence, the relationship of the cytokine concentration in BAL was to the presence of infection, and not the diagnostic category, and IL-1 activity was also significantly related to the lavage neutrophil count.

Other studies relating to serum or plasma cytokines have reported that prior to death there is a persistent and progressive increase in TNF$\alpha$ in plasma which is mirrored by changes in CRP and NEAPC, suggesting an enhanced level of inflammatory activity[71]. In six patients immunoreactive TNF$\alpha$ levels, measured in the last week of life, were as great as those reported in patients with ARDS. This group have also reported a downregulation of the TNF$\alpha$ secretory response of circulating monocytes to *Escherichia coli* LPS *in vitro*[72]. Downregulation occurred at the time of a clinical exacerbation with raised circulating levels of immunoreactive TNF$\alpha$ and was reversed by 14 days of antibiotic treatment for *Ps. aeruginosa*, at which time circulating levels of TNF$\alpha$ had decreased as previously reported. This may represent a protective mechanism to limit the systemic impact of a large but localized bacterial infection. Confirmation of this downregulation comes from *in vitro* studies with phytohaemagglutinin and zymosan[73,74]. In addition, zymosan also reduced IL-1$\beta$ secretion, adding further support to a homeostatic process of benefit to the host. The understanding of these potential mechanisms is further complicated by the demonstration that IL-1RA and IL-6 are elevated in the plasma of patients with undetectable IL-1$\alpha$, IL-1$\beta$, IL-8 or TNF$\alpha$ immunoreactivity[73].

Some clarification comes from the demonstration of variable levels of immunoreactive TNF$\alpha$ and IL-1$\beta$ in the plasma of patients with CF during a period of respiratory stability, but with a marked increase in those patients with a pulmonary and nutritional deterioration[75]. However, IL-6 was not detected as previously reported[73,76].

Increased mRNA for TNF$\alpha$ occurred in the peripheral blood mononuclear cells of patients with nutritional and pulmonary deterioration when compared with those of patients in a stable phase[75]. How this relates to the observations of plasma TNFα levels being elevated at the time of an exacerbation and reduced monocyte-induced secretion of TNFα is unknown. Apparently consistent results for TNFα and inconsistent results for various cytokines in plasma being related to the disease state need to be considered in light of negative reports. Absence of immunoreactive IL-1α, IL-1β, IL-6 and TNFα or IL-1RA in plasma was associated with detection of all at high concentration in sputum[76]. However, deteriorating pulmonary function was related to a raised plasma IL-1RA and longitudinal comparison suggested that IL-1RA concentration was greater in those with poorer pulmonary function, though this was a weak relationship. Supportive data of increased plasma IL-1RA clarify this finding except that the increase in IL-6 with IL-1RA was not consistent between the two research groups[73,76].

The difficulties of measuring cytokines in plasma and inferring pathophysiological significance from changes detected are further emphasized by the measurement of soluble IL-2 receptor (sIL-2R) in plasma as an index of the antigen-specific immune response and T cell function in particular[77]. In a cross-sectional survey of 115 children sIL-2R was raised, suggesting increased T cell activity, which might have been evident before clinical evidence of infection. The latter observation is hard to sustain because in stratified age groups significantly raised levels of sIL-2R were only present in those over the age of four. A link to infection occurred in children over the age of 12 years, where there was a significant increase in circulating sIL-2R in those with acute infection compared to those without, though there was no definition given of what constituted an acute infection. There was no difference in the younger groups, which may be related to the size of groups, ranging from 2 to 14 subjects in those with infection. There was, interestingly, no relationship to *Ps. aeruginosa* infection, or markers of disease activity: Shwachman score, lung function or IgM, IgG, IgA or IgE levels.

Thus, whichever compartment, either the circulation or bronchial epithelial lining fluid collected as BAL or sputum, there is still the problem of defining and understanding cytokine networks. Most of this difficulty is due to the simple questions being asked, which do not consider the temporal relationship of cytokine networks or receptor–inhibitor interactions which are largely unknown and at present possibly undefinable *in vivo* in patients with CF.

## THE METABOLIC IMPLICATIONS OF CYTOKINE FUNCTION

Many cytokines, including IL-1β, IL-6, TNFα and the interferons, have metabolic effects (Tables 2, 4 and 5). TNFα, also known as cachectin, is a potentially important factor in the deleterious systemic effects of chronic pulmonary infection. There is gathering evidence of such an effect and strong support comes from a comparison with acute infective states. Increased circulating concentrations of both bio- and immunoreactive TNF$\alpha$ have been reported in Gram-negative septicaemia[78], ARDS related to sepsis[79], chronic parasitic infections and in cerebral malaria[80,81]. Raised circulating concentrations of TNF$\alpha$ in animals have been associated with anorexia, weight loss and hypertriglyceridaemia[82].

Intravenous infusion of TNF$\alpha$ in man raises acute-phase proteins, increases resting energy expenditure (REE) and increases proteolysis, lipolysis and anorexia[83,84] (Table 4). Whether such effects are sustained in states associated with chronically elevated TNF$\alpha$ is unclear. In particular the overlapping effects of cytokines suggest that effects may be due to more than a single agent (Table 2).

In CF with chronic pulmonary infection, immunoreactive TNF$\alpha$ concentrations may be raised in plasma and have some biological activity[68]. Although TNF$\alpha$ concentrations may be reduced after two weeks' anti-pseudomonal antibiotic therapy they often remain increased compared to levels in healthy controls. This has important implications in that levels continue to increase when patients are clinically stable. Patients with CF tend to be underweight, with an elevated REE, and are often in negative energy and nitrogen balance, despite dietary supplementation and pancreatic enzyme replacement therapy[85]. Some of these features, including the cachexia and alterations in intermediary metabolism, could be due to the effects of TNF$\alpha$ and other metabolically active cytokines acting on peripheral tissues in an endocrine fashion or, secondarily, by induction of counter-regulatory hormone secretion[86] (Tables 2, 4 and 5). In addition, it is possible that the gene defect may also have an effect on energy expenditure and also that the work of breathing in patients with severely damaged lungs may also raise energy requirements[86,87].

Increased circulating immunoreactive TNF$\alpha$ was associated with measures of body wasting and abnormal intermediary metabolism in patients with CF[86]. REE ranged from normal to approximately 150% of predicted, confirming observations previously made in such patients. Statistically, significant relationships between circulating immunoreactive TNF$\alpha$, REE and arm muscle area suggested some element of causality between TNF$\alpha$ and cachexia.

The elevation of TNF$\alpha$ in the circulation was mirrored by raised levels of CRP, indicating a cytokine-mediated (IL-1$\beta$, IL-6 and TNF$\alpha$) systemic acute-phase response to severe pulmonary sepsis in these clinically stable patients (Table 2). This was also supported by earlier data from the same group showing similar patterns of changes in circulating CRP, TNF$\alpha$ and NEAPC[68]. Elevated levels of adrenaline, glycerol and non-esterified fatty acids, with relationships between TNF$\alpha$, adrenaline and non-esterified fatty acids, suggest a potential pathogenetic link between cytokine secretion, particularly TNF$\alpha$, and the systemic consequences of chronic localized pulmonary infection in CF. A hypothesis was developed that suggested mediators of the inflammatory response may well modulate the host metabolic response to injury and infection. If proven to be so, the poor nutritional state associated with increased morbidity and mortality in CF, and lung injury, also associated with a reduced survival, may be part of a single process, and new strategies of treatment aimed at reducing cytokine production or activity may help in the future management of CF.

## PROBLEMS WITH THE MEASUREMENT OF CYTOKINES

Cytokines can be detected in the secretions of the airways, bronchial tissue and the circulation. It remains unclear which compartment accurately reflects the pattern of activity of cytokines, though it is assumed to be the tissue compartment, which is the least accessible. Hence, cytokines have been measured in fluids from accessible locations, such as the circulation, bronchial epithelial lining fluid or sputum. The same criticism that changes may not accurately reflect those at the site of injury can be levelled at measurements made in both vascular and airway compartments.

Serum or plasma has the theoretical advantage of being the origin of various inflammatory cells and contains humoral signals up-regulating the inflammatory response systemically. This is a reasonable notion, but such cells are unlikely to be fully activated during the processes of margination and migration into the tissue compartment. In addition, the potential for back-diffusion into capillaries with greater permeability than usual is unknown. The analogous situation occurs in asthma, where a variety of mediators have been demonstrated in the circulation.

The detection of cytokines in sputum is potentially confounded by sputum not being homogeneous, even from the same patient over short periods of time. In addition, proteolytic enzymes and other constituents such as mucus may damage or non-specifically bind mediators.

However, the main factor causing discrepancies in the reported levels of cytokines is probably differences in the assay methods used. TNF$\alpha$ will be used as a representative cytokine, but there is no reason to believe that the problems to be discussed are unique to TNF$\alpha$. Bioassays for TNF$\alpha$ utilizing various cell lines have been described[88–94]. An inherent problem is that bioassays are less specific, may not reflect the physiologically relevant response to cytokine activity and may have high levels of inherent variation due to the effects of repeated passage on the cellular response to cytokines. Bioassays are also likely to be confounded by the presence of naturally occurring inhibitors to the action of cytokines. In addition, the results from different cell lines are not comparable. Hence, the major problem is one of poor reproducibility, non-specificity, high cost and a low capacity for processing samples.

Immunoassays have many advantages, chiefly of low cost, high reproducibility, a high volume through-put of samples and a high specificity based on the antibodies used. However, the specificity of an antibody is dependent upon the nature of the pure cytokine to which it was raised[92,93]. Due to the need to measure cytokines in clinical samples, immunoassays have been devised using local resources based on monoclonal and polyclonal antibodies as well as the use of commercially available assay kits. Inherent in this development has been a lack of standardization between laboratories which makes comparisons of data difficult. There are very wide discrepancies between laboratories for the measurement of TNF$\alpha$ in various body fluids. Such discrepancies are important as they may have implications for the understanding of the role of given cytokines in the pathophysiology of human disease and also the application of specific therapies aimed at reducing or altering the activity of a given cytokine.

These difficulties are evident when comparing the reported levels of TNF$\alpha$ in serum. In apparently healthy individuals TNF$\alpha$ ranges from $<10$ to 6400 pg/ml[95–100]. This wide variation, seen both in immuno- and bioassays, probably relates largely to differences in assay methods and sensitivities, although the collection of blood and handling of samples and the definition of a healthy population may be additional factors. Currently, there is apparent overlap between healthy individuals and patient groups.

High circulating levels of TNF$\alpha$ occur in various acute systemic bacterial and parasitic disorders[78–81]. However, in chronic inflammatory–infective states, such as CF, lower or undetectable levels are reported. The problem of comparing results between different laboratories is evident with TNF$\alpha$ levels in CF. TNF$\alpha$ was detected in plasma by both radioimmunoassay and enzyme-linked immunosorbent assay (ELISA) techniques[67,68]. With the latter assay using a monoclonal and a polyclonal antibody, both with neutralizing activity in the WEHI-164 clone 13 bioassay, TNF$\alpha$ was detectable both in healthy controls and in patients with CF and chronic pulmonary infection. However, these data have been questioned by workers unable to repeat these findings[69,76]

It is likely these differences in CF, as discussed earlier, are largely due to differences in the sensitivity of the assays, which is mainly dependent on the antibodies used and the protocol for the assay rather than discrepancies in clinical selection of patients. This view is supported by a similar finding in ARDS, where four antibody-based assays for TNF$\alpha$ gave large discrepancies in absolute levels measured and in detection levels between assays[101]. It is most likely that the different antibodies used in immunoassays have a confounding effect due to the variability in epitope specificity and affinity characteristics for sites on the TNF$\alpha$ molecule.

Some problems remain, however, particularly in CF, as not all laboratories have been able to substantiate the raised levels of TNF-$\alpha$ reported and there is no evidence that the TNF$\alpha$ in the circulation is from the lungs. This may be produced in other sites within the reticuloendothelial system, possibly in response to clearance of LPS–immune complexes or other immune complexes. However, downregulation of TNF$\alpha$ secretion by peripheral blood monocytes during periods of pulmonary exacerbation, with a return to normal responses to LPS after antibiotic treatment in patients with CF, suggests (with support by TNF$\alpha$ gene transcription studies and similar changes in IL-1$\beta$ secretion) that cytokine secretion is largely by the lung with downregulation of systemic circulating cells[72–74]. This may represent a general physiological protection against the indiscriminate production of systemically active cytokines, which would be detrimental to the host.

## SUMMARY

Cytokines are likely, by analogy with acute infectious states, to have a central role in the regulation of the host response to chronic pulmonary infection in CF. Much of this statement is speculative and is based on *in vitro* studies and animal model data, though measurement of various cytokines in serum and sputum tends to support such a role. Additionally, there is evidence to support the predicted role for cytokines in the metabolic changes associated with infection and possibly in the causation of cachexia in CF.

However, much of the data obtained in patients is contradictory. This is likely to be due to the inherent complexity of cytokine networks, the interaction of autocrine, paracrine and endocrine functions and the inhibitory role of soluble receptors, natural inhibitors and immunoglobulins. Further confounding factors are that measurements are made in material from different body compartments and using bio- and immunoassay methods with marked differences between laboratories for sensitivity, particularly in respect of immunoassays.

The future should yield more precise details of cytokine function in the cause of lung injury and metabolic changes that occur in CF with chronic pulmonary infection. Such understanding may indicate therapeutic interventions, such as cytokine receptor blockers, that augment or replace antibiotic treatment which has only a short-term impact on the inflammatory response.

## REFERENCES

1 Elborn JS, Shale DJ, Britton JR. Cystic fibrosis: current survival and population estimates to the year 2000. *Thorax* 1991; **46**: 881–5.

2 Bedrossian CWM, Greenberg SD, Singer DB, et al. The lung in cystic fibrosis: a quantitative study of pathologic findings amongst different age groups. *Hum Pathol* 1976; **7**: 195–204.
3 Oppenheimer EH, Esterly JR. Pathology of cystic fibrosis: review of the literature and comparison with 146 autopsied cases. *Prospect Pediatr Pathol* 1978; **2**: 241–78.
4 Cole PJ. Inflammation: a two-edge sword—the model of bronchiectasis. *Eur J Respir Dis* 1986: **69** (Suppl 147): 6–15.
5 Høiby N. Microbiology of lung infections in cystic fibrosis patients. *Acta Paediatr Scand Suppl.* 1982; **301**: 33–54.
6 Jankowskie R, Wayoff M, Lion C, et al. Virulence of *Haemophilus influenzae*. In: *Update of Haemophilus influenzae: How Virulence, Incidence and Resistance Affect Treatment* (ed R Rigelmann) Royal Society of Medicine Services, London, 1988, pp 41–8 (Publication 128).
7 Wilson R, Cole P. Pathogenic mechanisms during infection of the respiratory tract with special reference to *Haemophilus influenzae*. In: *Update of Haemophilus influenzae: Antimicrobials and the Host Response* (ed AJ Howard) Royal College of Medicine Sevices, London, 1988, pp 7–16 (Publication 138).
8 Döring G. The multifactorial virulence of *Pseudomonas aeruginosa*. In: *Cystic Fibrosis: Basic and Clinical Research* (eds N Høiby, SS Pedersen) Proceedings of the 17th Annual Meeting of the European Working Group for Cystic Fibrosis, Copenhagen, June 1991. Excerpta Medica, Amsterdam 1992, pp 93–100.
9 Döring G, Pfestorf M, Botzenhart K, Abdallah MA. Impact of proteases on iron uptake of *Pseudomonas aeruginosa* pyoverdin from transferrin and lactoferrin. *Infect Immun* 1988; **56**: 291–3.
10 Peters JE, Golloway DR. Purification characterisation of an active fragment of the LASA protein from *Pseudomonas aeruginosa* enhancement of elastase activity. *J Bacteriol* 1990; **172**: 2236–49.
11 Ramphal R, Carnay C, Fievre S, et al. *Pseudomonas aeruginosa* recognizes carbohydrate chains containing type 1 (Gal-Beta-1-3GlcNAc) or type 2 (Gal-Beta-1-AGlcMAc) disaccharide units. *Infect Immun* 1991; **59**: 700–4.
12 Döring G. Immunologic aspects of cystic fibrosis. *Chest* 1988; (Suppl 94): 109S–14S.
13 Pedersen SS, Høiby N, Shand GH, Pressler T. Antibody response to *Pseudomonas aeruginosa* antigens in cystic fibrosis. *Antibiot Chemother* 1989; **42**: 130–53.
14 Brett MM, Ghoneim ATM, Littlewood JM. Serum IgA antibodies against *Pseudomonas aeruginosa* in cystic fibrosis. *Arch Dis Child* 1990; **65**: 259–63.
15 Thanasekaraan V, Wiseman MS, Rayner RJ, et al. *Pseudomonas aeruginosa* antibodies in blood spots from patients with cystic fibrosis. *Arch Dis Child* 1989; **64**: 1599–603.
16 Cordon SM, Elborn JS, Rayner EJ, et al. IgG antibodies in early *Pseudomonas aeruginosa* infection in cystic fibrosis. *Arch Dis Child* 1992; **67**: 737–40.
17 Döring G, Goldstein W, Röll A, et al. Role of *Pseudomonas aeruginosa* exoenzymes in lung infections of patients with cystic fibrosis. *Infect Immun* 1985; **49**: 557–62.
18 Döring G, Obernesser H-J, Botzenhart K, et al. Proteases of *Pseudomonas aeruginosa* in patients with cystic fibrosis. *J Infect Dis* 1983; **147**: 744–50.
19 Döring G, Buhl V, Høiby N, et al. Detection of proteases of *Pseudomonas aeruginosa* in immune complexes isolated from sputum of cystic fibrosis patients. *Acta Path Microbiol Immunol Scand Sect C* 1984; **92**: 307–12.

20 Høiby N, Döring G, Schiøtz PO. The role of immune complexes in the pathogenesis of bacterial infections. *Annu Rev Microbiol* 1986; **40**: 29–53.
21 Theander TG, Kharazmi A, Pedersen BK, et al. Inhibition of human lymphocyte proliferation and cleavage of interleukin-2 by *Pseudomonas aeruginosa* proteases. *Infect Immun* 1988; **56**: 1673–7.
22 Nutman J, Berger M, Chase PA, et al. Studies on the mechanism of T-cell inhibition by the *Pseudomonas aeruginosa* phenzine pigment pyocyanin. *J Immunol* 1987; **138**: 3481–7.
23 Muhlradt PF, Tsai H, Conradt P. Effect of pyocyanine, a blue pigment from *Pseudomonas aeruginosa*, on separate steps of T-cell activation: interleukin 2 (IL-2) production, IL-2 receptor formation, proliferation and induction of cytolytic activity. *Eur J Immunol* 1986; **16**: 434–40.
24 Heath AW. Cytokines and infection. *Curr Opin Immunol* 1990; **2**: 380–4.
25 Horvat RT, Parmely MJ. *Pseudomonas aeruginosa* alkaline protease degrades human gamma interferon and inhibits its bioactivity. *Infect Immun* 1988; **56**: 2925–32.
26 Horvat RT, Clabaugh M, Duval-Jobe C, Parmely MJ. Inactivation of human gamma interferon by *Pseudomonas aeruginosa* proteases: elastase augments the effects of alkaline protease despite the presence of $\alpha_2$-macroglobulin. *Infect Immun* 1989; **57**: 1668–74.
27 Parmely M, Gale A, Clabaugh M, et al. Proteolytic inactivation of cytokines by *Pseudomonas aeruginosa*. *Infect Immun* 1990; **58**: 3009–14.
28 Novelli F, Giovarelli M, Reber-Liske R, et al. Blockade of physiologically secreted IFN-$\gamma$ inhibits human T lymphocyte and natural killer cell activation. *J Immunol* 1991; **147**: 1445–52.
29 Kagaya K, Watanabe K, Fukazawa Y. Capacity of recombinant gamma interferon to activate macrophages for *Salmonella*-killing activity. *Infect Immun* 1989; **57**: 609–15.
30 Speert DP, Thorson L. Suppression by human recombinant gamma interferon of *in vitro* macrophage nonopsonic and opsonic phagocytosis and killing. *Infect Immun* 1991; **59**: 1893–8.
31 Kunkel SL, Standiford T, Kasahara K, Strieter RM. Interleukin-8 (IL-8): the major neutrophil chemotactic factor in the lung. *Exp Lung Res* 1991; **17**: 17–23.
32 Elborn JS, Shale DJ. Lung injury in cystic fibrosis. *Thorax* 1990; **45**; 970–3.
33 Sibille Y, Reynolds HY. Macrophages and polymorphonuclear neutrophils in lung defence and injury. *Am Rev Respir Dis* 1990; **141**: 471–501.
34 Ozaki T, Maeda M, Hayashi H, et al. Role of alveolar macrophages in the neutrophil-dependent defence system against *Pseudomonas aeruginosa* infection in the lower respiratory tract. *Am Rev Respir Dis* 1989; **140**: 1595–601.
35 Nakamura H, Yoshimura K, McElvaney NG, Crystal RG. Neutrophil elastase in respiratory epithelial lining fluid of individuals with cystic fibrosis induces interleukin-8 gene expression in a human bronchial epithelial cell line. *J Clin Invest* 1992; **89**: 1478–84.
36 Rolfe MW, Kunkel SL, Standiford TJ, et al. Pulmonary fibroblast expression of interleukin-8: a model for alveolar macrophage-derived cytokine networking. *Am J Respir Cell Mol Biol* 1991; **5**: 493–501.
37 Cromwell O, Hamid Q, Corrigan CJ, et al. Expression and generation of interleukin-8, IL-6 and granulocyte–macrophage colony-stimulating factor by bronchial epithelial cells and enhancement by IL-1$\beta$ and tumour necrosis factor-$\alpha$. *Immunol* 1992: **77**; 330–7.

38 Borregaard N. Bactericidal mechanisms of the human neutrophil. *Scand J Haematol* 1984; **32**: 225–30.
39 Suter S. Lung inflammation and anti-inflammatory treatment. In: *Cystic Fibrosis, Basic and Clinical Research* (eds N Høiby, SS Pedersen) Proceedings of the 17th Annual Meeting of the European Working Group for Cystic Fibrosis, Copenhagen, June 1991. Excerpta Medica, Amsterdam, 1992, pp 177–82.
40 Suter S, Schaad UB, Tegner H, et al. Levels of free granulocyte elastase in bronchial secretions from patients with CF: effect of anti-microbial treatment against *Pseudomonas aeruginosa. J Infect Dis* 1986; **153**: 902–9.
41 Bruce MC, Poncz L, Klinger JD, et al. Biochemical and pathologic evidence for proteolytic destruction of lung connective tissue in CF. *Am Rev Respir Dis* 1985; **132**: 529–35.
42 Baker PJ. Regulation of magnitude of antibody response to bacterial polysaccharide antigens by thymus derived lymphocytes. *Infect Immun* 1990; **58**; 3465–70.
43 Pressler T, Mansa B, Jensen T, et al. Increased IgG2 and IgG3 concentration is associated with advanced *Pseudomonas aeruginosa* infection and poor pulmonary function in cystic fibrosis. *Acta Paediatr Scand* 1988; **77**: 576–82.
44 Cerami A, Beutler B. The role of cachectin/TNF in endotoxic shock and cachexia. *Immunol Today* 1988; **9**: 28–31.
45 Arnaout MA. Structure and function of the leukocyte adhesion molecules CD11/CD18. *Blood* 1990; **75**: 1037–50.
46 Springer TA. Adhesion receptors of the immune system. *Nature* 1990; **346**: 425–34.
47 Vedder NB, Winn RK, Rice CL, et al. A monoclonal antibody to the adherence-promoting leukocyte glycoprotein CD18, reduces organ injury and improves survival from hemorrhagic shock and resuscitation in rabbits. *J Clin Invest* 1988; **81**: 939.
48 Mulligan MS, Varani J, Warren JS, et al. Roles of $\beta_2$, integrins of rat neutrophils in complement- and oxygen radical-mediated acute inflammatory injury. *J Immunol* 1992; **148**: 1847–57.
49 Mulligan MS, Warren JS, Smith CW, et al. Lung injury after deposition of IgA immune complexes: requirements for CD18 and L-arginine. *J Immunol* 1992; **148**: 3086–92.
50 Lasky LA. Pectin cell adhesion molecules (LEC-CAMs): a new family of cell adhesion proteins involved with inflammation. *J Cell Biochem* 1991; **45**: 139–46.
51 McEver RP, Beckstead JH, Moore KL, et al. GMP-140, a platelet alpha-granule membrane protein, is also synthesized by vascular endothelial cells and is localized in Weibel–Palade bodies. *J Clin Invest* 1989; **84**: 92–7.
52 Butcher EC. Leukocyte–endothelial cell recognition: three (or more) steps to specificity and diversity. *Cell* 1991; **67**: 1033–6.
53 Picker LJ, Warnock RA, Burns A, et al. The neutrophil selectin LECAM-1 presents carbohydrate ligands to the vascular selectins ELAM-1 and GMP-140. *Cell* 1991; **66**: 921–33.
54 Le J, Vilcek J. TNF and IL-1: cytokines with multiple overlapping biological activities. *Lab Invest* 1987; **56**: 234–82.
55 Sherry B, Cerami A. Cachectin/tumor necrosis factor exerts endocrine, paracrine and autocrine control of inflammatory responses. *J Cell Biol* 1988; **107**; 1269–77.
56 Cerami A. Inflammatory cytokines. *Clin Immunol Immunopathol* 1992; **62**: S3–10.
57 Dinarello CA, Wolff SM. The role of interleukin-1 in disease. *New Eng J Med* 1993; **328**; 106–13.

58 Loetscher H, Pan YE, Lahm H, et al. Molecular cloning and expression of the 55 kd tumor necrosis factor receptor. *Cell* 1990; **61**; 351–9.
59 Schall TJ, Lewis M, Koller KJ, et al. Molecular cloning and expression of a receptor for human necrosis factor. *Cell* 1990; **61**; 361–70.
60 Dembic Z, Loetscher H, Gubler U, et al. Two human TNF receptors have similar extracellular, but distinct intracellular domain sequences. *Cytokine* 1990; **2**; 231–7.
61 Darbonne WC, Rice GC, Mohler MA, et al. Red blood cells are a sink for interleukin 8, a leukocyte chemotaxin. *J Clin Invest* 1991; **88**; 1362–9.
62 Sylvester I, Yoshimura T, Sticherling M, et al. Neutrophil attractant protein-1–immunoglobulin G immune complexes and free anti-NAP-1-antibody in normal human serum. *J Clin Invest* 1992; **90**; 471–81.
63 Fomsgaard A, Svenson M, Bendtzen K. Auto-antibodies to tumour necrosis factor in healthy humans with inflammatory diseases and Gram-negative bacterial infections. *Scand J Immunol* 1988; **30**: 219–23.
64 Dinarello CA. Interleukin-1 and interleukin-1 antagonism. *Blood* 1991; **77**: 1627–52.
65 Carter DB, Deibel MR, Dunn CJ, et al. Purification, cloning, expression and biological characterization of an interleukin-1 receptor antagonist protein. *Nature* 1990; **334**: 633–8.
66 Ohlsson K, Bjork P, Bergenfeldt M, et al. IL-1ra reduces mortality from endotoxin shock. *Nature* 1990; **348**: 550–2.
67 Suter S, Schaad UB, Roux-Lombard P, et al. Relation between tumour necrosis factor-$\alpha$ and granulocye elastase-$\alpha$1-proteinase inhibitor complexes in plasma of patients with cystic fibrosis. *Am Rev Respir Dis* 1989; **140**: 1640–4.
68 Norman D, Elborn JS, Cordon SM, et al. Plasma tumour necrosis factor-$\alpha$ in cystic fibrosis. *Thorax* 1991; **46**: 91–5.
69 Brown MA, Morgan WJ, Finley PR, Scuderi P. Circulating levels of tumour necrosis factor and interleukin-1 in cystic fibrosis. *Pediatr Pulmonol* 1991; **10**: 86–91.
70 Wilmott RW, Kassab JT, Kilian PL, et al. Increased levels of interleukin-1 in bronchoalveolar washings from children with bacterial pulmonary infections. *Am Rev Respir Dis* 1990; **142**: 365–8.
71 Elborn JS, Cordon SM, Parker D, et al. The host inflammatory response prior to death in patients with cystic fibrosis and chronic *Pseudomonas aeruginosa* infection. *Resp Med* 1993; **87**: 603–7.
72 Elborn JS, Norman D, Delamere FM, Shale DJ. In vitro tumour necrosis factor-$\alpha$ secretion by monocytes from patients with cystic fibrosis. *Am J Respir Cell Mol Biol* 1992; **6**: 207–11.
73 Denis M, Bédard M, Francoeur C, Cantin A. Local and systemic release of cytokines in CF. *Pediatr Pulmonol* 1993; Suppl 9: 287.
74 Belli DC, Schlegel S, Roux P, et al. Influence of IV antibiotherapy on inflammatory mediators in cystic fibrosis children. *Pediatr Pulmonol* 1993; Suppl 9: 288.
75 Wilson CB, Franklin T, Smith AL, et al. Increased TNF$\alpha$ and IL-1$\beta$ production in CF patients with clinical deterioration. *Pediatr Pulmonol* 1993; Suppl 9: 119–20.
76 Kronborg G, Hansen MB, Svenson M, et al. Cytokines in sputum and serum from patients with cystic fibrosis and chronic *Pseudomonas aeruginosa* infection as markers of destructive inflammation in the lungs. *Pediatr Pulmonol* 1993; **15**: 292–7.

77 Dagli E, Warner JA, Besley CR, Warner JO. Raised serum soluble interleukin-2 receptor concentrations in cystic fibrosis patients with and without evidence of lung disease. *Arch Dis Child* 1992; **67**: 479–81.
78 Waage A, Brandzaeg P, Halstensen A, et al. The complex pattern of cytokines in serum from patients with meningococcal septic shock. *J Exp Med* 1989: **169**: 333–8.
79 Marks JD, Marks CB, Luke JM, et al. Plasma tumour necrosis factor in patients with septic shock. *Am Rev Respir Dis* 1990; **141**: 94–7.
80 Scuderi P, Sterling KE, Lam S, et al. Raised serum levels of tumour necrosis factor in parasitic infections. *Lancet* 1990; **ii**: 1364–5.
81 Grau GE, Taylor TE, Molyneux ME, et al. Tumour necrosis factor and disease severity in children with falciparum malaria. *N Engl J Med* 1989; **320**: 1586–91.
82 Oliff A, Defo-Jones D, Boyer M, et al. Tumours secreting human TNF/cachectin induce cachexia in mice. *Cell* 1987; **50**: 155–63.
83 Starnes HF, Warren RS, Heevanandam M, et al. Tumor necrosis factor and the acute metabolic response to tissue injury in man. *J Clin Invest* 1988; **82**: 1321–5.
84 Van Der Poll T, Sauerwein HP. Tumour necrosis factor-$\alpha$: its role in the metabolic response to sepsis. *Clin Sci* 1993; **84**: 247–56.
85 Ramsey B, Farrell PM, Pencharz PB. Nutritional assessment and management in cystic fibrosis. *Am J Clin Nutr* 1992; **455**: 108–16.
86 Elborn JS, Cordon SM, Western PJ, et al. Tumour necrosis factor-$\alpha$, resting energy expenditure and cachexia in cystic fibrosis. *Clin Sci* 1993; **85**: 563–8.
87 O'Rawe A, McIntosh I, Dodge JA, et al. Increased energy expenditure in cystic fibrosis is associated with specific mutations. *Clin Sci* 1992; **82**: 71–6.
88 Flick DA, Gifford GE. Comparison of *in vitro* cell cytotoxic assays for tumour necrosis factor. *J Immunol Methods* 1984; **68**: 167–75.
89 Klostergaard J. A rapid, extremely sensitive, quantitative microassay for cytotoxic cytokines. *Lymphokine Res* 1985; **4**: 309–17.
90 Kramer SM, Carver ME. Serum-free in vitro bioassay for the detection of tumour necrosis factor. *J Immunol Methods* 1986; **93**: 201–6.
91 Espevik T, Nissen-Meyer J. A highly sensitive cell line, WEHI 164 clone 13, for measuring cytotoxic factor/tumor necrosis factor from human monocytes. *J Immunol Methods* 1986; **95**: 99–105.
92 Meager A, Leung H, Woolley J. Assays for tumour necrosis factor and related cytokines. *J Immunol Methods* 1989; **116**: 1–17.
93 Fomsgaard A, Warsaae H, Bendtzen K. Detection of tumour necrosis factor from lipopolysaccharide-stimulated human mononuclear cells by enzyme-linked immunosorbent assay and cytotoxicity bioassay. *Scand J Immunol* 1988; **27**: 143–7.
94 Mathews N, Neale ML. Cytotoxicity assays for tumour necrosis factor and lymphotoxin. In: *Lymphokines and Interferons: A Practical Aproach* (eds Clemens MJ, Morris AG and Gearing AJH) IRL Press. Oxford, 1987, pp. 221–5
95 McLaughlin P, Davies H, Aikiwa A. Tumour necrosis factor in normal plasma (letter). *Lancet* 1990; **336**: 1014–15.
96 Freeman R. *In vitro* production of TNF in blood samples (letter). *Lancet* 1990; **336**: 312–13.
97 Murch S, Macdonald T. In vitro production of cytokines in serum (letter). *Lancet* 1990; **336**: 687–8.
98 Maury C. Monitoring the acute phase response: comparison of tumour necrosis factor (cachectin) and C-reactive protein responses in inflammatory and infectious diseases. *J Clin Pathol* 1989; **43**: 1078–82.

99 Levine B, Kalman J, Mayer L, et al. Elevated circulating levels of TNF in severe chronic heart failure. *N Eng J Med* 1990: **323**: 236–41.
100 Girardin E, Grau GE, Dayer J-M, et al. Tumour necrosis factor and interleukin-1 in the serum of children with severe infectious purpura. *N Eng J Med* 1988; **319**: 397–400.
101 Parsons PE, Moore FA, Moore EE, et al. Studies on the role of tumor necrosis factor in adult respiratory distress syndrome. *Am Rev Respir Dis* 1992; **146**: 684–700.

## Chapter Fifteen

# Lung and Heart–Lung Transplantation for Cystic Fibrosis

Thomas M. Egan
*University of North Carolina, Chapel Hill, North Carolina, USA*

## INTRODUCTION

Despite recent advances in our understanding of the genetic defect in cystic fibrosis (CF), the disease remains the most common lethal genetic disease of Caucasians. Notwithstanding the advent of innovative therapies based on a better understanding of the pathophysiology of the CF gene defect, it is estimated that 95% of patients with CF will succumb from end-stage pulmonary disease[1]. In the last decade, lung transplantation has emerged as a palliative therapy for patients with a variety of end-stage lung diseases[2–5].

As candidates for lung transplantation, patients with CF pose considerable technical challenges. CF lungs are routinely colonized with a variety of multiply resistant organisms that have contributed to the destruction of the organ. The frequent lung infections result in extensive intrathoracic adhesions that are often vascular and a proliferation of systemic bronchial vasculature with encasement of major airway and well-vascularized lymph nodes. In other respects, CF patients are potentially ideal candidates for lung transplantation. They are frequently young, with life-threatening disease confined to one organ system. Even before the genetic defect was established, it was apparent that

*Cystic Fibrosis—Current Topics, Volume 2.* Edited by J. A. Dodge, D. J. H. Brock and J. H. Widdicombe

the CF pulmonary epithelial abnormality evidenced by an altered potential difference[6] was not manifested in the epithelium of heart–lung grafts in CF patients[7], providing some assurance that the pulmonary abnormalities observed in CF patients were unlikely to recur following transplantation.

## HISTORY OF LUNG AND HEART–LUNG TRANSPLANTATION

The lung possesses several unique features that pose special problems for transplantation. The lung has a very delicate architecture that subserves its function as a huge membrane interface between blood and air, but the fragile nature of this membrane can contribute to significant pulmonary dysfunction from even a minor insult. The lung is the only solid organ currently transplanted that is in constant contact with the outside environment, rendering it particularly susceptible to infection. Because conventional donors are brain dead but are maintained intubated and ventilated, most donor lungs are contaminated with bacteria at the time of transplantation, and infection remains a significant reason for donor scarcity and early graft dysfunction. Also, because the lung is the only solid organ transplanted in which the systemic arterial blood supply is not routinely reconstituted, airway ischaemia can occur; this has been another major cause of graft failure.

The first recorded attempt at isolated lung transplantation was reported by Hardy from the University of Mississippi in 1963[8]. The first reported heart–lung transplant was by Cooley in 1968 in a $2\frac{1}{2}$-month-old child with atrial ventricular canal defect and pulmonary hypertension[9]. Despite numerous attempts, success eluded thoracic surgeons for a period of almost two decades. Major developments that ushered in a new era of successful lung and heart–lung transplantation included the introduction of the new immunosuppressive agent cyclosporine[10] and a better understanding of the effects of high-dose steroids on airway healing[11].

Shumway's team at Stanford University, which had been instrumental in the development and successful introduction of heart allotransplantation, had continued to work on the technical problems of heart–lung transplantation. Early experience with cyclosporine and primate heart–lung transplantation was encouraging[12]. This laboratory experience culminated in the first successful heart–lung transplant at Stanford by Reitz and colleagues in 1981[13].

At the University of Toronto, the combination of cyclosporine and azathioprine immunosuppression, coupled with avoidance of high-dose steroids and bronchial omentopexy[14,15], resulted in the first demonstration of consistent long-term survival in dogs after single lung transplantation[16]. This laboratory experience culminated in the first successful isolated single lung transplant for pulmonary fibrosis at the University of Toronto in November 1983[17]. With experience, isolated single lung transplantation was shown to be reasonable palliation for patients with pulmonary fibrosis[18,19].

A large population of patients remained for whom single lung replacement was judged inappropriate for their disease process—specifically, patients with infectious end-stage lung disease or patients with obstructive pulmonary disease. To circumvent the necessity of heart transplantation in heart–lung transplant recipients, the Lung Transplant Group at the University of Toronto developed a technique for double lung transplant, initially as an en bloc procedure[20]. The first successful double lung transplant using this technique was performed in 1986 in a patient with emphysema[21]. The first reported pulmonary transplant for CF was in September 1984, when a CF patient underwent heart–lung transplant at Harefield[22].

With experience, it became clear that the en bloc double lung transplant procedure was fraught with serious, sometimes lethal, airway complications[23]. Additional morbidity and mortality were encountered when the procedure was extended to patients with other forms of lung disease, such as CF. To address the issue of ischaemic airway complications, Noirclerc and colleagues in Marseille introduced the technique of bilateral bronchial anastomoses[24]. By substantially reducing the amount of ischaemic donor airway, the incidence of airway complications was reduced. Subsequently, Pasque and others at Washington University described the ‘bilateral lung transplant’ procedure[25].

This newer approach offers several advantages. First, the transverse incision (Figure 1) provides excellent exposure of all aspects of the pleural spaces and still allows for cannulation of the major vessels for the institution of cardiopulmonary bypass. For patients with CF, this approach means that the vascular adhesions that are so commonly found in the pleural spaces can be adequately visualized and safely divided using electrocautery. Additionally, the rich network of bronchial arteries in the posterior hilum can be accessed so that bleeding can be controlled. An additional benefit of this procedure is the ability to avoid cardiopulmonary bypass in many instances. By the sequential removal and subsequent transplantation of a lung on each side, cardiopulmonary bypass with its requirement for anticoagulation and subsequent bypass-induced coagulopathy can often be avoided. This has substantial advantages, particularly in patients with CF.

Controversy remains as to what constitutes the most appropriate transplant procedure for patients with CF. Proponents of heart–lung transplantation argue that the incidence of airway complications following heart–lung transplantation is less than that following double lung transplantation. Although this is true for the older technique of en bloc double lung transplantation, the bilateral sequential technique has a substantially reduced incidence of airway complications and would appear to confer several advantages to the recipient. First, if the heart is not transplanted, potential recipients are not exposed to

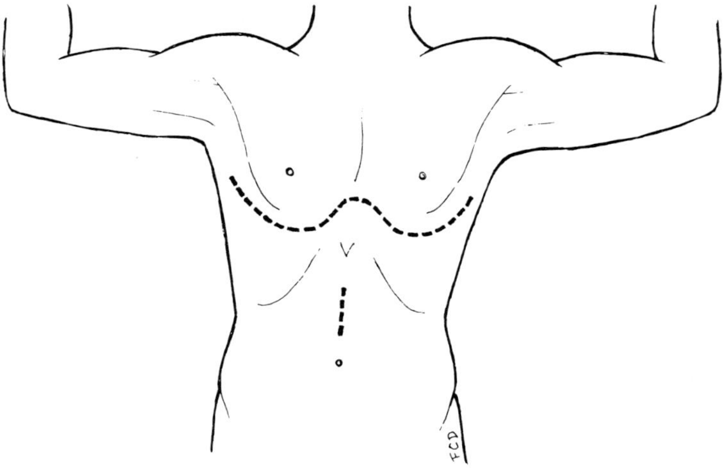


**Figure 1** Incisions for double lung transplant procedure. The small midline laparotomy incision is used to mobilize the omentum, while the transverse anterior chest incision provides excellent exposure of both pleural spaces. (Reproduced from Egan and Detterbeck[34], with permission)

the added risks of cardiac transplantation and the development of graft atherosclerosis. Although episodes of acute cardiac rejection are observed less frequently after heart–lung transplantation than after isolated heart transplantation[26], there are complications of heart–lung transplantation related to the cardiac graft to which patients are not exposed if they undergo bilateral lung replacement. Delayed cardiac arteriosclerosis is observed after heart–lung transplantation as well as after isolated heart transplantation[27], and cardiac denervation consequent to heart–lung transplant delays heart rate response in exercise, which may reduce exercise performance following this procedure[28]. Avoiding cardiopulmonary bypass should result in less peri-operative blood loss. Bleeding has been less problematic with cardiopulmonary bypass for heart–lung transplantation since the introduction of aprotinin, which has reduced the need for blood transfusion after repeat open cardiac surgery[29]. To address the issue of donor organ scarcity, some heart–lung transplant surgeons champion the so-called 'domino procedure', in which CF recipients of heart–lung grafts donate their native heart to recipients awaiting cardiac transplantation[22].

Initial experience with heart–lung transplantation for CF patients in North America was discouraging, with a one-year actuarial survival of 42% reported for 33 CF patients who underwent heart–lung transplant at 14 centres in North America between October 1983 and August 1990[30]. Heart–lung transplantation for CF patients has been more popular in European centres. In the USA, the current organ allocation system prioritizes status I cardiac recipients (potential recipients for heart transplantation maintained on mechanical assist devices or requiring intravenous inotropic support). Additionally, the large number of successful cardiac transplant programmes renders far fewer heart–lung grafts available in the USA, making a bilateral lung transplant procedure a more logical choice for patients with CF.

## TECHNIQUE OF HEART–LUNG TRANSPLANTATION

Heart–lung transplantation is usually performed through a median sternotomy, although some centres have adopted the 'clamshell' incision popularized for bilateral lung transplant. The operation entails removal of the native heart and both lungs and replacement with a heart–lung graft en bloc (Figure 2). Details

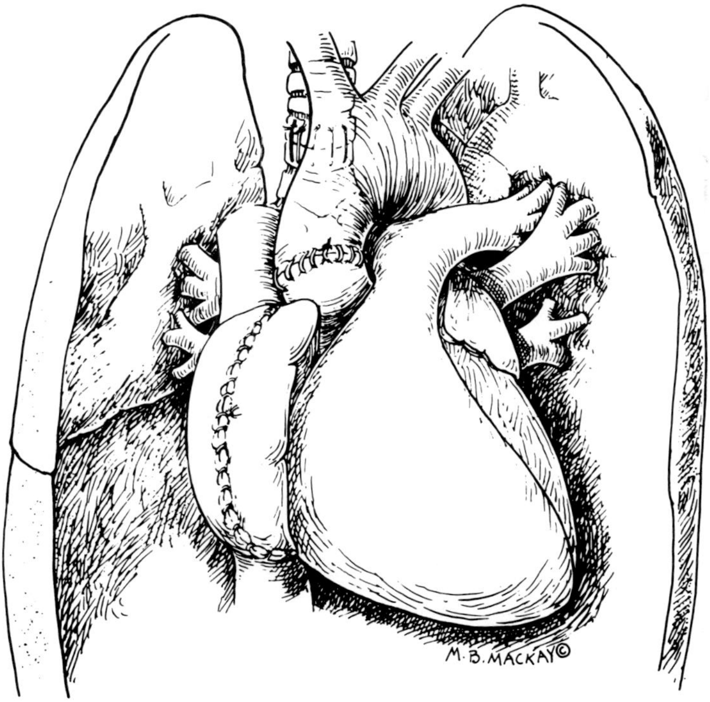


**Figure 2** Dashed lines indicate suture lines for heart–lung transplant procedure; a tracheal anastomosis, ascending aortic anastomosis and right atrial anastomosis are depicted. (Copyrighted figure, reproduced by permission of Margot B. Mackay)

of the operative procedure are outlined in detail elsewhere[31,32]. In brief, the heart and lungs are mobilized through a median sternotomy. After institution of cardiopulmonary bypass, the heart is excised, followed by the native lungs. Generous pleuropericardial windows are constructed posterior to phrenic nerve pedicles. Care must be taken not to injure the phrenic nerves. The heart is excised at the level of the right atrium. The recipient airway is generally excised to the level of the carina. In patients with CF, this dissection in the posterior mediastinum is fraught with significant bleeding problems. An incision in the posterior pericardium facilitates this dissection. The donor heart–lung block is positioned by placing each atelectatic lung through its pleural pericardial window into the appropriate thorax. The donor trachea is trimmed back to within one ring of the carina, and the most posterior tracheal anastomosis is performed. The remaining right atrial and aortic anastomoses are performed in a manner similar to that used in cardiac transplantation. Bleeding remains a significant complication of this procedure in CF patients when aprotinin is not utilized[33].

## TECHNIQUE OF DOUBLE LUNG TRANSPLANTATION

The currently employed bilateral lung transplant procedure has been described elsewhere in some detail[34]. One of the features of the procedure is the preoperative assessment of each lung's function, determined by a quantitative radionucleide perfusion scan. The use of a double lumen endotracheal tube facilitates the explantation of each lung separately. In general, the lung with the least perfusion is removed first to reduce the requirement for institution of cardiopulmonary bypass.

The 'clamshell' bilateral anterior thoracosternotomy results in excellent exposure of the pleural spaces, particularly at the apices, where dense pleural adhesions are often present in patients with CF (Figure 3). The skin incision, which is made in the submammary fold, can be extended posteriorly as far as the latissimus dorsi muscle. Should cardiopulmonary bypass be required, the ascending aorta can easily be cannulated through this incision, and by opening the pericardium the right atrium is accessible for venous drainage. Recipient pneumonectomy is carried out by dividing the native pulmonary artery distal to its first division. The pulmonary veins are divided outside of the pericardium, the inferior pulmonary ligaments and other adhesions are taken down using electrocautery, and finally the bronchus is divided. We routinely clamp the bronchial divisions distal to bronchial division into upper and lower lobe sections to minimize the egress of purulent material from the lung at the time of division of the airway. Once the lung is removed, the open airway and pleural space are irrigated with warm Betadine solution.

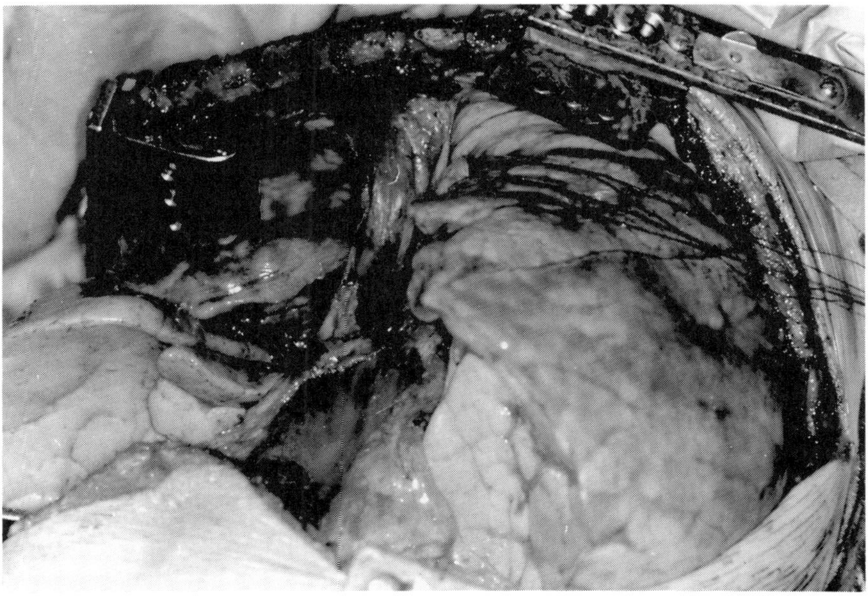

**Figure 3** Surgical exposure of both pleural spaces afforded by the anterior bilateral thoracotomy 'clamshell' incision. Although the left lung is not ventilated, it has not collapsed because of the obstructive nature of the pulmonary disease. (Reproduced from Egan and Detterbeck[34], with permission)

The double lung block is separated into its constituent lungs by staple division of the left main stem bronchus and apportioning the posterior wall of the left atrium and atrial cuffs between the two lung blocks.

The donor bronchus is prepared by excising donor airway back to within two rings of the upper lobe take-off. Minimizing the length of ischaemic donor airway is important in reducing airway complications. Support has been growing for a 'telescoping' airway anastomosis, first described by Trinkle and colleagues from the University of Texas[35]. However, we have had excellent results with end-to-end airway anastomosis using polyglycolic acid suture, and we routinely employ omentopexy. We have found that airway healing is superior when omentopexy is used[36]. The recipient pericardium around the pulmonary vein stumps is opened and a Satinsky clamp is placed on the left atrium. Amputation of the pulmonary vein stumps results in the creation of a left atrial cuff which is sutured to the left atrial cuff of the donor lung. A clamp is then placed on the recipient pulmonary artery, and the stumps of the upper and lower divisions of the pulmonary artery are excised. Care must be taken to align this anastomosis properly, since rotational deformity can easily be produced and can result in a technical problem. Once the vascular anastomoses are completed, the vasculature of the implanted lung is de-aired. Ventilation of the newly transplanted lung usually provides sufficient pulmonary function to allow for explantation of the second native lung in the same manner as described above for the first implant. Both pleural spaces are drained. The incision is closed by reapproximating the sternal ends with wire and reapproximating the divided pectoral muscle with running suture. The incision has been well tolerated, and some centres have begun to use this operative approach for heart–lung transplantation in CF patients[33].

## TRANSPLANT PROCEDURE IN CYSTIC FIBROSIS

As experience has been gained in lung and heart–lung transplantation, increasing numbers of CF patients have been availed of this palliation. A total of 1349 heart–lung transplants and 1665 isolated lung transplants (521 double lung and 1144 single lung) have been reported to the International Registry of the Society for Heart and Lung Transplantation[37]. This is a voluntary registry that collects data from transplant centres around the world. CF accounted for 18% of the paediatric heart–lung transplants and 17% of the adult heart–lung transplants performed and reported to the Registry. In contrast, CF is the most common indication for paediatric double lung transplant, accounting for more than 60% of the double lung transplants reported to the Registry in recipients under the age of 18. CF accounted for 38% of the adult double lung transplants reported to the Registry. It would appear that the opportunity to perform heart–lung transplant for this disease is diminishing; and as experience with double lung transplant accumulates, it will likely become the transplant procedure of choice for patients with CF.

Only 50 heart–lung transplants were performed in the USA in 1992, compared with more than 500 isolated lung transplants. Despite acceptable success rates with transplantation of CF patients in experienced centres, emphysema continues to be the leading indication for isolated lung transplantation at present[37]. Since approximately 400 deaths occur each year in the USA among patients with CF[38], it is clear that there are not nearly enough pulmonary donors to meet the demand for lung transplantation in CF patients in the USA.

## CURRENT INDICATIONS FOR TRANSPLANTATION IN CYSTIC FIBROSIS

While selection criteria vary from centre to centre, there is general agreement concerning the criteria listed in Table 1. Although predicting life expectancy is difficult in any chronic illness, a recent study from the Hospital for Sick

**Table 1** Selection criteria for lung transplantation in CF

| |
|---|
| Age <50 years |
| Life expectancy 18–24 months |
| No significant renal or hepatic disease |
| No evidence of malignancy >5 years |
| Ambulatory and able to participate in rehabilitation programme |
| Ability to understand and comply with a complex medical regimen |
| Psychological stability |
| Previous pleural procedures acceptable |

Children in Toronto may help identify appropriate CF candidates for transplant[39]. During a 12-year period, a cohort of 673 patients was followed. One hundred and ninety patients died during this study. Cox proportional hazards regression analysis was used to compute the relative risk of death within one or two years from prior measurements of pulmonary function, blood gases and nutritional status. Among the laboratory measurements, the forced expiratory volume in 1 s ($FEV_1$) was the most significant predictor of mortality in this study, but age and sex were also significant for predicting risk. The study identified a risk of mortality within two years of 50% for CF patients younger than 18 years of age with an $FEV_1$ of <30% predicted. Older patients had a somewhat reduced risk of death within two years if their $FEV_1$ was <30% predicted. For patients with an $FEV_1$ of <20% predicted, the risk of death within two years increased to 70% for patients under the age of 18 and 58% for patients younger than 44 years of age. The risks of death were higher in female patients with equivalent pulmonary function. Weight-for-height was also a significant predictor of death. A weight : height ratio of <70% predicted was associated with increased risk of mortality. A partial pressure of arterial oxygen of <55 mmHg on room air, or a partial pressure of arterial carbon dioxide >50 mmHg, was associated with two-year mortality rates in excess of 50%. These data have helped to identify candidates for transplant with CF who are at an increased risk of death. Decreasing pulmonary functions, oxygen dependence, inability to maintain weight and increasing need for hospitalization all serve to identify CF patients with an increased risk of mortality.

Since renal insufficiency is a significant cause of post-lung transplant morbidity, adequate renal function is judged to be important for successful transplant outcome. Long-standing aminoglycoside therapy causes problems for some candidates with CF, since the perioperative use of aminoglycoside antibiotics is virtually mandatory, in our experience. We have no experience with combined liver and heart–lung or double lung transplants, but there is a limited clinical experience among patients with CF and end-stage liver and lung disease[40,41]. Given the current donor shortage, it is difficult to justify the increased risk that the combined procedure would entail. We do not consider diabetes mellitus an absolute contraindication among CF patients because diabetes itself does not seem to adversely affect prognosis in CF patients[42], but we would be reluctant to transplant a patient with diabetes that is difficult to control.

We have recently analysed our CF referrals for lung transplantation (Ciriaco et al., submitted for publication). Over a $3\frac{1}{2}$-year period, we have seen 95 patients with CF for consideration of lung transplantation. Seventy-four of the 95 were considered acceptable; of these, seven refused transplantation at our institution. Of the 67 patients who were listed, 11 died on the waiting list. The relatively high ratio of acceptability speaks to the notion that patients with CF are being referred for transplant late in the course of their disease. It would be preferable to follow patients with CF while they are too well for transplant in order to identify patients who are appropriate to list. As more patients are listed, waiting time increases, and ultimately growing numbers of patients will die on the lung transplant waiting list.

This aspect of lung transplantation for CF is an emotional one that has occasioned desultory remarks concerning lung transplant efforts in these patients. In an analysis of paediatric referrals for heart–lung transplant, Warner noted that of 27 patients referred for consideration, only 10 were transplanted, with six of 10 ultimately surviving[43]. Warner questions whether the benefit of successful outcome seen in only 22% of the referrals is worth the effort and resources expended, particularly in light of the risk of death on the waiting list (29%). Nevertheless, lung transplantation is currently the only therapy that can improve quality and quantify of life for appropriately selected patients with end-stage lung disease due to CF.

## RESULTS OF TRANSPLANTATION IN CYSTIC FIBROSIS

As experience has been gained in the technical aspects of thoracic organ transplant, survival for heart–lung and isolated lung transplant procedures has improved. Current anticipated actuarial one-year survival is in excess of 60% for heart–lung transplantation and is approximately 70% for double lung transplant[37]. Despite the increased risks associated with purulent lung disease, nutritional deficiency and intrathoracic adhesions associated with CF recipients, centres that have accumulated experience with these patients have demonstrated no difference in mortality between CF recipients and non-CF recipients. The published results from a variety of transplant centres in Europe and North America are summarized in Table 2.

The first reported application of heart–lung transplant for end-stage pulmonary disease (distinct from pulmonary vascular disease) came from

**Table 2** Summary of reported results in CF lung and heart–lung transplants

| Centre | *n* | Procedure | Operative survival (%) | Actuarial survival (%) 1 year | 2 year |
|---|---|---|---|---|---|
| Papworth[41] | 42 | Heart–lung | 83 | 78 | 69 |
| Harefield[40] | 79 | Heart–lung | 77[a] | 69 | 52 |
| University of Toronto[44] | 17 | Double lung | 65 | 58 | 58 |
| Stanford[33] | 15 | Heart–lung and double lung | 93 | 76 | 76 |
| Montreal–Marseille[45] | 25 | Double lung | 76 | 64 | 56 |
| University of North Carolina[b] | 39 | Double lung | 100 | 83 | 66 |

[a]18 deaths within two months of surgery.
[b]Unpublished data.

Papworth Hospital, Cambridge[5]. This report included one patient with CF. The experience at Papworth has continued to grow. Their most recent report outlines results in 42 CF patients undergoing heart–lung transplant. There were five deaths within 30 days. The actuarial one-year survival was 78%. Causes of late death were infectious in three patients before six months and related to the development of bronchiolitis obliterans in six other patients beyond six months. Actuarial survival in CF and non-CF patients is identical in the Cambridge experience out to four years[41].

The largest published series of heart–lung transplants for CF comes from Harefield Hospital in the UK, where Yacoub and colleagues have reported on 79 CF patients who underwent heart–lung transplantation[40]. There were 18 deaths within the first two months, with six deaths related to infection and five to multiple organ failure. Haemorrhage accounted for four deaths in this group of patients, underscoring the technical difficulties imposed by these patients. One-year actuarial survival was 69%.

The University of Toronto Lung Transplant Group has published its experience with bilateral lung transplantation in CF[44]. During a three-year period, 17 patients underwent double lung transplant. There were six operative deaths, four of which were caused by bacterial infection. The actuarial survival reported in this series was 58% at 12 months.

Shennib and Noirclerc reported the combined experience from the Montreal General Hospital and Ste-Marguerite Hospital in Marseille, France, where 25 patients underwent double lung transplant for CF[45]. All four intraoperative deaths were related to bleeding from adhesions. Actuarial survival at one year was 64%. An intriguing aspect of this report is that the experience spanned the evolution of airway anastomotic techniques for double lung transplant. Two patients in this series underwent tracheal anastomosis with an en bloc double lung transplant procedure, 15 other patients had en bloc double lung transplant with bibronchial anastomoses, and the last eight patients had sequential single bilateral lung transplant as described earlier in this chapter.

Starnes and his colleagues from Stanford University reported on 15 patients who underwent transplantation for CF[33]. Thirteen recipients received heart–lung transplant, while the two most recent recipients received double lung transplant. One-year actuarial survival for all patients was 76%.

At the University of North Carolina, our initial published series of 28 patients included eight patients with CF[4]. To date, 39 patients with CF have undergone double lung transplant. Two of these patients developed acute early graft failure; both were retransplanted and both survived. No operative deaths have occurred in this series. Three deaths within six months of surgery have occurred; two deaths were related to *Pseudomonas cepacia* pneumonia, and one patient died from unexplained increase in intracranial pressure three months after transplant. Actuarial survival at one year is 83%. Postoperative pulmonary function has been dramatically improved in recipients. Spirometry for transplanted CF patients, shown in Figure 4, is consistent with reports from other centres after heart–lung[33,40,46] or double lung[44] transplantation for CF.

An important component of our programme is mandatory involvement in a pulmonary rehabilitation regimen by all candidates with end-stage parenchymal lung disease awaiting lung transplantation. Patients undergo aerobic exercise in a monitored setting three to five times a week. Involvement

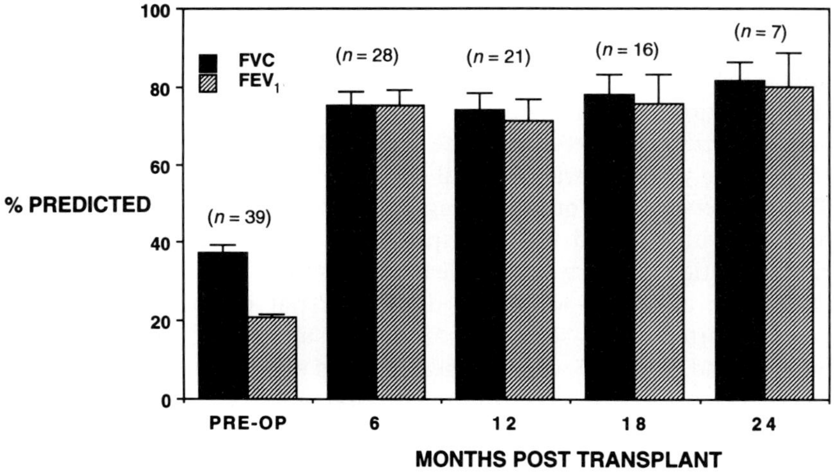


**Figure 4** $FEV_1$ and FVC expressed as percentage predicted ( ± s.e.m.) before double lung transplant and at intervals after transplant for 39 CF recipients at the University of North Carolina at Chapel Hill

of CF patients in a programme of physical exercise has been reviewed[47,48] and is believed to be beneficial for CF patients for a variety of reasons, including increasing ventilator muscle endurance. For our patients with CF awaiting transplantation, we have demonstrated an improvement in 6 min walk and lower extremity ergometry while awaiting transplant[49], even though these patients have end-stage lung disease.

## INFECTIOUS COMPLICATIONS FOLLOWING LUNG TRANSPLANTATION IN CYSTIC FIBROSIS

Infection is a cause of serious morbidity and mortality after lung transplantation among all types of recipients. At the University of Pittsburgh, the prevalence of bacterial pneumonia occurring in the first two weeks after lung and heart–lung transplant procedures is 35%[50]. Two-thirds of recipients of pulmonary transplant at the University of Toronto experience some sort of infectious complication, with pulmonary infection the most common[51]. In our experience, approximately 50% of transplant recipients require antibiotic therapy for bacterial pulmonary infection (bronchitis or pneumonia)[52]. This incidence is the same among patients with CF and those with other indications for lung transplantation.

The transplanted lung is probably more susceptible to infection than an intact native lung. Mucociliary clearance is impaired after lung transplantation[53,54], which may be a function of altered mucous viscosity[55]. Airway denervation also leads to hypersensitivity to noxious stimuli[56], increasing the risk of bronchospasm. Postoperative pain after transplant also undoubtedly plays a role in the impairment of airway clearance. These factors contribute to a high risk of graft infection following lung transplantation. Colonization of the airway, nasopharynx and sinuses with resistant organisms is another factor increasing the risk of graft infection for CF patients. For these reasons, CF recipients are maintained on prophylactic antibiotics for a longer duration than are non-CF patients, and prophylaxis is continued for varying periods postoperatively ranging from 6 to 16 days.

At Papworth Hospital, Cambridge, the incidence of infectious complications after transplantation in CF patients was no different from the incidence of infectious complications after heart–lung transplantation for other reasons[46]. A similar incidence of infection between CF and non-CF recipients of lung transplants was also reported by the Stanford group[33].

Four of five early postoperative deaths at the University of Toronto were related to sepsis, with four deaths in this series the result of *Ps. cepacia* sepsis[44]. *Ps. cepacia* has emerged as a particularly lethal organism following lung transplantation[57]. At the University of Toronto, where the incidence of *Ps. cepacia* is higher than at other centres, a recent report suggests that

*Ps. cepacia* is the main predictor of poor outcome following double lung transplant for CF. Of 10 patients who were known to have *Ps. cepacia* pre transplant, three died as a direct result of *Ps. cepacia* infection. Five other patients acquired *Ps. cepacia* post transplant, and four of these died[57]. At the University of North Carolina, five patients with *Ps. cepacia* have undergone lung transplantation. Two of these died within six months from disseminated *Ps. cepacia* pneumonia, one has never grown *Ps. cepacia* following her transplant, one developed obliterative bronchiolitis requiring retransplant 14 months after her initial transplant and ultimately died from cytomegalovirus (CMV) pneumonia, and one patient had a successful outcome but committed suicide 10 months post transplant. A sixth patient developed *Ps. cepacia* pneumonia three months post double lung transplant but never grew the organism prior to transplant.

Reports about the transmissibility of *Ps. cepacia* from patient to patient present conflicting evidence. It is clear that *Ps. cepacia* can be transmitted from one CF patient to another[58], but transmission between patients is rare, even after prolonged social exposure[59]. Further epidemiological studies are required to determine the impact of this pathogen on lung transplant programmes. Currently, the presence of *Ps. cepacia* is considered a relative contraindication to transplant at some centres because of the higher risk of death following transplant in this cohort of patients.

Some programmes surgically drain the sinuses of CF patients prior to lung transplantation in an attempt to reduce the burden of bacteria[60]. This practice is based on a study that suggested that surgical drainage and administration of intrasinus antibiotics decreased exacerbations of pulmonary infections in CF patients with severe lung diseases[61]. We have chosen not to perform sinus drainage procedures routinely in our CF patients. Some of our CF patients have required postoperative treatment of sinus infection, and this is more frequent in CF patients than in non-CF patients. Performing this procedure after a transplant has the benefit of allowing the use of general anaesthesia with endotracheal intubation to protect the airway from soiling.

The incidence of other infectious complications is no different among CF recipients of lung transplantation. A marked reduction has been seen in *Pneumocystis* pneumonia in transplant recipients with the prophylactic use of trimethoprin–sulphamethoxazole[50]. Other antibiotics that are of use prophylactically include nystatin, which minimizes the incidence of oral *Candida*, and low-dose acylovir, which is useful for HSV prophylaxis. The ideal prophylactic regimen for CMV disease has yet to be established for lung transplant recipients. In our experience, CMV disease is very common after lung transplantation, but is effectively treated in most instances with gancyclovir. CMV pneumonia has been the cause of one late death among 39 lung transplants for CF at the University of North Carolina.

The importance of other infectious agents in CF patients is controversial. Although we are concerned about transplantation and immunosuppression in patients who harbour mycobacterial organisms, we have not seen this mycobacterial disease recur in two patients, one colonized with *Mycobacterium avium intracellulare* and one with *M. chelonae*. However, granulomatous inflammation in the lungs was not demonstrated by histology at explantation for either of the patients colonized in our series. Similarly, we have not considered colonization with *Aspergillus*, a contraindication to lung transplantation, but we do concur with other centres[40,41] that aspergillomas involving the chest wall or breaching the visceral pleura are contraindications because of the risk of extensive pleural *Aspergillus* contamination at the time of surgery.

## OTHER COMPLICATIONS OF LUNG TRANSPLANTATION

Aside from the early complications of graft dysfunction and infection, which account for the largest number of early deaths following lung transplantation[37], recipients of lung transplants or heart–lung transplants are at risk for the development of bronchiolitis obliterans and lymphoproliferative disease, which are major causes of morbidity and mortality for long-term survivors. Bronchiolitis obliterans is an inflammatory process of small airways leading to obstruction and destruction of pulmonary bronchioles[62]. The aetiology remains obscure, but bronchiolitis obliterans is presumed to be a manifestation of chronic rejection (Figure 5).

While some authors have attempted to demonstrate a relationship between CMV infection[63] or the number of episodes of acute rejection[64] and the subsequent development of obliterative bronchiolitis, the disease process is increasingly common as time elapses following transplant. According to Madden et al.[40], who reported the largest series of heart–lung transplants for CF, the cumulative probability of having this complication at one, two and three years after surgery was 17%, 23% and 48%, respectively. The development of bronchiolitis obliterans leads to a number of different clinical scenarios. Some patients have a decrement in pulmonary function which stabilizes, occasionally in response to augmented immunosuppression[65]. Other patients develop rapidly progressive obstructive pulmonary disease leading to death or requiring retransplant, while still others have a more insidious course of deteriorating pulmonary function. Some observers have noted that bronchoalveolar lavage (BAL)-derived lymphocytes from patients with obliterative bronchiolitis may demonstrate donor antigen-specific reactivity (using the primed lymphocyte test) to class I to class II antigens. Furthermore, the pattern of the reactivity correlated with the pattern of progression of the

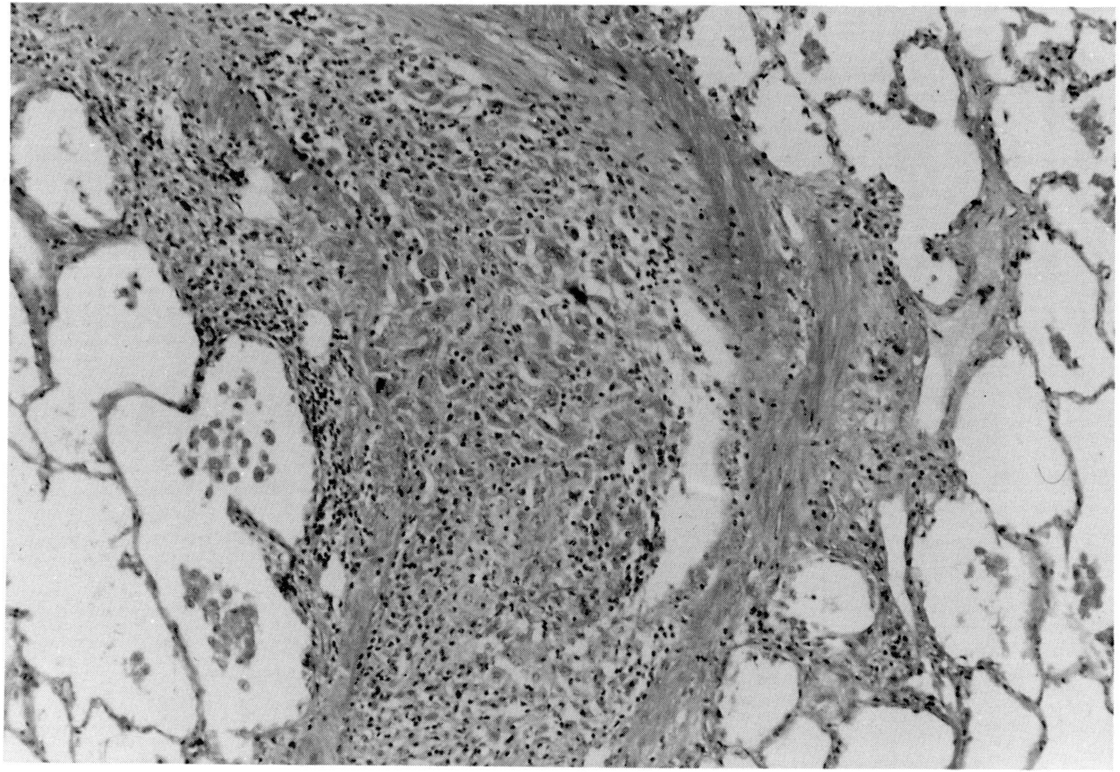

**Figure 5** Open lung biopsy of a CF patient 13 months after double lung transplant, demonstrating obliterative bronchiolitis. Note the inflammatory granulation tissue filling the lumen of a bronchiole. (Reproduced from Egan[78], with permission)

bronchiolitis (stable versus progressive), implying that distinct immunopathogenetic events may be responsible for the development and progression of obliterative bronchiolitis[66]. In our experience, the development of obliterative bronchiolitis predisposes patients with CF to recurrent bouts of infectious bronchiolitis, usually with *Pseudomonas* species.

To better define and classify patients who develop this most common long-term complication of lung transplantation, a classification system was recently proposed[67]. This classification system, which is summarized in Table 3, uses clinical variables to determine departure from baseline $FEV_1$ as a basis for grading the severity of bronchiolitis obliterans syndrome (BOS). Of note, the diagnosis of BOS does not require histological confirmation, and indeed the histological presence of bronchiolitis obliterans can occasionally be observed in patients with no demonstrable decrement in pulmonary function. It is anticipated that classification of patients with respect to severity of obliterative bronchiolitis will allow for better interpretation of clinical trials that might be forthcoming to reduce the incidence and severity of BOS following transplantation.

Following any solid organ transplant, patients are at increased risk for a variety of neoplastic disorders, including lymphoproliferative disorders. This is the most common type of neoplastic disorder associated with transplantation and is thought to occur in approximately 5% of recipients of heart–lung allografts[68]. There is a poorly understood relationship between Epstein–Barr virus and the development of some post-transplant lymphoproliferative disorders (PTLD)[68]. Occasionally, patients with PTLD respond to antiviral therapy or reduction in immunosuppression[40], but this therapeutic strategy places the graft at risk and may increase the risk of the development of obliterative bronchiolitis. It is hoped that the development of more specific immunosuppressive therapies will reduce the incidence of PTLD in recipients of all solid organ transplants in the future.

**Table 3** Proposed staging system for bronchiolitis obliterans syndrome[67]

| Grade | Pulmonary function text characteristics |
|---|---|
| 0 | No significant abnormality: $FEV_1$ 80% or more of baseline value |
| 1 | Mild obliterative bronchiolitis syndrome: $FEV_1$ 66–80% of baseline value |
| 2 | Moderate obliterative bronchiolitis syndrome: $FEV_1$ 51–65% of baseline value |
| 3 | Severe obliterative bronchiolitis syndrome: $FEV_1$ 50% or less of baseline value |

*Subclassifications*
a. Without pathological evidence of obliterative bronchiolitis
b. With pathological evidence of obliterative bronchiolitis

## QUALITY OF LIFE FOLLOWING LUNG TRANSPLANTATION FOR CYSTIC FIBROSIS

For appropriately selected patients with end-stage lung disease, it would hardly be surprising to establish that restoration of near-normal lung function would result in improved quality of life. However, not all patients evaluated for transplantation ultimately receive a graft, and not all transplant recipients have a successful outcome. The Cambridge group has utilized a general health status questionnaire—the Nottingham Health Profile—in an attempt to quantify the impact of heart–lung transplantation on patients with CF. There was improvement in all six dimensions of the health profile after heart–lung transplant for CF; differences reached statistical significance in physical mobility, energy, sleep, social isolation and emotional reactions[41,69]. The areas of daily living most affected by health status before heart–lung transplant for CF were: looking after the home, social life, sex life, hobbies and holidays, according to these investigators[41]. Perhaps the most convincing testament to the utility of transplant procedures for this disorder comes from recipients themselves. One 34-year-old recipient of a heart–lung transplant writes: 'for the person with CF who has a successful transplant, the quality of life is often considerably better postop than even at the best of times preop. Although chest physical therapy and nebulized antibiotics are still used, they are prophylactic. Most of the time, consuming treatments are not now required simply to stay alive. ... There have been few drawbacks to having one of the most remarkable operations.'[70] Another young woman writes: 'It is hard to take in the magnitude of the miracle and change in lifestyle the transplant has meant to me. I may still die a pulmonary death, someday, but the victory over CF is sweet.'[71]

## THE FUTURE OF LUNG TRANSPLANTATION

Three critical issues hinder more widespread utilization of lung transplantation for patients with end-stage CF lung disease. The first is the inadequate supply of donor organs. The number of cadaver organ donors in Europe and the USA is remarkably consistent[72] and is woefully inadequate to meet the growing demand for organs. In the experience of the Montreal–Marseille combined programme, the number of patients with CF who died waiting for transplant equalled the number of patients who received organs[45]. Among 95 patients referred for evaluation to the University of North Carolina, 11 who were deemed acceptable candidates died waiting for a graft to become available. Waiting time has increased annually and now averages over a year for CF patients at our institution. Strategies to increase the number of pulmonary donors include increasing the number of donors in the population in general, maximizing retrieval of suitable lungs from currently identified organ donors, relaxing the criteria for lung donation (which entails increasing the risk of primary graft dysfunction post transplant), or considering other tactics to identify potential sources of lungs not currently used for transplantation. Although xenotransplantation offers a way to ameliorate the donor shortage in the future, applicability awaits a better understanding of the immune mechanisms responsible for hyperacute rejection[73]. Xenotransplantation does offer the potential for genetic engineering to modify the donor tissue, potentially making it less susceptible to rejection. Living relation donation of a pulmonary lobe has been achieved technically[74], but is not practical for large numbers of CF patients because of the requirement for bilateral lung replacement and because most CF patients will survive to adulthood with their disease before transplantation is an option.

It is conceivable that lungs may be retrieved from donors after cessation of circulation. Some laboratory data are available that support this notion[75–77]. If this strategy is practical, then there are potentially large numbers of accident victims, suicide victims and other casualties that might provide lungs suitable for transplantation.

A second vexing issue that threatens to detract from lung transplant efforts in CF is the disconcerting development of obliterative bronchiolitis in large numbers of recipients. Clearly, more research is needed to better understand this process and develop strategies to prevent it or reduce its severity in transplant recipients. Finally, there are increasing numbers of patients who become colonized with *Ps. cepacia* and other pathogens that increase the risk of transplantation. As donor organs become more scarce in relation to the numbers on the waiting list, ethical debates will arise concerning the advisability of transplanting patients who are at higher risk of lethal complications. Studies of *Ps. cepacia* in particular are necessary to develop antibiotic therapies that are efficacious for these patients.

## SUMMARY

In the last decade, lung transplantation has emerged as a valuable and effective palliative therapy for CF patients with end-stage lung disease. Dramatic improvements have been seen in operative survival and operative techniques so that this lifesaving therapy can be offered to many patients with CF who previously had been considered inappropriate candidates, e.g. patients with previous thoracotomy or pleurodesis. A major limitation to more widespread application of this therapy is the shortage of suitable pulmonary donors. To prevent this devastating complication, research must be directed at a better understanding of the immune processes responsible for the development of obliterative bronchiolitis. Ultimately, the goal of CF researchers is to prevent the devastating bronchiectasis that is the hallmark of this disease; but until this goal is reached, lung transplantation offers an opportunity for improved quantity and quality of life for patients with CF pulmonary disease.

## REFERENCES


1 Scanlin TF. Cystic fibrosis. In: *Pulmonary Diseases and Disorders*, 2nd edn (ed AP Fishman) McGraw-Hill, New York, 1988, pp 1273–94.
2 Egan TM, Kaiser LR, Cooper JD. Lung transplantation. *Curr Probl Surg* 1989; **26**: 675–751.
3 Trulock EP, Cooper JD, Kaiser LR, et al. The Washington University–Barnes Hospital experience with lung transplantation. *JAMA* 1991; **266**: 1943–6.
4 Egan TM, Westerman JH, Lambert CJ Jr, et al. Isolated lung transplantation for end stage lung disease: a viable therapy. *Ann Thorac Surg* 1992; **53**: 590–6.
5 Penketh A, Higenbottam T, Hakim M, Wallwork J. Heart and lung transplantation in patients with end stage lung disease. *Br Med J* 1987; **295**: 311–14.
6 Knowles M, Gatzy J, Boucher R. Increased bioelectric potential difference across respiratory epithelia in cystic fibrosis. *N Engl J Med* 1981; **305**: 1489–95.
7 Wood A, Higenbottam T, Jackson M, et al. Airway mucosal bioelectric potential difference in cystic fibrosis after lung transplantation. *Am Rev Respir Dis* 1989; **140**: 1645–9.
8 Hardy JD, Webb WR, Dalton ML, Walker GR. Lung homotransplantation in man. *JAMA* 1963; **186**: 1065–74.
9 Cooley DA, Bloodwell RD, Hallman GL, et al. Organ transplantation for advanced cardiopulmonary disease. *Ann Thorac Surg* 1969; **8**: 30–46.
10 Stiller CR, Keown PA. Cyclosporine therapy in perspective. *Prog Transplant* 1984; **1**: 11–45.
11 Lima O, Cooper JD, Peters WJ, et al. Effects of methylprednisolone and azathioprine on bronchial healing following lung transplantation. *J Thorac Cardiovasc Surg* 1981; **82**: 211–15.
12 Reitz BA, Burton NA, Jamieson SW, et al. Heart and lung transplantation: autotransplantation and allotransplantation in primates with extended survival. *J Thorac Cardiovasc Surg* 1980; **80**: 360–72.
13 Reitz BA, Wallwork JL, Hunt SA, et al. Heart–lung transplantation: successful therapy for patients with pulmonary vascular disease. *N Engl J Med* 1982; **306**: 557–64.
14 Morgan E, Lima O, Goldberg M, et al. Successful revascularization of totally ischemic bronchial autografts with omental pedicle flaps in dogs. *J Thorac Cardiovasc Surg* 1982; **84**: 204–10.
15 Lima O, Goldberg M, Peters WJ, et al. Bronchial omentopexy in canine lung transplantation. *J Thorac Cardiovasc Surg* 1982; **83**: 418–21.
16 Saunders NR, Egan TM, Chamberlain D, Cooper JD. Cyclosporine and bronchial healing in canine lung transplantation. *J Thorac Cardiovasc Surg* 1984; **88**: 993–9.
17 The Toronto Lung Transplant Group. Unilateral lung transplantation for pulmonary fibrosis. *N Engl J Med* 1986; **314**: 1140–5.
18 The Toronto Lung Transplant Group. Experience with single lung transplantation for pulmonary fibrosis. *JAMA* 1988; **259**: 2258–62.
19 Grossman RF, Frost A, Zamel N, et al. Results of single-lung transplantation for bilateral pulmonary fibrosis. *N Engl J Med* 1990; **322**: 727–33.

20 Dark JH, Patterson GA, Al-Jilaihawi AN, et al. Experimental en bloc double-lung transplantation. *Ann Thorac Surg* 1986; **42**: 394–8.
21 Patterson GA, Cooper JD, Dark JH, Jones MT, the Toronto Lung Transplant Group. Experimental and clinical double lung transplantation. *J Thorac Cardiovasc Surg* 1988; **95**: 70–4.
22 Yacoub MH, Banner NR, Khaghani A, et al. Heart–lung transplantation for cystic fibrosis and subsequent domino heart transplantation. *J Heart Transplant* 1990; **9**: 459–67.
23 Patterson GA, Todd TR, Cooper JD, et al. Airway complications after double lung transplantation. *J Thorac Cardiovasc Surg* 1990; **99**: 14–21.
24 Noirclerc MJ, Metras D, Vaillant A, et al. Bilateral bronchial anastomosis in double lung and heart–lung transplantations. *Eur J Cardiothorac Surg* 1990; **4**: 314–17.
25 Pasque MK, Cooper JD, Kaiser LR, et al. Improved technique for bilateral lung transplantation: rationale and initial clinical experience. *Ann Thorac Surg* 1990; **49**: 785–91.
26 Baldwin JC, Oyer PE, Stinson EB, et al. Comparison of cardiac rejection in heart and heart–lung transplantation. *J Heart Transplant* 1987; **6**; 352–6.
27 Billingham ME. Cardiac transplant atherosclerosis. *Transplant Proc* 1987; **19** (Suppl 5): 19–25.
28 Traill TA. Physiology and function of the transplant allograft. In: *Heart and Heart–Lung Transplantation* (eds WA Baumgartner, BA Reitz, SC Achuff) Saunders, Philadelphia, 1990, pp 266–78.
29 Royston D, Taylor KM, Bidstrup BP, Sapsford RN. Effect of aprotinin on need for blood transfusion after repeat open-heart surgery. Lancet 1987; **ii**: 1289–91.
30 Frist WH, Fox MD, Campbell PW, et al. Cystic fibrosis treated with heart–lung transplantation: North American results. *Transplant Proc* 1991; **23**: 1205–6.
31 Reitz BA. Heart and lung transplantation. In: *Heart and Heart–Lung Transplantation* (eds WA Baumgartner, BA Reitz, SC Achuff) Saunders, Philadelphia, 1990, pp 319–46.
32 Jamieson SW, Kaye MP. Operative procedure and postoperative management. In: *Heart and Heart–Lung Transplantation* (ed J Wallwork) Saunders, Philadelphia, 1989, pp 481–90.
33 Starnes VA, Lewiston N, Theodore J, et al. Cystic fibrosis: target population for lung transplantation in North America in the 1990s. *J Thorac Cardiovasc Surg* 1992; **103**: 1008–14.
34 Egan TM, Detterbeck FC. Technique and results of double lung transplantation. *Chest Surg Clin N Am* 1993; **3**: 89–111.
35 Calhoon JH, Grover FL, Gibbons WJ, et al. Single lung transplantation: alternative indications and technique. *J Thorac Cardiovasc Surg* 1991; **101**: 816–25.
36 Egan TM, Paradowski LJ, Detterbeck FC, Mill MR. Is bronchial omentopexy helpful in human lung transplantation? (abstract). *Chest* 1992; **102** (Suppl): 74S.
37 Registry of the International Society for Heart and Lung Transplantation: 10th official report—1993. *J Heart Lung Transplant* 1993; **12**: 541–8.
38 FitzSimmons SC. The changing epidemiology of cystic fibrosis. *J Pediatr* 1993; **122**: 1–9.
39 Kerem E, Reisman J, Corey M, et al. Prediction of mortality in patients with cystic fibrosis. *N Engl J Med* 1992; **326**: 1187–91.
40 Madden BP, Hodson ME, Tsang V, et al. Intermediate-term results of heart–lung transplantation for cystic fibrosis. *Lancet* 1992; **339**: 1583–7.

41 Dennis C, Caine N, Sharples L, et al. Heart–lung transplantation for end stage respiratory disease in cystic fibrosis patients at Papworth Hospital. *J Heart Lung Transplant* 1993; **12**: 893–902.
42 Reisman J, Corey M, Canny G, Levison H. Diabetes mellitus in patients with cystic fibrosis: effect on survival. *Pediatrics* 1990; **86**: 374–7.
43 Warner JO. Heart–lung transplantation: all the facts. *Arch Dis Child* 1991; **66** (Suppl): 1013–16.
44 Ramirez JC, Patterson GA, Winton TL, et al. Bilateral lung transplantation for cystic fibrosis. *J Thorac Cardiovasc Surg* 1992; **103**: 287–94.
45 Shennib H, Noirclerc M, Ernst P, et al. Double-lung transplantation for cystic fibrosis. *Ann Thorac Surg* 1992; **54**: 27–32.
46 de Leval MR, Smyth R, Whitehead B, et al. Heart and lung transplantation for terminal cystic fibrosis: a $4\frac{1}{2}$-year experience. *J Thorac Cardiovasc Surg* 1991; **101**: 633–42.
47 Stanghelle JK. Physical exercise for patients with cystic fibrosis: a review. *Int J Sports Med* 1988; **9** (Suppl): 6–18.
48 Canny GJ, Levison H. Exercise response and rehabilitation in cystic fibrosis. *Sports Med* 1987; **4**: 143–52.
49 Arnold CD, Westerman JH, Downs AM, Egan TM. Benefits of an aerobic exercise program in CF patients waiting for double lung transplantation. *Pediatr Pulmonol* 1991; **6** (Suppl): 287.
50 Dauber JH, Paradis IL, Dummer JS. Infectious complications in pulmonary allograft recipients. *Clin Chest Med* 1990; **11**: 291–308.
51 Maurer JR, Tullis DE, Grossman RF, et al. Infectious complications following isolated lung transplantation. *Chest* 1992; **101**: 1056–9.
52 Flume PA, Egan TM, Paradowski LJ, et al. Infectious complications of lung transplantation: impact of cystic fibrosis. *Am J Resp Crit Care Med* 1994; **149**: 1601–7.
53 Edmunds LH, Stallone RJ, Graf PD, et al. Mucus transport in transplanted lungs of dogs. *Surgery* 1969; **66**: 15–22.
54 Dolovich M, Rossman C, Chambers C, et al. Muco-ciliary function in patients following single lung or lung/heart transplantation (abstract). *Am Rev Respir Dis* 1987; **135**: A363.
55 Brody JS, Klempfner G, Staum MM, et al. Mucociliary clearance after lung denervation and bronchial transection. *J Appl Physiol* 1972; **32**: 160–4.
56 Glanville AR, Burke CM, Theodore J, et al. Bronchial hyper-responsiveness after human cardiopulmonary transplantation. *Clin Sci* 1987; **73**: 299–303.
57 Snell GI, de Hoyos A, Krajden M, et al. *Pseudomonas cepacia* in lung transplant recipients with cystic fibrosis. *Chest* 1993; **103**: 466–71.
58 LiPuma JJ, Dasen SE, Nielson DW, et al. Person-to-person transmission of *Pseudomonas cepacia* between patients with cystic fibrosis. *Lancet* 1990; **336**: 1094–6.
59 Gladman G, Connor PJ, Williams RF, David TJ. Controlled study of *Pseudomonas cepacia* and *Pseudomonas maltophilia* in cystic fibrosis. *Arch Dis Child* 1992; **67**: 192–5.
60 Lewiston N, King V, Umetsu D, et al. Cystic fibrosis patients who have undergone heart–lung transplantation benefit from maxillary sinus antrostomy and repeated sinus lavage. *Transplant Proc* 1991; **23**: 1207–8.
61 Umetsu DT, Moss RB, King VV, Lewiston NJ. Sinus disease in patients with severe cystic fibrosis and relation to pulmonary exacerbation. *Lancet* 1990; **335**: 1077–8.
62 Theodore J, Starnes VA, Lewiston NJ. Obliterative bronchiolitis. *Clin Chest Med* 1990; **11**: 309–21.

63 Duncan AJ, Dummer JS, Paradis IL, et al. Cytomegalovirus infection and survival in lung transplant recipients. *J Heart Lung Transplant* 1991; **10**: 638–46.
64 Scott JP, Higenbottam TW, Clelland C, et al. The natural history of obliterative bronchiolitis and occlusive vascular disease of patients following heart–lung transplantation. *Transplant Proc* 1989; **21**: 2592–3.
65 Glanville A, Baldwin J, Burke C. Obliterative bronchiolitis after heart–lung transplantation: apparent arrest by augmented immunosupession. *Ann Intern Med* 1987; **107**: 300–4.
66 Reinsmoen NL, Bolman RM, Savik K, et al. Are multiple immunopathogenetic events occurring during the development of obliterative bronchiolitis and acute rejection? *Transplantation* 1993; **55**: 1040–4.
67 Cooper JD, Billingham M, Egan T, et al. A working formulation for the standardization of nomenclature and for clinical staging of chronic dysfunction in lung allografts. *J Heart Lung Transplant* 1993; **12**: 713–16.
68 Nalesnik MA, Makowka L, Starzl TE. The diagnosis and treatment of post-transplant lymphoproliferative disorders. *Curr Probl Surg* 1988; **25**: 365–472.
69 Caine N, Hathaway T, Dennis C, et al. Quality of life of cystic fibrosis patients before and after heart–lung transplantation (abstract). *Pediatr Pulmonol* 1991; **6** (Suppl): 288.
70 Oakman P. My heart–lung transplant. *J R Soc Med* 1993; **86** (Suppl 20): 34–5.
71 Gibson DL. Lung transplantation for cystic fibrosis: a patient's perspective. *Pediatr Pulmonol* 1992; Suppl 8: 213–14.
72 *1993 Annual Report of the US Scientific Registry of Transplant Recipients and the Organ Procurement and Transplantation Network—Transplant Data: 1988–1991.* UNOS, Richmond, VA, and the Division of Organ Transplantation, US Department of Health and Human Services, Bethesda, MD, 1993.
73 Platt JL, Bach FH. The barrier to xenotransplantation. *Transplantation* 1991 **52**: 937–47.
74 Starnes VA, Lewiston NJ, Luikart H, et al. Current trends in lung transplantation: lobar transplantation and expanded use of single lungs. *J Thorac Cardiovasc Surg* 1992; **104**; 1060–6.
75 Egan TM, Lambert CJ Jr, Reddick RL, et al. A strategy to increase the donor pool: the use of cadaver lungs for transplantation. *Ann Thorac Surg* 1991; **52**: 1113–21.
76 Egan TM, Ulicny KS Jr, Lambert CJ Jr, Wilcox BR. Effect of a free radical scavenger on cadaveric lung transplantation. *Ann Thorac Surg* 1993; **55**: 1453–9.
77 Ulicny KS Jr, Egan TM, Lambert CJ Jr, et al. Cadaver lung donors: effect of preharvest ventilation on graft function. *Ann Thorac Surg* 1993; **55**: 1185–91.
78 Egan TM. Lung transplantation in cystic fibrosis. *Semin Respir Infect* 1992; **7**: 227–39.

Chapter Sixteen

# Prevention and Treatment of Liver Disease in Cystic Fibrosis

Carla Colombo and Maria Letizia Petroni[a]
*Department of Paediatrics and [a]Istituto di Scienze Biomediche (Ospedale San Paolo), University of Milan, Italy*

## INTRODUCTION

With improved survival of patients with cystic fibrosis (CF), the characteristic form of associated liver disease has become more frequently recognized. The pathognomonic lesion, focal biliary cirrhosis, is present in 25–30% of CF patients and is characterized by accumulation of eosinophilic material in intrahepatic bile ducts, chronic inflammatory cell infiltrate, bile duct proliferation and fibrosis. These lesions initially have a focal distribution, but during the course of the disease they tend to progress, ultimately leading to multilobular biliary cirrhosis and portal hypertension. Preservation of hepatic function until late stage is characteristic, thus explaining the long natural history of this potentially severe complication of CF[1,2].

Chronic liver disease, despite not being a major direct cause of death in CF patients[3], has been suggested to have a negative prognostic impact even in the absence of hepatic decompensation: hepatomegaly has been recognized as a risk factor for early death[4], which may be favoured by deterioration of nutritional status induced by liver disease itself[5].

While lacking a specific treatment, therapeutic options have so far included supportive care and treatment of the complications of cirrhosis and portal

*Cystic Fibrosis—Current Topics, Volume 2.* Edited by J. A. Dodge, D. J. H. Brock and J. H. Widdicombe

hypertension; more recently, liver transplantation for CF patients with end-stage liver disease and mild respiratory involvement has been proposed[6].

With the future perspective of gene therapy for CF lung disease[7], hepatobiliary complications are likely to become an increasingly important cause of morbidity and mortality. For these reasons the development of effective strategies for treatment and prevention of liver disease has been included among the priorities to be achieved in CF research.

## PATHOGENESIS OF LIVER DISEASE

There is increasing evidence that liver disease is a direct consequence of the basic defect of CF[8]. Reduced hydration, due to the chloride channel defect, results in hyperviscosity and low solubility of biliary secretions. Obstruction of bile ductules may induce a series of events (such as retention of hepatotoxic bile acids, production of inflammatory cytokines and free radicals, lipid peroxidation), which in turn can aggravate and perpetuate liver damage. A close association between cirrhosis and the presence of mucous plugs in the bile ductules has been reported by an autopsy survey, providing further evidence on the role of dehydrated secretions in the pathogenesis of CF-associated liver disease[9].

## THE CYSTIC FIBROSIS BASIC DEFECT AND THE LIVER

A series of studies dealing with the definition of CFTR function at the hepatobiliary level as well as with the impact of the CF secretory abnormality on bile flow are available or currently in progress.

First, the crucial role of chloride channels in the process of bile formation has been suggested by *in vitro* studies. Recently, measurement of membrane chloride conductance in isolated rat bile duct epithelial cells using whole-cell patch-clamp recording techniques has clearly shown that two separate $Ca^{2+}$ and cAMP-regulated chloride channels participate in the control of fluid and electrolyte transport across biliary epithelium[10]. In the rat, the cAMP-regulated channel is stimulated by forskolin and is DIDS insensitive, showing therefore the typical characteristics of chloride conductance associated with CFTR expression[11]. In order to establish whether this channel is indeed caused by endogenous expression of CFTR at the hepatobiliary level, this protein was looked for in sections of rat liver. Immunoblot and immunoperoxidase staining revealed that CFTR is detectable in bile duct epithelial cells, but in no other cells of the liver, including hepatocytes[12,13]. The existence in man of a similar CFTR localization in the apical membrane of bile duct epithelial cells has been recently demonstrated[13A].

The fact that CFTR expression occurs exclusively in intrahepatic biliary epithelial cells is in agreement with the pathology of CF-associated liver disease, which suggests a primary abnormality in biliary function.

Finally, phenotypic expression of the CF defect within the intrahepatic biliary duct epithelium has been explored using a recently developed model system: expression of ΔF508 and G542X genotypes has been demonstrated in immortalized intrahepatic bile duct epithelial cell lines from CF patients[14].

All these data indicate that the biliary tract epithelium is affected similarly to the secretory epithelial cells in airway and pancreas and that CFTR may function as an apical cAMP-dependent chloride channel. Abnormalities of this channel are important in the pathogenesis of liver disease in CF. Perhaps other functions of CFTR (e.g. regulation of water movement through the channel and/or chloride–bicarbonate exchange) may contribute as well, but this will need further clarification.

## THERAPEUTIC OPTIONS

With remarkable advances in the global treatment of CF patients over the last two decades, the expectant management policy so far adopted for hepatobiliary complications has become no longer acceptable. As has been recently proposed for CF lung disease[8], a multifaceted therapeutic approach targeted at the different steps of the physiopathological process of CF-associated liver disease can now be identified (Table 1).

### SOMATIC GENE THERAPY

Specific therapy for CF-associated liver disease requires somatic gene transfer. Strategies for liver-directed gene therapy have so far focused exclusively on the hepatocyte as a target cell and therefore would not be appropriate for targeting affected bile duct epithelial cells *in vivo* in CF-associated liver disease. New strategies should therefore be developed. Recent experimental studies in the rat have indicated that it may be feasible to deliver recombinant viruses specifically to the biliary tract by a non-surgical approach, i.e. endoscopic retrograde cholangiography[13]. Recombinant adenoviruses expressing the human CFTR gene were infused retrograde into the rat biliary tract through the common bile duct: gene expression was successfully achieved in virtually all cells for the whole duration of the experiment (21 days).

Retrograde biliary delivery of recombinant adenoviruses to the human biliary tract could also be theoretically applicable as a strategy to prevent liver disease in CF patients at risk.

**Table 1** Therapeutic approaches to liver disease associated with cystic fibrosis

| Abnormality | Solution | Approach |
|---|---|---|
| Abnormal CFTR gene<br>Abnormal CFTR protein | Provide normal gene | Liver-targeted gene therapy |
| Abnormally viscous biliary secretion | Decrease viscosity | Choleretic agents<br>UDCA* |
| Retention of hepatotoxic bile acids | Replace them with non-toxic bile acids | UDCA* |
| Free radical production<br>Lipid peroxidation | Increase antioxidant activity | $\beta$-Carotene<br>Vitamin E |
| Massive<br>Steatosis | Correct pancreatic insufficiency | Pancreatic enzymes |
| | Improve nutritional status | Hypercaloric diet |
| Multilobular biliary cirrhosis | Prevent complications of portal hypertension | UDCA?<br>Sclerotherapy of varices |
| Liver failure | Replace the liver | Liver transplantation |

* UDCA: Ursodeoxycholic acid.

This is an exciting approach which, however, raises a number of questions and problems. The assessment of the potential efficacy of gene therapy for liver disease in the murine animal model of CF is not feasible, since these animals apparently do not develop hepatobiliary disease[15]. It will probably be necessary to develop other animal models to assess whether this strategy can be considered in humans. It is therefore unlikely that it will be applied in the near future.

## EMPIRICAL THERAPIES

While waiting for liver-targeted gene therapy to be developed, therapeutic and prophylactic strategies should be aimed at counteracting the subsequent pathogenetic events of CF-associated liver disease.

First of all, bile viscosity should be reduced by administering a choleretic agent; this would prevent mucus plugging and bile sedimentation within the portal bile ductules.

Second, changes in biliary bile acid composition can be induced by medical treatment. Endogenous bile acids are detergent and cytotoxic *in vitro*; at high concentrations, they can damage cell membranes. Retention of these hepatotoxic bile acids is therefore considered to have a prominent role in determining liver cell injury during cholestasis[16].

The cytotoxic effects of different bile acids are related to the physicochemical properties of each compound and increase with the degree of hydrophobicity. Hydrophobicity is inversely related to the number of hydroxyl groups in the bile acid steroid nucleus: monohydroxy bile acids are more hydrophobic and hepatotoxic than di- and trihydroxy bile acids. Hydrophobicity is also influenced by conjugation: free bile acids are more hydrophobic than glycine conjugates, which in turn are more hydrophobic than taurine conjugates[17].

In CF, the hydrophobicity of the bile acid pool may be relatively high, due to the net predominance of the more hydrophobic glycoconjugated over tauroconjugated bile acids[1]. This is a consequence of bile acid malabsorption[18], which causes increased fecal losses of taurine in CF patients. Taurine deficiency has therefore been indicated as a possible mechanism contributing to liver damage in these patients[19].

A different but complementary pathogenetic mechanism involves increased free radical production and decreased lipid-soluble antioxidant activity, leading to oxidative damage to liver cell membranes. Deficiencies in vitamin E and β-carotene as well as in essential fatty acids may combine with hydrophobic bile acids and hepatic copper accumulation to cause free radical injury during cholestasis in CF patients[20]. No information is available on the effects of antioxidant supplementation in CF-associated liver disease, although preliminary data suggest that β-carotene supplementation improves overall antioxidant status in essential fatty acid deficient CF patients[21].

## BILE ACID THERAPY

The hydrophilic, non-toxic ursodeoxycholic acid (UDCA) has been in clinical use for the dissolution of cholesterol gallstones for at least two decades, and only more recently it has been employed in the treatment of chronic cholestatic liver diseases, such as primary biliary cirrhosis, primary sclerosing cholangitis and several forms of paediatric cholestasis[22,23]. The rationale for its use in liver diseases was initially to displace detergent endogenous bile acids from the enterohepatic circulation, replacing them with a non-toxic compound[24]. However, the finding that the pool size of the major endogenous hydrophobic bile acids remains basically unchanged during UDCA treatment[25] has recently led to a search for other possible mechanisms of action of UDCA in chronic liver diseases.

A cytoprotective effect at the level of the canalicular membrane has been suggested: there is growing experimental evidence that UDCA can stabilize cell membranes and protect them from disruption by detergent bile acids[24,26]

The beneficial effects of UDCA observed in chronic cholestatic liver diseases may also be accounted for by a choleretic effect of UDCA[23]: this latter mechanism of action has not yet been extensively explored in humans. The choleretic potency of the conjugated form of UDCA is probably not greater than that of the two primary bile acids, cholic and chenodeoxycholic acids. In contrast, unconjugated UDCA is able to induce a bicarbonate-rich choleresis in the rat: this hypercholeresis has been explained by ductular absorption and recycling of the protonated bile acid, i.e. the 'cholehepatic' shunt[27]. No such effect has been so far demonstrated in man. In addition, UDCA was shown to be secreted in bile almost exclusively in the conjugated form during its chronic administration to patients with cholestatic liver diseases[24,30].

Although the role of the choleretic properties of UDCA in determining its effectiveness in chronic liver diseases of adults is probably not relevant, its flushing effect may be particularly important in CF patients with liver disease, whose bile ducts are plugged by abnormal viscid secretions resulting in local bile stasis.

## TREATMENT WITH UDCA IN CYSTIC FIBROSIS ASSOCIATED LIVER DISEASE

In recent years, the efficacy of UDCA treatment in chronic liver diseases has been the object of a large number of studies[22,23]. Although it remains to be established whether UDCA therapy can alter the natural history of chronic cholestatic liver diseases, it is presently considered the most effective treatment for cholestasis of mild and moderate degree[24].

Several uncontrolled studies have been carried out to evaluate the efficacy of UDCA treatment in CF-associated liver disease[28-39] and the results from the first controlled studies are becoming available[40-42]. All studies have evaluated the effects of treatment on standard liver function tests, whereas only a few have explored the effects on quantitative liver function, histological findings, fat absorption and nutritional status.

**Table 2** Studies on UDCA therapy for CF-associated liver disease

| Reference | Design | Patients (no.) | Dose (mg/kg per day) | Duration (months) |
|---|---|---|---|---|
| 28 | Open | 9 | 10–15[a] | 6 |
| 29 | Open | 9 | 15–20 | 6 |
| 40 | Placebo-controlled | 38 | 10 | 6 |
| 31 | Open | 22 | 10–20[a] | 12 |
| 33 | Open | 13 | 15–20 | 12 |
| 41 | Randomized, UDCA versus no treatment | 12 | 20 | 6 |
| 38 | Open | 10 | 10–15 | 24 |
| 39 | Open | 30 | 20 | 24 |
| 42 | Placebo-controlled | 55 | 15[b] | 12 |

[a]Taurine supplementation to all patients.
[b]Taurine supplementation evaluated in a double-blind fashion.

Most of these studies are short term and were performed in a limited number of patients (Table 2). Daily doses of UDCA ranged from 10 to 20 mg/kg per day, which were well tolerated, with no significant side-effects. During UDCA treatment, a few patients complained of diarrhoea and abdominal pain, which were generally mild and transient and did not require permanent changes in treatment schedule.

Progression of liver disease and anecdoctal deterioration of liver function during UDCA administration have been reported in adult patients with chronic cholestatic liver diseases[43,44]. Indeed, patients with late-stage liver disease either respond poorly to treatment or may even deteriorate on UDCA. One of the CF patients enrolled in the Italian multicentre trial, with advanced liver disease at entry, developed jaundice and deterioration of liver biochemistry after a few months of treatment with UDCA; she was withdrawn from the study and candidated to liver transplantation[42].

## EFFECTS OF UDCA ON SYMPTOMS

Improvement in symptoms related to cholestasis such as jaundice, pruritus and fatigue has been suggested by several studies on UDCA treatment in chronic cholestatic liver diseases of adults[22,23]. These symptoms are only rarely observed in CF patients with liver disease[1,2]. Watson and colleagues have recently reported on complete resolution of jaundice and satisfactory biochemical improvement in an infant with CF after one month of treatment with UDCA (25 mg/kg per day)[36]

## EFFECTS OF UDCA ON SERUM LIVER ENZYMES

Improvement in serum liver enzyme levels has been uniformly documented by all studies on UDCA treatment in different forms of chronic cholestatic conditions, with a decrease in enzyme concentrations ranging from 30% to 70% of pretreatment values[22–24]. In CF-associated liver disease biochemical abnormalities may be intermittent and even absent in cases with advanced cirrhosis[2]. In CF patients with deranged liver biochemistry, UDCA treatment was always followed by a consistent and sustained improvement in indices related to cytolysis and cholestasis[28–42], which subsequently deteriorated when UDCA was discontinued[31]. These beneficial effects have been confirmed in two multicentre placebo-controlled trials[40,42].

The biochemical response is dose dependent in CF patients[34], who need higher doses than those commonly used in adults with other chronic cholestatic liver diseases (usually in the range of 10–15 mg/kg per day). In a dose–response study, UDCA was administered to nine of our patients in daily doses ranging from 5 to 20 mg/kg for consecutive periods of two months, according to a replicated Latin square design. Serum levels of liver enzymes decreased in a dose-dependent fashion. Biliary UDCA enrichment increased with increasing doses, attaining values similar to those observed in adults with other chronic liver diseases (>40%) only with the highest dose. These data indicate that in CF patients with liver disease doses of UDCA of 20 mg/kg per day or greater are needed to compensate for poor intestinal absorption[18]. Based on our data, a dose–response study testing the effect of doses up to 40 mg/kg per day is in progress in the USA.

An additional observation from our dose–response study was that during treatment serum concentrations of UDCA were highly variable and not related with the percentage of UDCA in bile or with the dose of UDCA administered, thus suggesting that serum UDCA levels cannot be used to evaluate either the degree of biliary enrichment or compliance to treatment[34].

The significance of improvement in serum liver function tests is still unclear, since none of the biochemical parameters so far available has been shown to be of prognostic significance. Furthermore, in a few patients with primary biliary cirrhosis clinical and histological progression of liver disease has been reported despite adequate biochemical response.[44]

Serum liver enzyme levels do not normalize in all CF patients with liver disease, and this is also true for more sensitive markers of cholestasis, such as serum levels of the biliary and liver fractions of alkaline phosphatase isoenzymes[45]. In the group of 22 patients with CF-associated liver disease treated with UDCA by Galabert et al., after one year of treatment the biliary and the liver fraction were still abnormally elevated in 86% and in 90% of cases, respectively[31].

## EFFECTS OF UDCA ON QUANTITATIVE LIVER FUNCTION

Several dynamic tests, which can provide information on different aspects of liver function, have been used in order to evaluate disease progression in chronic cholestasis[46]. In experimental models of chronic cholestasis[47] as well as in patients with primary biliary cirrhosis[48] these tests have been able to provide valuable information on prognosis. Their use has also been advocated to monitor the effects of UDCA therapy in patients with chronic cholestatic liver disease[49]. In CF-associated liver disease, the focal distribution of hepatic lesions may limit sensitivity of dynamic liver function tests, which may become abnormal only in very advanced stages of the disease. Indeed, in CF patients with advanced liver disease Cotting et al. have reported a small but significant improvement in the microsomal capacity (assessed by the aminopyrine breath test) and also in hepatic excretory function (evaluated by BSP retention) after UDCA treatment[29]. However, the effects of UDCA administration on quantitative liver function induced by UDCA were less consistently maintained than the effects on serum liver enzymes[32,35]. In addition, treatment had no apparent effect on functional liver cell mass (cytosolic function)[29], as indicated by galactose elimination capacity.

It is unlikely, though, that patients with advanced liver disease may experience a substantial functional improvement and this view is supported by a randomized study from Ireland[41]. In this study, the effects of a six-month period on UDCA versus no treatment were evaluated in 12 CF patients with advanced liver disease. The improvement in liver biochemistry was confirmed, but no significant effect was shown on hepatocellular function, as assessed by hepatic clearance of indocyanine green[41].

Additional data on larger numbers of patients and on a wider disease spectrum are needed before a definitive conclusion on the usefulness of dynamic tests of liver function in CF can be made.

## EFFECTS OF UDCA ON HEPATOBILIARY SCINTIGRAPHY

Evaluation of hepatic excretion of technetium-labelled iminodiacetic acid derivatives ($^{99m}$Tc-HIDA) represents a non-invasive means of quantifying liver function and bile secretion in CF patients[50,51]. Therefore hepatobiliary scintigraphy, when available, can be used to monitor the response to UDCA treatment[33].

By means of hepatobiliary scintigraphy, we have obtained evidence of improved hepatic excretory function and biliary drainage, which may be mediated by a choleretic effect of UDCA[24]. After one year of treatment, the time to visualization of the intestine decreased substantially in all the patients in whom it was abnormal; we also observed a substantial reduction of intrahepatic bile duct dilatation associated to a lesser grade of intrahepatic retention and to a more rapid biliary outflow of the isotope[33].

Similar results were obtained in a recent study in adult patients with primary biliary cirrhosis and primary sclerosing cholangitis: UDCA treatment resulted in quicker hepatic transit time and enhanced biliary excretion of endogenous bile acids, as assessed by hepatic handling of the taurocholate analogue $^{75}$Se-HCAT[52].

## EFFECTS OF UDCA ON HISTOLOGY

Histological features have prognostic significance in chronic liver diseases and their improvement could be considered a relevant endpoint of UDCA treatment. Controlled trials in primary biliary cirrhosis[53] and primary sclerosing cholangitis[54] have reported improvement in histology after treatment with UDCA, with a significant reduction in inflammation and bile duct proliferation, but not in fibrosis.

Liver biopsy has a limited role in CF-associated liver disease, due to the heterogeneous distribution of hepatic lesions[1,2]: the value of histology in assessing treatment efficacy is also probably limited by the actual possibility of large sampling error when repeated needle liver biopsies are performed. Accordingly, information on the effects of treatment on liver histology are very limited: preliminary data from a Swedish study in a small group of patients indicate only a marginal improvement in inflammation and fibrosis after two years of treatment with UDCA[38].

## EFFECTS OF UDCA ON NUTRITIONAL STATUS AND FAT ABSORPTION

With regard to the effect of UDCA treatment on nutritional status, an improvement in several nutritional parameters has been documented in young adults with CF and long-standing cholestasis associated with major nutritional problems[29,32,35]. These included body weight, body mass index, urine creatinine excretion (as an index of muscular mass), serum albumin and prothrombin time. However, no beneficial effect on growth and nutritional status has been so far documented in CF patients of paediatric age.

Despite the fact that UDCA is known to form mixed micelles less efficiently than primary bile acids[55], no substantial modification in the degree of steatorrhea has been reported following treatment with UDCA. In the multicentre placebo-controlled trial from Italy, deterioration of steatorrhea has been observed only in a few patients treated with UDCA; these patients may benefit from simultaneous taurine supplementation[42].

## LONG-TERM EFFECTS OF UDCA TREATMENT

The long-term benefit of UDCA treatment in preventing events related to morbidity and mortality in patients with chronic cholestatic liver diseases, including CF, has not yet been established. This important information will hopefully be obtained by the ongoing long-term studies on large cohorts of patients, aimed at evaluating the effects of UDCA treatment on clinically relevant endpoints such as survival, need for transplantation or occurrence of complications of cirrhosis and portal hypertension.

Ultrasonography is widely used in the follow-up of CF patients with liver disease[56] and it has also been employed in the long-term evaluation of UDCA treatment[31,37,39,42]. Changes in liver architecture and size of the portal vein are looked for in order to assess progression to cirrhosis and/or portal hypertension; however, these changes require a long period to be observed. The poor sensitivity of this technique, particularly in the early stages of CF-associated liver disease, represents an additional shortcoming.

Ultrasonography did not change significantly after one year of UDCA treatment[31,42]. Data on ultrasonographic follow-up of patients treated with UDCA for longer periods suggest that in patients with multilobular biliary cirrhosis treatment does not prevent development of portal hypertension[37]; in contrast, if treatment is started at the early stage of focal biliary cirrhosis, it may prevent its progression to multilobular biliary cirrhosis[37,39]. These data require confirmation on larger numbers of patients followed-up for longer periods of time.

### IS TAURINE SUPPLEMENTATION NEEDED DURING UDCA THERAPY?

Since CF patients with pancreatic insufficiency are often in a negative taurine balance, taurine supplementation has been recommended by some investigators during treatment with UDCA in CF-associated liver disease[28,31].

Long-term administration of unconjugated UDCA may critically increase taurine need for bile acid conjugation and may aggravate the degree of taurine deficiency, with possible detrimental effects on the efficiency of fat digestion in CF patients[57].

For these reasons, in the Italian multicentre trial, the effects of taurine supplementation during oral bile acid therapy were evaluated in double-blind fashion[42]: taurine supplementation alone had no effect on the biochemical expression of liver damage and no further improvement was observed when it was added to UDCA. However, patients who received taurine supplementation, with or without UDCA, showed a trend towards improvement in the degree of fat malabsorption and a significant increase in serum prealbumin levels, which are a sensitive indicator of nutritional status. These findings are in agreement with previous studies showing that taurine can improve the efficiency of fat absorption in CF patients with severe steatorrhea[57–60]. Therefore taurine supplementation is advisable in CF patients with severe pancreatic insufficiency and poor nutritional status during chronic administration of UDCA.

## PREVENTION OF CF-ASSOCIATED LIVER DISEASE

An unanswered question is whether prophylactic UDCA treatment may prevent the development of focal biliary cirrhosis. In order to do this, we first have to identify the subgroup of CF patients at greatest risk of developing liver disease. With this aim we have recently evaluated the role of different clinical and genetic variables as possible risk factors for the development of liver disease in a large cohort of CF patients[61].

We first assessed the relationship between liver disease and CF genotypes. A familial concordance for liver disease of 20% has been reported[62], suggesting that its clinical expression could be determined by specific gene mutations, as occurs for pancreatic insufficiency[63]. Genetic analysis in our group of 189 CF patients failed to reveal any significant difference in the allele frequencies of defined (ΔF508, 1717-1G-A, G542X, N1303K, W1282X, R553X) and undefined mutations of the CFTR gene in patients with and without liver disease; genotype frequencies were also not significantly different. CF patients with liver disease were found to carry mostly the severe mutations of the CF gene, which have been associated with pancreatic insufficiency and more severe disease[64].

Other studies have also reported a lack of association between a number of CFTR mutations and liver disease[62,65,66]; a study on a particularly large series of patients could not show any obvious association between 29 individual CFTR mutations and abnormal liver function tests. Again in this latter study, hepatic abnormalities were seldom detected in patients carrying mild missense mutations[66].

Overall these data suggest that liver disease is more likely to occur in patients with mutations that are associated with pancreatic insufficiency. It is also evident that mutation analysis will not provide a guideline for high-risk patients.

With regard to clinical variables, the risk for the development of liver disease was almost four-fold higher in our CF patients with a positive history of meconium ileus or its equivalent, than in patients unaffected by these complications (OR: 3.9043; 95% confidence interval: 1.666–9.149)[61].

Our results are in agreement with data from autopsy studies[9] which suggested an association between cirrhosis at postmortem and distal intestinal obstruction in the neonatal period or later in life. Meconium ileus and meconium ileus equivalent have been attributed to the lack of fluid in the small intestine due to defective chloride secretion by intestinal epithelia; the increased risk of developing liver disease in these patients may be related to the production of particularly viscous secretions also at the hepatobiliary level. The tendency to have a particularly high viscosity of biliary and intestinal secretions could be determined genetically and several of the severe mutations of the CFTR gene could be involved.

In the high-risk group of CF patients with a positive history of meconium ileus or its equivalent, UDCA treatment could therefore be attempted as a prophylactic strategy aimed at reducing the viscosity of bile and at improving biliary drainage. This prophylactic strategy may be theoretically feasible since liver disease is not a late complication of CF: a peak in prevalence during adolescence and a fall over the age of 20 have been reported[5]; in our series of 33 CF patients with liver disease, mean age at presentation of hepatic abnormalities was even lower (7.7 ± 6.0 years, unpublished data).

Large multicentre trials are required in order to establish the efficacy of UDCA treatment on prevention of liver disease in CF patients.

## CONCLUSIONS

CF-associated liver disease has become increasingly recognized as a major cause of morbidity in CF patients. This has also induced a change of attitude by physicians, from merely expectant management to a more aggressive multifaceted therapeutic approach, which also includes liver transplantation.

While waiting for specific, liver-targeted gene therapy to be developed, a number of empirical treatments are being actively investigated. Among these, treatment with the choleretic agent UDCA is the most promising. However, its impact on the natural history of the disease is still to be established.

## REFERENCES


1 Roy CC, Weber AM, Morin CL et al. Hepatobiliary disease in cystic fibrosis: a survey of current issues and concepts. *J Pediatr Gastroenterol Nutr* 1982; **1**: 469–78.
2 Colombo C, Apostolo MG, Assaisso ML, et al. Liver disease in cystic fibrosis. *Neth J Med* 1992; **41**: 119–22.
3 FitzSimmons SC. The changing epidemiology of cystic fibrosis. *J Pediatr* 1993; **122**: 1–9.
4 Williams SGJ, Hayller KM, Hodson ME, Westaby D. Prognosis in cystic fibrosis. *N Engl J Med* 1992; **325**: 1244–54.
5 Scott-Jupp R, Lama M, Tanner MS. Prevalence of liver disease in cystic fibrosis. *Arch Dis Child* 1991; **66**: 698–701.
6 Tanner MS. Current clinical management of hepatic problems in cystic fibrosis. *J R Soc Med* 1986; **79** (Suppl 12): 38–43.
7 Tizzano EF, Buchwald M. Cystic fibrosis. Beyond the gene to therapy. *J Pediatr* 1992; **120**: 337–49.
8 Collins FC. Cystic fibrosis: molecular and therapeutic implications. *Science* 1992; **256**: 774–9.
9 Maurage C, Lenaerts C, Weber AM, et al. Meconium ileus and its equivalent as a risk factor for the development of cirrhosis: an autopsy study in cystic fibrosis. *J Pediatr Gastroenterol Nutr* 1989; **9**: 17–20.
10 Fitz JG, Basavappa S, McGill J, et al. Regulation of membrane chloride currents in rat bile ducts epithelial cells. *J Clin Invest* 1993; **91**: 319–28.
11 Berger HA, Anderson MP, Gregory RJ, et al. Identification and regulation of cystic fibrosis transmembrane conductance regulator-generated chloride channel. *J Clin Invest* 1991; **88**: 1422–31.
12 Cohn JA, McGill J, Basavappa S, et al. Bile ducts epithelial cells are the predominant site of CFTR in liver (abstract). *Pediatr Pulmonol* 1992; Suppl 8: 249.
13 Yang Y, Raper SE, Cohn JA, et al. An approach for treating the hepatobiliary disease of cystic fibrosis by somatic gene transfer. *Proc Natl Acad Sci* 1993; **90**: 4601–5.

13A Cohn JA, Strong TV, Picciotto MR, et al. Localisation of the cystic fibrosis transmembrane conductance regulator in human bile duct epithelial cells. *Gastroenterology* 1993; **105**: 1857–64.
14 Mulberg AE, Grubman SA, Perrone RD, et al. Human intrahepatic biliary epithelial cell lines for the study of cystic fibrosis-related hepatobiliary disease (abstract). *Pediatr Pulmonol* 1993; Suppl 9: 221.
15 Snouwaert J, Brigman K, Latour A, et al. An animal model for cystic fibrosis made by gene targeting. *Science* 1992; **257**: 1083–8.
16 Hofmann AF, Popper H. Ursodeoxycholic acid for primary biliary cirrhosis. *Lancet* 1987; **ii**: 398–9.
17 Attili AF, Angelico M, Cantafora A, et al. Bile acid-induced liver toxicity: relationship to the hydrophobic–hydrophilic balance of bile acids. *Med Hypotheses* 1986; **19**: 57–69.
18 Weber AM, Roy CC. Bile acid metabolism in children with cystic fibrosis. *Acta Paediatr Scand* 1985; Suppl 317: 9–15.
19 Thompson GN. Excessive fecal taurine loss predisposes to taurine deficiency in cystic fibrosis. *J Pediatr Gastroenterol Nutr* 1988; **7**: 214–17.
20 Sokol RJ. Lipid peroxidation in cholestasis. In: *Paediatric Cholestasis: Novel Approaches to Treatment*. Proceedings of the 63rd Falk Symposium (ed MJ Lentze, J Reichen) Kluwer, Dordrecht, 1992, pp 75–80.
21 Kneepkens CMF, Lepage G, Roy CC. Role of $\beta$-carotene in cystic fibrosis. *Pediatr Pulmonol* 1993; Suppl 9: 169–70.
22 de Caestecker JS, Jazrawi RP, Petroni ML, Northfield TC. Ursodeoxycholic acid in chronic liver disease. *Gut* 1991; **32**: 1061–5.
23 Anonymous. Bile acid therapy in the 1990s. *Lancet* 1992; **340**: 1260–1.
24 Heuman DM. Hepatoprotective properties of ursodeoxycholic acid (editorial). *Gastroenterology* 1993; **104**: 1865–70.
25 Beuers U, Spengler U, Zwiebel FM, et al. Effect of ursodeoxycholic acid on the kinetics of the major hydrophobic bile acids in health and in chronic cholestatic liver disease. *Hepatology* 1992; **15**: 603–8.
26 Guldutuna S, Zimmer G, Imhof M, et al. Molecular aspects of membrane stabilization by ursodeoxycholic acid. *Gastroenterology* 1993; **104**: 1736–44.
27 Dumont M, Uchman S, Erlinger S. Hypercholeresis induced by ursodeoxycholic acid and 7-ketolithocholic acid in the rat: possible role of bicarbonate transport. *Gastroenterology* 1980; **79**: 82–9.
28 Colombo C, Setchell KDR, Podda M, et al. The effects of ursodeoxycholic acid therapy in liver disease associated with cystic fibrosis. *J Pediatr* 1990; **117**: 482–9.
29 Cotting J, Lentze M, Reichen J. Effects of ursodeoxycholic acid treatment on nutrition and liver function in patients with cystic fibrosis and longstanding cholestasis. *Gut* 1990; **31**: 918–21.
30 Nakagawa M, Colombo C, Setchell KDR. Comprehensive study of the biliary bile acid composition of the patients with cystic fibrosis and associated liver disease before and after UDCA administration. *Hepatology* 1990; **12**: 322–34.
31 Galabert C, Montet JC, Lengrand D, et al. Effects of ursodeoxycholic acid on liver function in patients with cystic fibrosis and chronic cholestasis. *J Pediatr* 1992; **121**: 138–41.
32 Reichen J, Paumgartner G, Cotting J, Lentze MJ. Effect of long-term ursodeoxycholate on liver function, nutritional state and serum bile acids in cystic fibrosis with long-standing cholestasis. In: *Bile Acids as Therapeutic Agents: From Basic Science to Clinical Practice*. Proceedings of the 58th Falk Symposium (eds G Paumgartner, A Stiehl, W Gerok) Kluwer, Dordrecht, 1991, pp 335–44.

33 Colombo C, Castellani MR, Balistreri WF, et al. Scintigraphic documentation of an improvement in hepatobiliary excretory function after treatment with ursodeoxycholic acid in patients with cystic fibrosis and associated liver disease. *Hepatology* 1992; **15**: 677–84.

34 Colombo C, Crosignani A, Assaisso ML, et al. Ursodeoxycholic acid therapy in cystic fibrosis associated liver disease: a dose–response study. *Hepatology* 1992; **16**: 924–30.

35 Cotting J, Dufour JF, Lentze MJ, et al. Ursodeoxycholate in the treatment of cholestasis in cystic fibrosis: a 2-year experience and review of the literature. In: *Paediatric Cholestasis: Novel Approaches to Treatment*. Proceedings of the 63rd Falk Symposium (eds MJ Lentze, J Reichen) Kluwer, Dordrecht, 1992, pp 345–54.

36 Watson JBG, Babu MVS, Shortt C, O'Halloran ET. Successful treatment of prolonged neonatal jaundice in an infant with cystic fibrosis. *Proceedings of the XIth International Cystic Fibrosis Congress*, Dublin, 1992, WS 18.

37 Colombo C, Crosignani A, Bertolini E, et al. Ursodeoxycholic acid treatment in hepatobiliary complications of cystic fibrosis. In: *Bile Acids and the hepatobiliary system: From Basic Science to Clinical Practice*. Proceedings of the 68th Falk Symposium, Basel, October 1992 (eds G Paumgartner, A Stiehl, W Gerok) Kluwer, Dordrecht, 1992, pp 283–8.

38 Lindblad A, Strandvik B. Long-term study of the effect of ursodeoxycholic acid on liver morphology and liver function in patients with cystic fibrosis (abstract). *Proceedings of the 18th European Cystic Fibrosis Conference* 1993; 89.

39 Nousia-Arvanitakis S, Fotoulaki M, Rafailides D, et al. Early detection and therapy of biliary cirrhosis in cystic fibrosis (abstract). *Proceedings of the 18th European Cystic Fibrosis Conference* 1993; 86–88.

40 Bittner P, Posselt HG, Sailer T, et al. The effect of treatment with ursodeoxycholic acid in cystic fibrosis and hepatopathy: results of a placebo-controlled study. In: *Bile Acids as Therapeutic Agents: From Basic Science to Clinical Practice*. Proceedings of the 58th Falk Symposium, Freiburg, Germany, October 1990 (eds G Paumgartner, A Stiehl, W Gerok) Kluwer, Dordrecht, 1991, pp 345–8.

41 O'Brien S, Fitzgerald MX, Hegarty JE. A controlled trial of ursodeoxycholic acid treatment in cystic fibrosis-related liver disease. *Eur J Gastroenterol Hepatol* 1992; **4**: 857–63.

42 Colombo C, Podda M, Battezzati PM, et al. Ursodeoxycholic acid for cystic fibrosis-associated liver disease: final report of a multicenter trial (abstract). *Hepatology* 1993; **18**: 142A.

43 Perdigoto R, Wiesner RH. Progression of primary biliary cirrhosis with ursodeoxycholic acid therapy. *Gastroenterology* 1992; **102**: 1389–91.

44 Vogel W, Kathrein H, Judmaier G, Braunsteiner H. Deterioration of primary biliary cirrhosis during treatment with ursodeoxycholic acid. *Lancet* 1988; **i**: 1163.

45 Schoenau E, Boeswalld W, Wanner R, et al. High-molecular-mass ('biliary') isoenzyme of alkaline phosphatase and the diagnosis of liver dysfunction in cystic fibrosis. *Clin Chem* 1989; **35**: 1888–90.

46 Reichen J, Krahenbuhl S, Wirth HP, Maier KP. Liver function in cholestatic liver disease: a critical appraisal. In: *Bile Acids and the Hepatobiliary System* (eds G Paumgartner, A Stiehl, W Gerok) Kluwer, Dordrecht, 1993, pp 258–70.

47 Gross JB, Reichen J, Zeltner T, Zimmermann A. The evolution of changes in quantitative liver function tests in a rat model of cirrhosis: correlation with morphometric measurement of hepatocyte mass. *Hepatology* 1987; **7**: 457–63.

48 Reichen J, Widmer T, Cotting J. Accurate prediction of death by serial determination of galactose elimination capacity in primary biliary cirrhosis: a comparison with the Mayo model. *Hepatology* 1991; **14**: 504–10.
49 Reichen J. Pharmacologic treatment of cholestasis. *Semin Liver Dis* 1993; **13**: 302–15.
50 Gaskin KJ, Waters DLM, Howman-Giles R, et al. Liver disease and common bile-duct stenosis in cystic fibrosis. *N Engl J Med* 1988; **318**: 340–6.
51 Nagel RA, Westaby D, Javaid A et al. Liver disease and bile duct abnormalities in adults with cystic fibrosis. *Lancet* 1989; **ii**: 1422–5.
52 Jazrawi RP, de Caestecker JS, Goggin PM, et al. Kinetics of hepatic bile acid handling in cholestatic liver disease: effect of ursodeoxycholic acid. *Gastroenterology* 1994; **106**: 134–142.
53 Poupon RE, Balkau B, Eschwège E, Poupon R and the UDCA-PBC Study Group. A multicenter controlled trial of ursodiol for the treatment of primary biliary cirrhosis. *N Engl J Med* 1991; **324**: 1548–54.
54 Beuers U, Spengler U, Kruis W, et al. Ursodeoxycholic acid for treatment of primary sclerosing cholangitis: a placebo-controlled trial. *Hepatology* 1992; **16**: 707–14.
55 Carey MC, Montet JC, Phillips MC, et al. Thermodynamic and molecular basis for dissimilar cholesterol-solubilizing capacities by micellar solutions of bile salts: cases of sodium chenodeoxycholate and sodium ursodeoxycholate and their glycine and taurine conjugates. *Biochemistry* 1981; **20**: 3637–48.
56 Graham N, Manhlre AR, Stead RJ, et al. Cystic fibrosis: ultrosonographic findings in the pancreas and hepatobiliary system correlated with clinical data and pathology. *Clin Radiol* 1985; **36**: 199–203.
57 Anonymous. Taurine supplementation in cystic fibrosis. *Nutr Rev* 1988; **46**; 257–8.
58 Smith LJ, Lacaille F, Lepage G, et al. Taurine decreases fecal fatty acid and sterol excretion in cystic fibrosis: a randomized double-blind trial. *Am J Dis Child* 1991: **145**: 1401–4.
59 Darling PB, Lepage G, Leroy C, et al. Effects of taurine supplements on fat absorption in cystic fibrosis *Pediatr Res* 1985; **19**: 578–82.
60 Colombo C, Arlati S, Curcio L, et al. Effect of taurine supplementation on fat and bile acid absorption in patients with cystic fibrosis. *Scand J Gastroenterol* 1988; **23** (Suppl 143): 517–23.
61 Colombo C, Apostolo MG, Ferrari M, et al. Analysis of risk factors for the development of CF associated liver disease. *J Pediatr* 1994; **24**: 393–99.
62 Duthie A, Doherty DG, Williams C, et al. Genotype analysis for ΔF 508, G551D and R553X mutations in children and young adults with cystic fibrosis with and without liver disease. *Hepatology* 1992; **15**: 660–4.
63 Kerem E, Corey M, Kerem B, et al. The relation between genotype and phenotype in cystic fibrosis: analysis of the most common mutation (ΔF 508). *N Engl J Med* 1990; **323**: 1517–22.
64 Tsui LC. The spectrum of cystic fibrosis mutations. *Trends Genet* 1992: **8**: 392–8.
65 Ferrari M, Colombo C, Sebastio G, et al. Cystic fibrosis patients with liver disease are not genetically distinct (letter). *Am J Hum Genet*, 1991; **48**: 815–16.
66 Kovesi T, Corey M, Tsui L-C, et al. The association between liver disease and mutations of the cystic fibrosis gene (abstract). *Pediatr Pulmonol* 1992; Suppl 8: 244.

# Index

*Index compiled by Liza Weinkove*